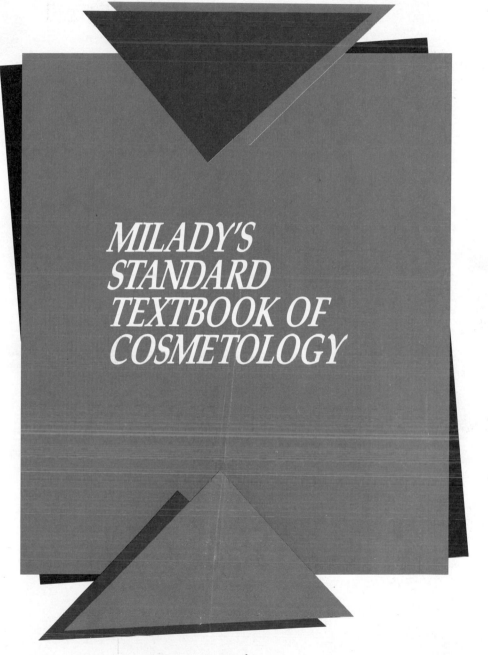

MILADY'S STANDARD TEXTBOOK OF COSMETOLOGY

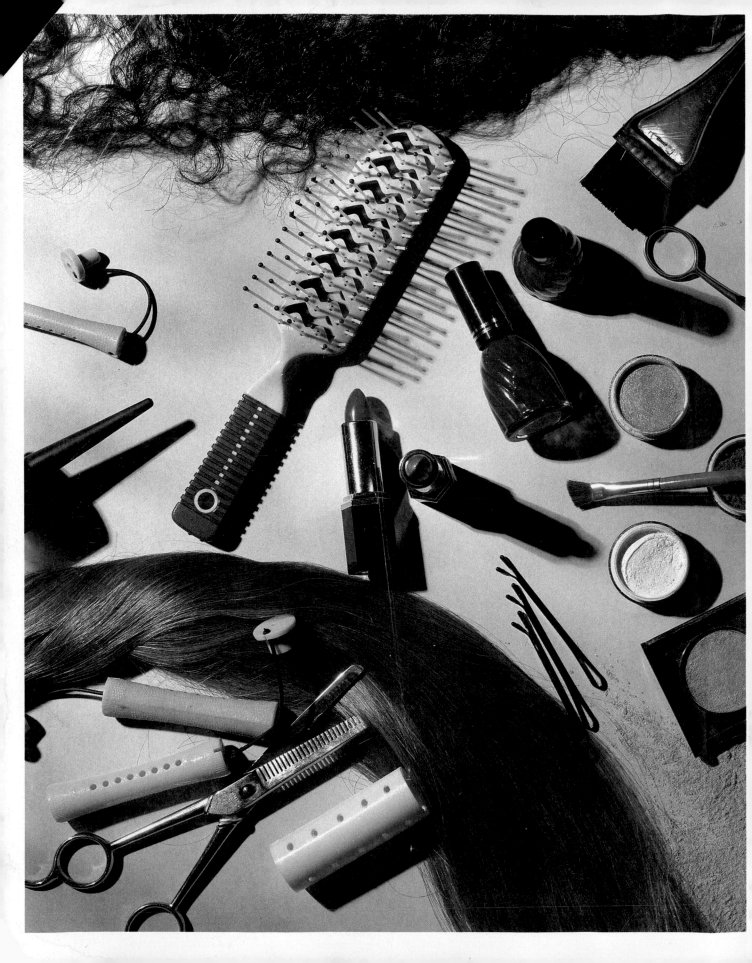

MILADY'S STANDARD TEXTBOOK OF COSMETOLOGY

Milady Publishing Company
(A Division of Delmar Publishers Inc.)
220 White Plains Road, Tarrytown, New York 10591

CREDITS

Publisher
Catherine Rossbach

Supervising Editor
Catherine Frangie

Development Editors
Joseph Miranda
Roz Sackoff

Editorial Assistants
Jacqueline Flynn
Linda Klein

Production Manager
John Mickelbank

Production Assistant
Lisa Mauro

Art Coordinator
John Fornieri

Art Assistants
Pat Genova
Roberto Williams

Manufacturing Coordinator
José Medina

Cover Photographer
Michael A. Gallitelli

Contributors to Cover Art
Linda Balhorn
Steven Landis
Garland Drake International
Tammy Bigan
John and Suzanne Chadwick

Photographers
Michael A. Gallitelli, on location
   at the Austin Beauty School,
   with Dino Petrocelli
Steven Landis,
   with direction from
   Vincent and Alfred Nardi
   of Nardi Salon
Eric Von Lockhart
Gillette Research Institute
New Image's Salon System

Artists
Edward Tadiello
Robert Richards
Judy Francis
Shizuko Horii
Jeanne A. Benas
Cynthia Saniewski
Randy Tibbot
Ron Young
CEM
Nelva Richardson
Gil Miret

Book Design
A Good Thing, Inc.

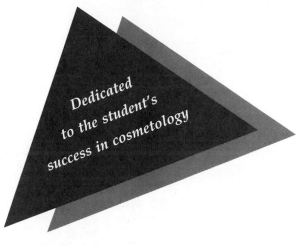

Dedicated
to the student's
success in cosmetology

Library of Congress Cataloging-in-Publication Data
Standard textbook of cosmetology.
    Milady's standard textbook of cosmetology. — [1991 ed.]
       p.   cm.
    ISBN 1-56253-001-1 : (hardcover) — ISBN 1-56253-003-8 (softcover)
    1. Beauty culture. I. Milady Publishing Company. II. Title.
    TT957.S77   1991
    646.7'2 — dc20
                                                    90-13361
                                                    CIP

Copyright © 1991
Milady Publishing Company
(A Division of Delmar Publishers Inc.)
220 White Plains Road
Tarrytown, NY 10591

ISBN: 1-56253-001-1 (Hardcover)
        1-56253-003-8 (Softcover)

Printed in the United States of America

10 9 8 7 6 5 4 3 2 1

Notice to the Reader

Contents

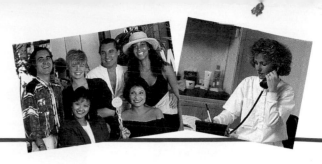

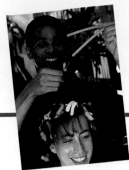
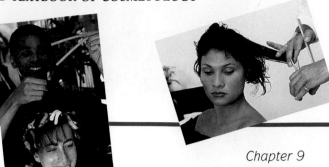
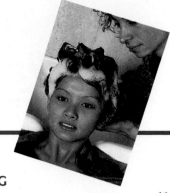

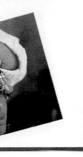
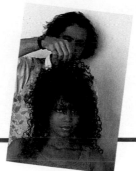
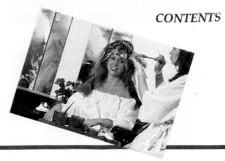

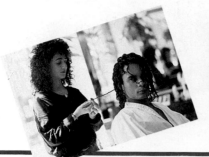
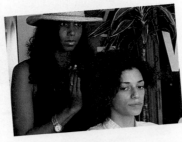
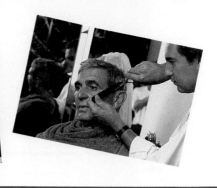

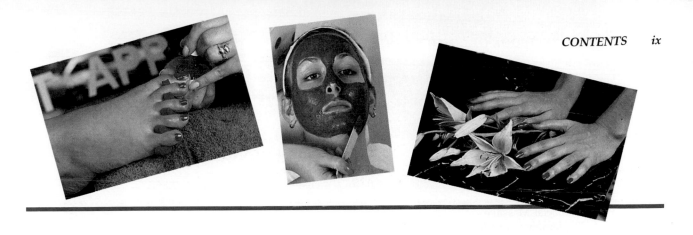

Chapter 16
MANICURING AND PEDICURING

Chapter 17
THE NAIL AND ITS DISORDERS

Chapter 18
THEORY OF MASSAGE

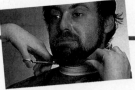

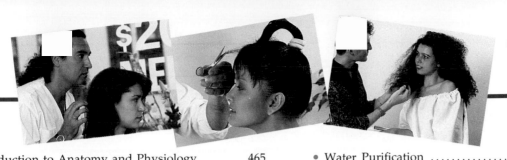

Preface

To The Student

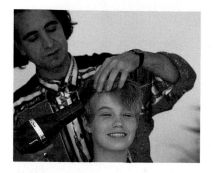

Congratulations! You have chosen a career filled with opportunity! Once you have trained to become a cosmetologist, you might open your own salon or manage a chain of salons. You may opt to specialize in an exciting area of cosmetology such as makeup artistry, hair coloring or nail technology. You may even team up with chemists to develop or market your own product line.

Whatever path you choose, you will play an important role in the lives of your clients. They will come to you for your advice and professional expertise, and you will share with them your experience and your artistic vision. As a cosmetologist, you'll be able to make that vision come to life.

Throughout this textbook, you'll see techniques that, with practice, you will gradually master. You'll be introduced to practicing cosmetologists who have used their cosmetology license as a passport to success. You'll meet business leaders, retail, hair coloring and cutting specialists, competition champions, people who specialize in chemical services, lecturers, educators and many creative, artistic cosmetologists who entered the profession for many of the same reasons as you!

You will learn from gifted and giving instructors who will share with you their skills and experiences. As you develop and realize your talents, you will have the opportunity to attend industry conventions, seminars and workshops where you'll learn the latest techniques. You'll meet industry leaders and be exposed to updated technology and scientific research. All of these experiences are opportunities to learn about the profession you have chosen and to excel in any of the facets you choose as a specialization.

You will build a network of people to turn to for career advice and encouragement. You will be able to take your career in cosmetology in any number of gratifying directions. Whichever direction you choose, we wish you success. Welcome and enjoy your journey!

To The Instructor

This edition of *Milady's Standard Textbook of Cosmetology* represents the most thorough modernization of appearance and content in the fifty-year history of this bestselling text. We have drawn upon the expertise of many industry leaders and educators, and they have worked with an entire staff of writers, editors, designers and artists in the development of this book. We hope we have made the subject easier for you to teach and that our book will please and motivate your students. If you have used *Milady's Standard* in the past, you will note the following exciting changes:

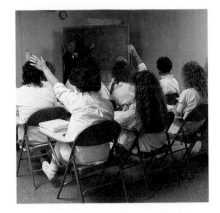

- A full-color design with 1,100 brand new illustrations and photographs
- Up-to-date methods and information with contemporary pictures
- A streamlined re-organization of chapters which ties theory and practice together more closely
- Illustrations of women and men from diverse cultural backgrounds and of varying ages
- Detailed, step-by-step procedures
- Highlighted safety cautions, particularly for the chemical services
- Key terms in boldface type with their pronunciations
- Motivational vignettes of industry leaders whose words describe business tips or human relations skills that helped them become successful
- Learning Objectives that are explained in the major topics of each chapter and then reinforced by the Review Questions
- Answers to the Review Questions provided in a separate booklet so the teacher has the choice of whether or not to make them available to the student
- A comprehensive Glossary and Index, combined to provide concise definitions of key terms along with pertinent page references so the student can find detailed explanations within the text
- A wide selection of supplementary materials for the student and for the teacher

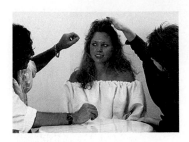

For The Student

- *Milady's Standard Theory Workbook and*
- *Milady's Standard Practical Workbook.* Feature word reviews, fill-in's, matching and multiple choice questions which increase students' comprehension and retention, help students learn practical procedures, and eliminate faulty practices. Each section refers to the pages in the text.
- *The Standard Hair Coloring Workbook.* Experiments and class projects provide students with hands-on experience in mixing colors and performing color services. To be used in conjunction with the Hair Coloring chapter in the text.
- *28 Styles for Student Practice.* Helps students perfect cutting and styling techniques and develop finger dexterity and artistic skills through mannequin practice.
- *Cosmetologists State Board Exam Review.* Helps students prepare for licensing examinations. Follows national testing exam requirements.
- *Preparing for the State Boards: Review Questions for Cosmetology.* A new, more challenging version for the Cosmetologists State Board Exam Review featuring situational problems.
- *Illustrated Practical Exam Review for Cosmetology.* This exam review consists of illustrated multiple-choice questions on practical procedures.
- *Milady's Cosmetology Word Puzzles.* Add fun and help build students' cosmetology vocabulary with word search puzzles and crossword puzzles.
- *Students' Illustrated Cosmetology Dictionary.* This pocket-sized reference defines terms in cosmetology and related subjects in simple, non-technical language.
- *Smart Tutor/Smart Tester.* A computer software program using multiple choice, fill-in, true-false, and matching questions in random order on all subjects found in *Milady's Standard Textbook of Cosmetology*.

For The Instructor

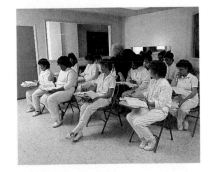

- *Answers to Milady's Standard Theory Workbook and*
- *Answers to Milady's Standard Practical Workbook.* Provides solutions to all workbook problems.
- *The Creative Teacher: An Instructor's Guide for Milady's Standard Textbook of Cosmetology.* Lecture notes on specific topics, plus teaching tips, oral quizzes, individual and group activities, points to emphasize, and additional sources of information for each chapter.
- *Projects for Cosmetology.* Projects and experiments help students learn by seeing and doing.
- *Competency Checklists to Accompany Milady's Standard Textbook of Cosmetology.* Helps ensure that students develop the basic skills and knowledge required for employability in the salon.
- *Lesson Plans for Cosmetology.* Lesson plans with objectives, materials and facilities needed, suggested visual aids, motivational devices, leading questions, and student assignments.
- *Competency-Based Curriculum for Cosmetology.* Curricula for 1,000, 1,500 and 2,000 hour programs includes practical skills divided into task performance, student and client preparation. Theory section includes all cosmetology subjects.
- *8 Cosmetology Review Exams.* Each 100 multiple-choice question test can be issued to students at specific intervals during the course, reviewing previous lessons, improving retention, and helping teachers discover students' weaknesses. Includes answer key.

Acknowledgments

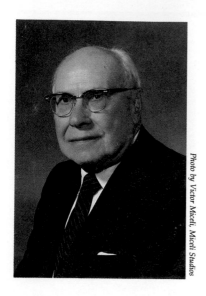

Photo by Victor Miceli, Miceli Studios

Many cosmetologists and educators have contributed to the development of this book over the years since its initial publication in 1938. *Milady's Standard Textbook of Cosmetology* owes its creation to the lifetime dedication of Nicholas F. Cimaglia, founder of Milady Publishing Company. Mr. Cimaglia was also one of the founders of the National Association of Accredited Cosmetology Schools, the Teacher's Educational Council and helped form the National Accrediting Commission for Cosmetology Arts and Sciences.

The standard set by N. F. Cimaglia has been carried on in the beauty education industry by his son Thomas Severance and by two gentlemen whose tireless efforts have established the success of *Milady's Standard Textbook of Cosmetology:* Jacob Yahm, the Father of Accreditation in our industry and a driving force behind the National Interstate Council of State Boards of Cosmetology; and Arnold DeMille, founding editor of the *National Beauty School Journal* (now *Beauty Education*) and continuing education specialist.

The current staff of Milady Publishing Company surveyed many instructors as they shaped and refined this edition of your textbook. We held focus groups, solicited written critiques and reviewed drafts of the book with industry experts. We wish to extend our enormous gratitude to the following people who contributed to our efforts.

- Gary Ahlquist
Tensorlon
San Diego, CA

- Kenneth Anders
Kenneth's Design Group
Columbus, OH

- Jan Austin
Austin Beauty School
Albany, NY

- Emma Ayala
Emma's Beauty School
Mayaguez, PR

- Giselle Bahamonde
Austin Beauty School
Albany, NY

- Linda Balhorn
Chicago, IL

- Mark Beck
The Massage Clinic
Twin Falls, ID

- Olive Lee Benson
Olive's
Boston, MA

- Kathleen Bergant
Milwaukee Area Technical College
Milwaukee, WI

- Karen Bilbo
Creative Hairdressers Inc.
Falls Church, VA

- Charlotte Blanchard
Austin Beauty School
Albany, NY

- Jan Bragulla
Creative Nail Design, Inc.
Carlsbad, CA

- Doris Brantly
South Carolina State Board of Cosmetology
Columbia, SC

● Sam Brocato
Brocato International
Lockworks USA
Baton Rouge, LA

● Burmax Co.
Hauppauge, NY

● Margaret Clevinger
Columbine Beauty Schools
Wheatridge, CO

● Denise Corbo
Manassas Park High School
Manassas Park, VA

● Louise Cotter
Adrian Creative Images
Orlando, FL

● Van Council
Van Michael Salon
Atlanta, GA

● Nina Curtis
International Dermal Institute
Marina del Rey, CA

● Joseph Dallal, M.Sc.
Zotos International, Inc.
Darien, CT

● Elizabeth Daniels
Total Beauty Enterprises
Hempstead, NY

● Darla Del Duca
South Vocational Technical
High School
Pittsburgh, PA

● Michael Dick
Santa Cruz Beauty College
Santa Cruz, CA

● Peggy Dietrick
Laredo Beauty College
Laredo, TX

● Janice Dorian
Mansfield Beauty School
Quincy, MA

● Nancy Dugan
Plastic Surgery Center
Montclair, NJ

● Rosalyn Duncan
Debbie's School of Beauty Culture
Houston, TX

● Mary Eiring
Moraine Park Technical College
Fond Du Lac, WI

● Leslie Edgerton
Nu-Tech Hair Salons
Ft. Wayne, IN

● Frederick Ford
Career Beauty School
Florissant, MO

● Wadad Frangie
Austin Beauty School
Albany, NY

● Anne Fretto
Career Academy
Seal Beach, CA

● Balmer Galindez
Bronx, NY

● Ray Gambrell
South Carolina State Board
of Cosmetology
Greenwood, SC

● Lavonne Gearheardt
Ohio State Board of Cosmetology
Columbus, OH

● Joel Gerson
New York, NY

● Fino Gior
Advanced Electrolysis Center
Great Neck, NY

● Pat Goins
Pat Goins Beauty School
Bossier City, LA

● Jerry Gordon
J. Gordon Designs
Chicago, IL

● Aurie Gosnell
National Interstate Council
Aiken, SC

● Barbara Griggs
Creative Nail Design
Pasadena, MD

● Scheryl Hanson
Lancaster School of Cosmetology
Lancaster, PA

● Juanita Harris
International Beauty Schools
Cumberland, MD

● Michael Hill
Arkansas State Board
of Cosmetology
Fayetteville, AR

● Linda Howe
Pittsburgh Beauty Academy
New Kensington, PA

● Harvey Huth
Albany, NY

● Evelyn Irvine
Virginia Board for Cosmetology
Newport News, VA

● Sandra Isaacs
Chino, CA

● Charlotte Jayne
Garland Drake International
Newport Beach, CA

● Dan Jeans
Ritter/St. Paul Beauty College
St. Paul, MN

● Glenda Jemison
Franklin Beauty Schools
Houston, TX

● Michele Johnson
Tipton, MI

● Janit Kangas
South Carolina State Department
of Education
Columbia, SC

● Tama Kieves
Denver, CO

● Lenny La Cour
Chicago, IL

● Barbara Lane
Sheridan Vo-Tech
Hollywood, FL

● Carole Laubach
San Jacinto College
Pasadena, TX

● Linnea Lindquist
Minneapolis Technical College
St. Paul, MN

● Dottie Lineberry
Chantilly High School Cosmetology
Center
Chantilly, VA

● Marc London
Pasadoula Beauty Academy
Moss Point, MS

● Rhonda Lyon
Gi Gi Laboratories
City of Commerce, CA

● Rocky Lyons
Lyons Salons
Miami, FL

● Charles Lynch
International Beauty School
Lancaster, PA

● Lois Dorian Malconian
Mansfield Beauty Academy
Quincy, MA

• Thomas Marks
Southern Nevada Vo-Tech
Las Vegas, NV

• Thia Masciana
International Haircolor Exchange
Torrance, CA

• Geri Mataya
Uptown Hair Design
Pittsburgh, PA

• Adele McNiven
Kelowna, British Columbia

• Victoria Melesko
Clairol Incorporated
New York, NY

• Damien Miano
La Dolce Vita Salon
New York, NY

• Carol Micciche
Lancaster Beauty School
Lancaster, PA

• Arnold Miller
Matrix Essentials, Inc.
Solon, OH

• Lynn Mills
Don's Beauty School
San Mateo, CA

• Beth Minardi
Minardi Minardi Image Makers
New York, NY

• Carmine Minardi
Minardi Minardi Image Makers
New York, NY

• Vincent and Alfred Nardi
Nardi Salon
New York, NY

• Florence A. Neblett
National Institutes of Cosmetology
Washington, DC

• Stanley K. Nielson
Sevier Valley Technical School
Richfield, UT

• Pat Nix
Indiana State Board of Cosmetology
Examiners
Booneville, IN

• Andres Nizetich
Andres Salon
San Pedro, CA

• Debra Norton
Arkansas State Board
of Cosmetology
Little Rock, AR

• Patricia Oberhausen
Richmond Northeast High School
Columbia, SC

• Mark Padgett
Zotos International, Inc.
Darien, CT

• Patrick Poussard
Brooklyn, NY

• Joe O'Riorden
East Coast Salon Owner's
Association
Marlboro, MA

• Larry Oskin
Creative Hairdressers Inc.
Falls Church, VA

• Lynn Parentini
Esthetic Research Group
Long Island City, NY

• Carol Phillips
Huntington Beach, CA

• Stan Campbell Place
Maybelline
Gahana, OH

• Lynn Plant
Zotos International, Inc.
Darien, CT

• Horst Rechelbacher
Aveda Corporation
Minneapolis, MN

• Tom Ross
Ohio State Board of Cosmetology
Columbus, OH

• Thelma Ruffe, R.N.
Old Bridge, NJ

• Margaret Ruffin
Derma-Clinic Academy of Skincare
Atlanta, GA

• Sue Sansom
Arizona State Board of Cosmetology
Phoenix, AZ

• Paul Scillia
Roman Academy of Beauty Culture
Hawthorne, NJ

• Nikki Schwartz
American Beauty Academy
Houston, TX

• Serge
Bruno Dessange
New York, NY

• Joan Sesock
Austin Beauty School
Albany, NY

• Keiko Shino
Garland Drake International
Newport Beach, CA

• Gianni Siniscalchi
Gianni Hair and Skin Care
Montclair, NJ

• Heather Slack
Arts of Nails and Beauty Academy
Winter Haven, FL

• Patricia Spencer
Riverside Community College
Riverside, CA

• Rosemary Steffish
Lancaster Beauty School
Lancaster, PA

• Judith Stewart
PJ's College of Cosmetology
Carmel, IN

• Michael Stinchcomb
Yves Claude Salon
New York, NY

• Jack Storey
Scruples Inc.
Lakeville, MN

• Stephanie Tebow
Pro-Tech College
Carterville, IL

• Edward Tezak
Warren Occupational
Technical Center
Golden, CO

• Alma Tilghman
North Carolina Board of
Cosmetology
Beaufort, NC

• Veda Traylor
Arkansas State Board of
Cosmetology
Mayflower, AR

• Peggy Turbyfill
Mike's Barber and Beauty Salon
Hot Springs, AR

• Martha Weller
University of New Mexico-Gallup
Gallup, NM

• Lois Wiskur
South Dakota Cosmetology
Commission
Pierre, SD

• Arnold Zegarelli
Zegarelli Inc.
Pittsburgh, PA

• Zotos International, Inc.
Darien, CT

INTRODUCTION

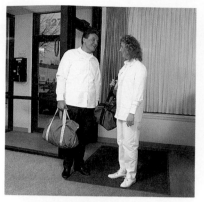
Welcome to the
cosmetology profession.

Here you are at the threshold of opportunity. You have a chance for glamour, excitement, and other untold rewards. Welcome to the world of cosmetology! Apply yourself and there are no limits to the possibilities. Your license to practice cosmetology is an unlimited passport to the world.

Whether you like working with hair, skin, or nails, your certification provides you with the opportunity to select a career path to suit you. To get the most out of your passport, make the most of your education. Every lesson has something to teach you, something that may start you on your way. Your license unlocks countless doors, but it is what *you learn* that can really launch your career.

The World of Cosmetology

As you begin your journey, you may not know whether you prefer working with hair, skin, or nails. Even if you do have something in mind, leave yourself open to other possibilities. Let your learning guide you. Enter each classroom with an open mind and a wholehearted desire to learn as much as you can.

Some of the most well-known people in the beauty world began just as you are beginning. A broad beauty education gave them the chance to enthusiastically explore different avenues of cosmetology until they found the path that suited them. Why not give yourself that chance as well? You have so many possibilities. Here are just some of the many vocations that you may be tempted to try upon graduation. No matter what area interests you, take the time to read the following sections. Each one has helpful information suggested by some of the most accomplished professionals in the beauty world today.

MAKEUP ARTIST

Are you artistically inclined? Do you like blending, shading, creating? A makeup artist "paints faces," explains one top artist in the field. "He or she brings out beauty without making it look like a disguise." Makeup artists most frequently apply cosmetics to enhance a client's appearance, but they can create *any* image a particular job calls for.

As a makeup artist, you can establish yourself in a salon with a private clientele, become makeup director for a prestigious department store, represent a line of cosmetics, work in television and movie production, find a position with a fashion magazine, or work behind the scenes in theater production. You can operate as an independent freelancer, which allows you to create your own schedule, or you can find full-time employment with one company.

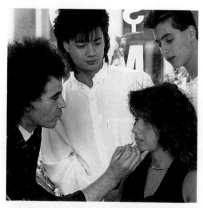
Makeup artist.

Advice from the Experts

"Makeup artistry is so much more than just fashion and taste. It's a lot of training," advises a top talent in the field. "If you don't learn as much as you can, eventually it corners you." Pay strict attention in *all* your classes. Concentrate on chemistry and anatomy.

After beauty school, consider continuing your education in the fine arts, with an emphasis on drawing and painting courses. Theater experience will also prove helpful, especially a study of stage lighting.

Work in a salon for at least six months after school. Consider volunteering your services to community theaters, fashion shows, and department stores in your area. Volunteer work will afford you experience and help you build a resume as well as contacts, that is, people you meet who may be important to your career. Start to develop a portfolio that you can present to potential employers. In this portfolio, compile before and after photographs of makeovers you have performed, along with any awards or certificates you may have earned.

SKIN CARE SPECIALIST/ESTHETICIAN

Are you drawn by the allure of a radiant complexion and the secrets of different creams and lotions? An *esthetician* offers treatments to perfect the look and health of skin.

As an esthetician you can work in a salon, teach, travel throughout the world giving demonstrations at beauty shows, or become a consultant to a cosmetic company. You can work exclusively for one company or you can be a freelancer.

Advice from the Experts

Consider attending a beauty school that specializes in or emphasizes facial treatments. "Devote yourself to your training," advises an esthetician who lectures worldwide. "It's such a short training period and once you start work, it's difficult to get away to take classes."

Read as much as you can about skin care. "Since I was always reading, I could sound authoritative when I spoke to clients," continues the skin care expert. Attend seminars where you can meet and learn from the specialists in your area of interest. Subscribe to professional publications that list events and classes you can participate in to supplement your education. Study the different skin care products on the market so that you understand what they are supposed to do and how you can use them.

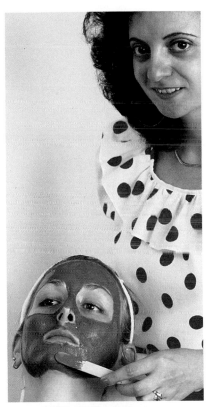

Skin care specialist/ esthetician.

COSMETIC CHEMIST

Are you curious and creative? Do you like experimenting? Cosmetic chemists supply the beauty world's expanding needs by creating new products through research and experimentation.

"Every business has its tools," explains one cosmetic chemist. "I help make the tools that cosmetologists use." He continues, "I get a profile from the marketing company that shows what type of product they want to market. Then I go through my mental and physical library to bring together that product."

As a cosmetic chemist you can work for a cosmetic manufacturer or become a consultant to several companies.

Advice from the Experts

Learn everything you can in cosmetology school. "I draw from everything I've ever studied," confirms one highly paid cosmetic chemist. Pay close attention to your marketing courses. An understanding of the commercial marketplace will help to direct your scientific exploration. It is also important to acquire a chemistry education in addition to what you learn in beauty school. You should consider continuing your education in a college.

After completing your schooling, apply for an internship with a cosmetic company working on a panel that studies new products. If you can't get into a company this way, apply for a position in the manufacturer's marketing department.

PUBLISHING

Do you like to write? You can use your cosmetology license to enter the publishing world. With a beauty background, you can write articles, books, brochures, columns, educational manuals— even produce videos. "You get to wear the latest, trendiest hairstyles, clothes, and accessories *and* you get to do what you love," says one cosmetologist turned beauty writer.

As a writer with a cosmetology license, you can work for a publishing company, freelance, travel and review major beauty shows, or develop a lifestyle that combines it all.

Advice from the Experts

Master the technical basics of cosmetology. "You need to really understand *why* a certain procedure works better in order to write about it," explains one cosmetology editor with a major publishing firm. "It's the way to open doors. Then, you can go on to let your creativity out."

Fine-tune your writing skills by taking writing courses and reading as much as possible to see how things are written.

Keep current with what's happening in your industry by attending seminars. "You can use this knowledge to determine what to write, because you'll know what's needed," advises the publishing expert. "Be up on the latest information because you can bet your audience will be."

Practice networking; create contacts by being open and friendly with other people. These contacts might have a hot tip for you or remember your name when a position opens.

HAIR COLORIST

Do you have an exacting eye for pigment? Do flattering shades jump out at you? A hair colorist picks out the best color and process to enhance a client's hair. The colorist mixes the dye, applies it, and evaluates the resulting shade.

"Hair coloring is such a creative part of the industry," says one noted hair colorist. "There's so many different ways to arrive at a color. It's not like haircutting where there's only one way."

As a hair colorist you can establish a specialized color department within a salon, become a color trainer (teaching at salons), work for a hair color manufacturer, or become a *platform artist*, demonstrating your technique at national and international shows.

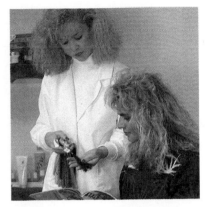

Hair colorist.

Advice from the Experts

Persevere and pay attention in beauty school. Take advantage of opportunities to work with your teachers. For example, ask if you can assist with a coloring. Observe other teachers or students doing color as often as you can. Attend classes and shows in your area. Most important, keep practicing. "Don't be afraid to make mistakes," advises one hair colorist. "You're going to make mistakes. It's the first ten thousand that are the toughest. Just keep going."

SALON OWNER

Do you have great ideas for how things *should* be done? Do you like varied responsibilities and challenges? Running your own salon allows you to set a standard for the quality of service you bring to the marketplace. You can choose the products and services to provide, and establish the level of skill you demand from your staff. You can exercise creativity, versatility, and independence in this position if you don't mind making decisions and putting in long hours.

Advice from the Experts

In beauty school you must learn everything you possibly can, paying particular attention to sales courses. When you graduate, take a job as a cosmetologist. "Never come right out and own a salon," says one salon owner of eighteen years. "A school environment is totally different from a salon. You absolutely need to work for a while first."

Owning a salon means assuming responsibility for paying bills, payrolls, and taxes as much as it means doing nails and giving haircuts and perms. You must develop business skills beyond what you learn in beauty school. Attend college business classes or seminars. You might even want to attend business school. You should also contact your local small business bureau and obtain literature about businesses in your area. Talk to local salon owners and learn what you can from their experience.

In addition to business expertise, you need people skills to run a salon. You will be in the public's eye and you will be managing a staff of employees. Take some courses that build upon your social skills and suggest successful techniques for resolving conflicts.

RETAIL SPECIALIST

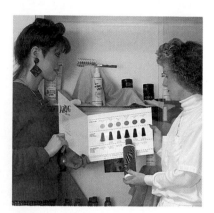

Retail specialist.

Do you have a flair for selling? Do you communicate well and enjoy working with people? With a cosmetology license, you can become a retail specialist working with salons and manufacturers to promote their products' sales. "Retailing is nothing more than good communication," explains one retail specialist who lectures nationwide. "All you need to do is understand people enough to sell your product, your service and yourself."

As a retail specialist, you can work in a salon, spa, or department store as a product manager handling the merchandising of inventory. Retail specialists also work as trainers, honing the sales techniques of a particular cosmetic company, or traveling throughout the country presenting general sales seminars. "Being a retail specialist is a great security," advises a self-made retail specialist. "Even as a stylist, every salon will want to hire you. You know a lot about sales, and salons today have to focus on sales."

Advice from the Experts

Get the best technological understanding you can at beauty school. To really sell a product, you need to know how to work with it and why it stands out as a product you recommend.

Work for a salon after beauty school. Time "in the trenches" gives you the experience you will need to market yourself to companies as an authority whom they can trust. Read about selling strategies. Spend time observing people. "If you don't understand people, you don't understand the business," advises one retail specialist, who recommends drawing from past work experience and practicing people skills daily.

COMPETITION CHAMPION

Are you a perfectionist? Do you get excited working toward a goal and winning? Competition champions compete for prizes and prestige in various cosmetology world championships. Here, "the best" display their individual talents and techniques. You must have dedication, good work habits, and utmost skill to enter this honored realm that holds so many rewards.

"The commitment reflects on your everyday lifestyle," explains one champion who has competed for years. "As you train to be a winner, you bring back that attitude to the salon. You have no limit to what you can do."

Competition champions often establish their own salons. Their reputation as distinguished artists attracts a following and adds to the prosperity of their business endeavors. Champions can also work as trainers, coaching the next generation of competitors.

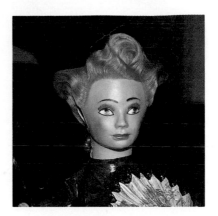
Competition winner.

Advice from the Experts

In beauty school, make sure you cultivate your styling skills as perfectly as possible. Pay close attention to details. Make sure everything is balanced and immaculate. "Your combing should be spotless," advises one champion who now trains competitors. "Walk around the client and look at your work from different angles."

To enter competitions, you may need to hire a world champion trainer, spend time creating and perfecting your skills, and search for the right model. But for those dedicated to the path, the reward can be exhilaration and prestige.

EDUCATIONAL SPECIALIST

Do you like to teach? Do you enjoy seeing people grasp new information? The beauty industry abounds in teaching opportunities. For example, an educational consultant who works for a product manufacturer might conduct seminars for a salon staff, demonstrating how to use various products. Other consultants work for manufacturers of ingredients that are sold to cosmetic companies. They give presentations to the marketing departments of cosmetic companies to demonstrate how an ingredient can improve or enhance a product.

Other educational specialists write curriculums and training manuals that teach consultants to teach. As an educational specialist, you might work for a major manufacturer or travel around the country training industry professionals to teach.

Advice from the Experts

Concentrate on all your courses in beauty school. "All skills become cumulative," explains one educational specialist on board with a major manufacturer. "You may not like to do manicures, but it's always another skill you can pose to an employer to get your foot in the door of a job you want." Since marketing goes hand in hand with the educational specialist's objectives, consider adding some business courses to your training.

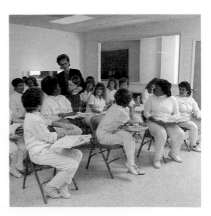
Educator.

Yet another way to begin your career is by working in a major department store training sales clerks to demonstrate and sell cosmetics. Then, prepare your resume and mail it to every manufacturer you can think of, outlining your skills, experience, and the type of position you are seeking.

The list of career opportunities is endless. The beauty industry continues to grow in order to accommodate the vivid imaginations and abilities of the artists. Welcome to this wonderful world of possibilities where, if you can imagine your ideal career, with a little perseverance, you can probably spend your life doing it!

1

YOUR PROFESSIONAL IMAGE

LEARNING OBJECTIVES

After completing this chapter, you should be able to:

1. Demonstrate guidelines to maintain a healthy body and mind.
2. List the qualities of effeclive physical presentation.
3. Define personality.
4. List the qualities of effective communication.
5. Demonstrate good humun relations and a professional attitude.
6. Define professional ethics.

Introduction

Good health is a basic element for living. Without it, one cannot work efficiently or enjoy the pleasures of life. As a cosmetologist, you should be a living example of good health so that you increase your value to yourself, to your employer, and to the community.

Your Personal and Professional Health

To be a successful cosmetologist, you should follow a set of guidelines to help you maintain a healthy body and mind.

REST

Adequate sleep is essential for good health. Without it you cannot function efficiently. The body should be allowed to recover from the fatigue of the day's activities and should be replenished with a good night's sleep. The amount of sleep needed to feel refreshed varies from person to person. Some people function well with 6 hours of sleep; others need 8 hours.

EXERCISE

Exercise ensures the proper functioning of organs such as the heart and lungs, strengthens muscles and bones, and improves circulation. An adequate fitness program includes exercises to accomplish aerobic strength, flexibility, and endurance.

RELAXATION

Relaxation is important as a change of pace from your day-to-day routine. Going to a movie or a museum, reading a book, watching television, or dancing are ways for you to "get away from it all." When you return to work, you will feel refreshed and eager to attend to your duties.

NUTRITION

What you eat affects your health, appearance, personality, and performance on the job. The nutrients in food supply the body with energy and ensure proper body functions. A balanced diet should include a variety of foods so that you obtain important vitamins and minerals. Drink plenty of water daily. Try to avoid sugar, salt, caffeine, and fatty or highly refined and processed foods and "fast" foods.

PERSONAL HYGIENE

Personal hygiene is the daily maintenance of cleanliness and healthfulness. The basics include daily bathing or showering, using deodorant, brushing your teeth and using mouthwash to freshen your breath during the day, and having clean and well-groomed hair and nails.

PERSONAL GROOMING

Personal grooming is an extension of personal hygiene. A well-groomed cosmetologist is one of the best advertisements for a salon. If you present a poised and attractive image, your client will have confidence in you as a professional. Many salon owners and managers consider appearance, personality, and poise to be as important as technical knowledge and manual skills. To begin, wear fresh undergarments daily and a freshly laundered, well-tailored uniform. Some salons do not require standard uniforms, but they may have a specific dress code. For example, some salons require that all their personnel wear the same color clothing. Select your outfits so that you reflect the image of the salon. Avoid obtrusive or excessive jewelry. A wristwatch will help you keep to your schedule.

The Female Cosmetologist

The female cosmetologist should wear stylish shoes that fit and are still comfortable at the end of a long day. Your makeup should be flattering and suited to the environment of your salon. (Fig. 1.1)

The Male Cosmetologist

In addition to the general guidelines discussed, the male cosmetologist should keep facial hair neatly trimmed and groomed. (Fig. 1.2)

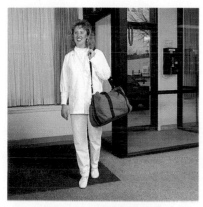

1.1 — A well-groomed female cosmetologist.

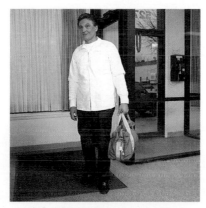

1.2 — A well-groomed male cosmetologist.

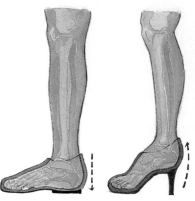

1.3 – For comfort and to help maintain good posture, wear well-fitted, low-heeled shoes.

CARE OF THE FEET

As a cosmetologist you will spend a great deal of time on your feet. Proper foot care will help you maintain a good posture and a cheerful attitude. Sore feet or poor-fitting shoes can cause great discomfort. (Fig. 1.3)

Shoes

Try to wear shoes with low, broad heels and with cushioned insoles. They give you support and balance, which help to maintain good posture and offset fatigue that can result from hours of standing. It also helps if you can stand on a carpeted or cushioned surface.

Daily Foot Care

After bathing, apply cream or oil and massage each foot for 5 minutes. Remove the cream or oil and apply an antiseptic foot lotion. Regular pedicures that include cleansing, removal of calloused skin, massage, and toenail trims will keep your feet at their best. When your feet ache, podiatrists recommend that you soak your feet alternately in warm and cool water. See a podiatrist if corns, bunions, ingrown toenails, or other foot disorders exist.

People Skills

When you think about the importance of people skills in the salon, don't overlook self-development. Arnold Zegarelli, a consultant and hairstyling director for the Regis Corporation and styles director for Hornes Salon in Pittsburgh, Pennsylvania, offers this advice to help you grow personally and professionally:

"Always keep in mind your role, purpose, function, and goal," says Zegarelli. "As an authority in the personal-appearance business, your role is to set a good example by looking fashionable, speaking professionally, and being as knowledgeable as possible. Your purpose is to be dedicated to helping clients look and feel their best. Your function is simple. You are in demand for your services and should perform them willingly, courteously, and diligently. Selling is not something you do *to* people, it's something you do *for* them. Goals are highly personal. Just remember, it is better to aim at a star than to shoot down a well. You're bound to hit a higher mark."

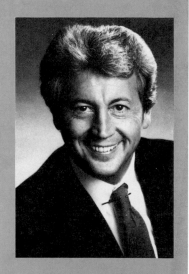

To help you achieve the above, Zegarelli offers these 11 suggestions: Know yourself. Visualize your desired self-image. Exercise self-discipline. Maintain a positive mental attitude. Develop your mind, body, and soul. Understand where you have been and decide where you're going. Know your priorities. Compromise when you must, but minimize your losses. Respond, don't react. Ask yourself if you're willing to pay the price for your goals. Respect others' points of view.

HEALTHY LIFESTYLE

You should practice stress management through relaxation, rest, and exercise and avoid substances that can negatively affect your good health, such as cigarettes, alcohol, and drugs.

Physical Presentation

Your posture, walk, and movements all make up your physical presentation. People form opinions about you by the way you present yourself. Do you stand straight or slouch; do you walk confidently or do you drag your feet? Your physical presentation is part of your professional image.

GOOD POSTURE

Good posture not only improves your personal appearance by presenting your figure to advantage and creating an image of confidence, it also prevents fatigue and many other physical problems. (Figs. 1.4, 1.5) Because you will be spending most of your time on your feet when working as a professional cosmetologist, good posture should be developed as early as possible through regular exercise and self-discipline.

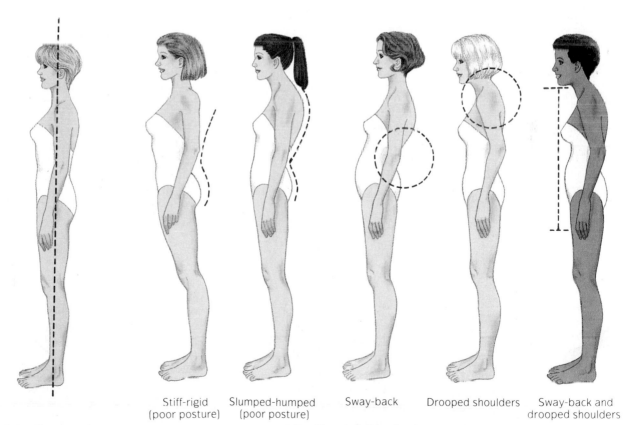

Stiff-rigid
(poor posture)   Slumped-humped
(poor posture)   Sway-back   Drooped shoulders   Sway-back and
drooped shoulders

1.4—Good posture.   1.5—Five defective body postures.

PHYSICAL PRESENTATION ON THE JOB

To prevent muscle aches, back strain, discomfort, fatigue, and other problems and to maintain an attractive image, it is very important to practice good physical presentation while performing work activities. (Figs. 1.6, 1.7)

Checkpoints of Good Posture

- Crown of head reaching upward while chin is kept level with the floor.
- Neck is elongated and balanced directly above the shoulders.
- Chest up; body is lifted from the breastbone.
- Shoulders are level, held back and down, yet relaxed.
- Spine is straight, not curved laterally or swayed from front to back.
- Abdomen is flat.
- Hips are level (horizontally) and protrude neither forward nor back.
- Knees are slightly flexed and positioned directly over the feet with the ankles firm.

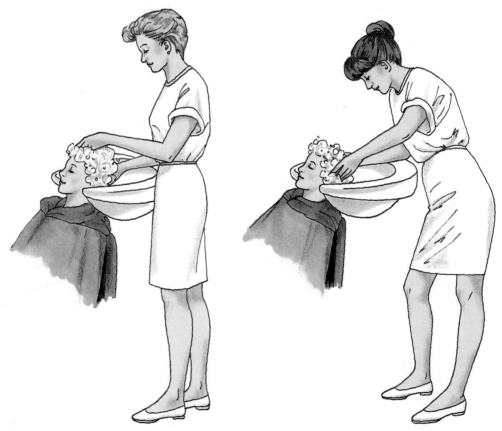

1.6—To avoid back strain, maintain good posture when giving a shampoo.

1.7—Poor posture.

Basic Stance for Women

- Place most of your weight on your right foot and point your toes straight ahead in a straight line.
- Place your left heel close to the heel or instep of your right foot and point the toes slightly outward.
- Bend your left knee slightly inward. (Fig. 1.8)

Basic Stance for Men

- Place your feet apart, but not wider than your shoulder width.
- Distribute your weight evenly over both feet.
- Your knees should be neither rigid nor bent.
- Your toes should point straight ahead or one or both feet should point slightly outward.
- For a more relaxed stance, bend one knee slightly while shifting some of your weight to the opposite foot. (Fig. 1.9)

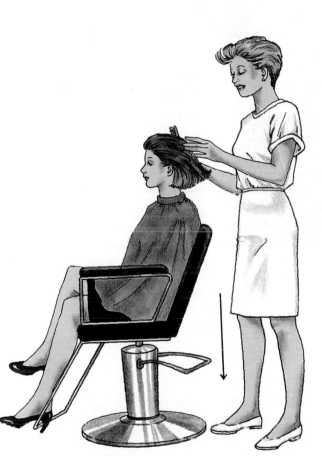

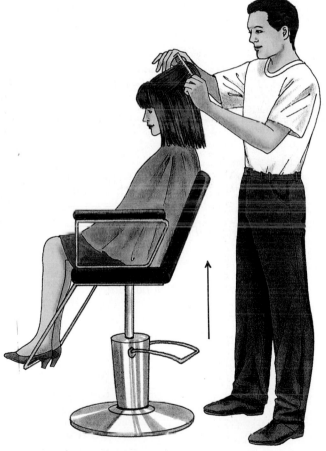

1.8 — Basic stance for the female cosmetologist, and the correct chair position for working on a client comfortably.

1.9 — Basic stance for the male cosmetologist, and the correct chair position for working on a client comfortably.

CORRECT SITTING TECHNIQUE

To sit attractively, use your thigh muscles and support from your hands and arms to lower your body smoothly into a chair. Do not fall or flop into a chair. When lowering your body, keep your back straight. Do not bend at the waist or reach with the buttocks. When seated, slide to the back of the chair by placing both hands on the front edge of the chair at the sides of your hips. Raise your body slightly and slide back. Do not wiggle or inch back.

When giving a manicure, assume a correct sitting position. Sit with the lower back against the chair, leaning slightly forward. If a stool is used, sit on the entire stool. Keep your chest up and rest your body weight on the full length of your thighs. (Figs. 1.10, 1.11)

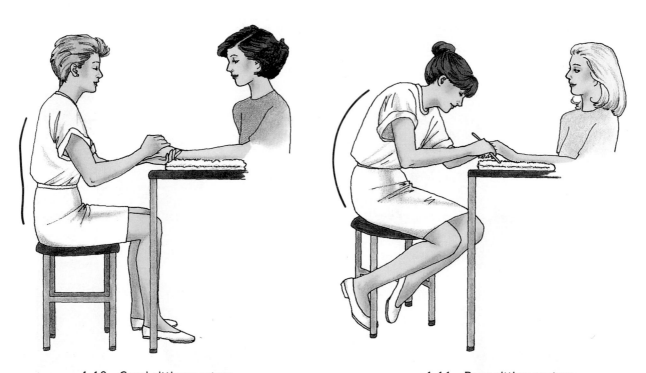

1.10—Good sitting posture.   1.11—Poor sitting posture.

Tips for a Proper Sitting Position

1. Keep your feet close together.
2. Keep your knees close together.
3. Place your feet out slightly farther than your knees.
4. Do not push your feet under the chair.
5. Keep the entire sole of your foot on the floor.

Personality

Your personality plays an important part in your personal and professional life. Personality can be defined as the outward reflection of your inner feelings, thoughts, attitudes, and values. Your personality is expressed through your voice, speech, and choice of words, as well as through your facial expressions, gestures, actions, posture, clothing, grooming, and environment. It is the total effect you have on other people.

DESIRABLE QUALITIES FOR EFFECTIVE CLIENT RELATIONS

Emotional Control
Learn to control your emotions. Discourage and do not reveal negative emotions such as anger, envy, and dislike. An even-tempered person is always treated with respect.

Positive Approach
Be pleasant and gracious. A smile of greeting and a word of welcome should be ready for each client and co-worker. A good sense of humor is also an important part of maintaining a positive attitude. A sense of humor enriches your life and cushions the disappointments. When you are able to laugh at yourself, you will have gained the ability to accept and deal positively with difficult situations.

Good Manners
Good manners reflect your thoughtfulness of others. Saying "thank you" and "please," treating other people with respect, exercising care of other people's property, being tolerant and understanding of other people's shortcomings and efforts, and being considerate of those with whom you work all express good manners. Courtesy is one of the keys to a successful career.

Mannerisms
Gum chewing and nervous habits such as tapping your foot or playing with your hair and personal items detract from your effectiveness. Yawning, coughing, and sneezing should be concealed when in the presence of others. Control body language that reveals negative communication, for example, sarcastic or disapproving facial grimaces. Pleasant facial expressions and attractive gestures and actions should be your goal.

Effective Communication

Communication includes your listening skills, voice, speech, manner of speaking, and conversational skills. Your ability to communicate will have a great influence on your effectiveness as a cosmetologist. A cosmetologist needs good communication skills for the following reasons:

- To make contacts
- To meet and greet clients
- To understand a client's needs, likes, dislikes, and desires (Fig. 1.12)
- To be self-promoting
- To sell services and products (Fig. 1.13)
- To build business
- To talk on the telephone
- To carry on a pleasant conversation
- To interact with the salon staff

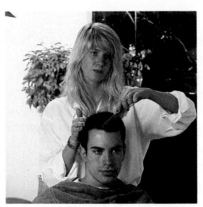

1.12—Cosmetologist communicating with client.

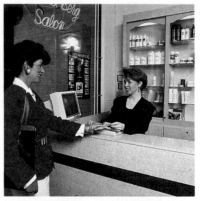

1.13—The cosmetologist as salesperson.

Human Relations and Your Professional Attitude

Human relations is the psychology of getting along well with others. Your professional attitude is expressed by your own self-esteem, confidence in your profession, and by the respect you show others.

Good habits and practices acquired during your school training lay the foundation for a successful career in cosmetology. The following are guidelines for good human relations that will help you to gain confidence and deal successfully with others.

1. Always greet a client by name, with a pleasant tone of voice. Address a client by his or her last name (Mrs. Smith, Mr. Jones, Miss Allen) unless the client prefers first names and if it is customary to use first names in your salon.

2. Be alert to the client's mood. Some clients prefer quiet and relaxation, others like to talk. Be a good listener and confine your conversation to the client's needs. Never gossip or tell off-color stories. (Fig. 1.14)

3. Topics of conversation should be carefully chosen. Friendly relations are achieved through pleasant conversations. Let your client be the guide in the topic of conversation. In a business setting it is best to avoid discussing controversial topics such as religion and politics, topics that relate to your personal life such as personal problems, or subjects relating to other people such as another client's behavior, poor workmanship of fellow workers or competitors, or information given to you in confidence.

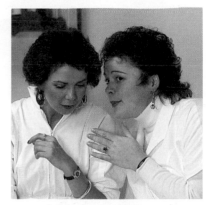

1.14—Nobody likes a person who gossips.

4. Make a good impression by looking the part of the successful cosmetologist, and by speaking and acting in a professional manner at all times.

5. Cultivate self-confidence, and project a pleasing personality.

6. Show interest in the client's personal preferences. Give your undivided attention. Maintain eye contact and concentrate totally on your client.

7. Use tact and diplomacy when dealing with problems you may encounter.

8. Be capable and efficient in your work.

9. Be punctual. Arrive at work on time and keep appointments on schedule. Plan each day's schedule so that you manage your time effectively.

10. Develop your business and sales abilities. Use tact when suggesting additional services or products to clients.

11. Avoid saying anything that sounds as if you are criticizing, condemning, or putting down a client's opinions.

12. Keep informed of new products and services so you can answer clients' questions intelligently.

13. Continue to add to your knowledge and skills.

14. Be ethical in all your dealings with clients and others with whom you come in contact.

15. Always let the client see that you practice the highest standards of sanitation.

16. Avoid criticizing your competitors.

17. Deal with all disputes and differences in private. Take care of all problems promptly.

People Skills

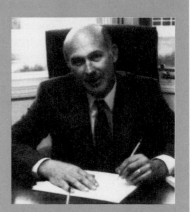

The East Coast Salon Owners' Association is not for owners only. President Joe O'Riorden, who is headquartered in Marlboro, Massachusetts, works with members' stylists and has trained some who are making substantial incomes by helping them to improve their communication skills. O'Riorden also lectures in schools, and his pointers on "people skills" are ones that you can use immediately, your first day on the job.

"First, take a course in public speaking," says O'Riorden. "Learn to listen, but not judgmentally. Try to view the world through your client's eyes. Also, it's alienating to talk to a client as she looks at you in the mirror. If it's important, look her in the eye when you say it.

"Ninety percent of communication is nonverbal, and the nonverbal can contradict what you say. You can't talk high fashion if you're wearing jeans. Conversely, the biggest thing is to ask the client questions to be certain that you understand *her,* especially those questions that are prompted by nonverbal clues. Knowing the right questions to ask can be your greatest asset."

To Be Successful . . .

1. Be punctual. Get to work on time and keep all appointments. Being punctual gains the admiration and confidence of your clients, your manager, and your co-workers.
2. Be courteous. Courtesy plays an important part in bringing clients to the salon and in keeping them as regular customers.
3. Set a good example for your profession. Your own neat, attractive, and fashionable appearance expresses your pride in yourself and your profession. Clients have confidence in the cosmetologist who looks the part.
4. Be efficient and skillful. Practice your skills so that you can give services efficiently and gently. Clients appreciate the cosmetologist who cares about their comfort and is skillful when giving services.
5. Practice effective communications. Speaking well of others and being able to give sincere compliments will be an asset in your career as a professional cosmetologist. Being a good listener and being efficient and courteous when speaking on the telephone or with clients during the service will help you build a successful business.

To be successful, you should extend courtesy to all with whom you come in contact. This includes state board members and inspectors, who are contributing to the higher standards of cosmetology.

To be successful, you must know the laws, rules, and regulations that govern cosmetology, and you must comply with them. By complying, you are contributing to the health, welfare, and safety of your community.

Professional Ethics

Ethics is defined as the study of standards of conduct and moral judgment. Codes of ethics for various professions are established by boards or commissions. In cosmetology, each state has a board or commission that sets standards that all cosmetologists who work in that state must follow. However, ethics goes beyond a set of rules and regulations. In the field of cosmetology, ethics is also a code of behavior by which you conduct yourself. Much of what was discussed in the previous section is directly related to an informal code of ethical standards.

Ethics deal with proper conduct and business dealings with employers, clients and co-workers, and others with whom you come in contact. Ethical conduct helps to build the client's confidence in you. Having your clients speak well of you to others is the best form of advertising and helps you build a successful business. The following are rules of ethics you should practice:

1. Give courteous and friendly service to all clients. Treat everyone honestly and fairly; do not show favoritism.
2. Be courteous and show respect for the feelings, beliefs, and rights of others.
3. Keep your word. Be responsible and fulfill your obligations.
4. Build your reputation by setting an example of good conduct and behavior.
5. Be loyal to your employer, managers, and associates.
6. Obey all provisions of the state cosmetology laws.
7. Practice the highest standards of sanitation to protect your health and the health of your co-workers and clients.
8. Believe in the cosmetology profession. Practice it faithfully and sincerely.
9. Do not try to sell your clients a product or service they do not need or want.
10. As a student:

    • Be loyal to, and cooperate with, school personnel and fellow students.
    • Comply with school and clinic rules and regulations.

Questionable practices, extravagant claims, and unfulfilled promises violate the rules of ethical conduct and cast an unfavorable light on cosmetology. Unethical practices affect the student, the cosmetologist, the school or salon, and the entire industry.

Review Questions

YOUR PROFESSIONAL IMAGE
1. List the guidelines you should follow to maintain a healthy body and mind.
2. Define physical presentation.
3. Define personality.
4. What does communication consist of?
5. Define good human relations.
6. How is your professional attitude expressed?
7. What is professional ethics?

2

BACTERIOLOGY

LEARNING OBJECTIVES

After completing this chapter, you should be able to:

1. List the various types and classifications of bacteria.
2. Describe how bacteria grow and reproduce.
3. Describe the relationship of bacteria to the spread of disease.

Introduction

Bacteriology (bak-teer-i-**OL**-o-jee), *sterilization* (ster-i-li-**ZAY**-shun), and *sanitation* (san-i-**TAY**-shun) are subjects of practical importance to you as a cosmetologist, because they have a direct bearing on your well-being as well as on your clients' welfare. To protect individual and public health, every cosmetologist should know when, why, and how to use good sterilization and sanitation practices.

In order to understand the importance of sanitation and sterilization, a basic understanding of how *bacteria* (bak-**TEER**-i-ah) affect our daily lives is most helpful.

Bacteriology

Bacteriology is the science that deals with the study of *micro-organisms* (meye-kroh-**OR**-gah-niz-ems) called bacteria.

As a cosmetologist, you should understand how the spread of disease can be prevented and what precautions you must take to protect your health and your clients' health. Once you have an understanding of the relationship between bacteria and disease, you will understand the need for school and salon cleanliness and sanitation.

State boards of cosmetology and health departments require that a business that serves the public must follow certain sanitary precautions. Contagious diseases, skin infections, and blood poisoning are caused either by infectious bacteria being transmitted from one individual to another, or by the use of unsanitary implements (such as combs, brushes, hairpins, clippies, rollers, etc.). Dirty hands and fingernails are other sources of infectious bacteria.

Bacteria are minute, one-celled vegetable micro-organisms found nearly everywhere. They are especially numerous in dust, dirt, refuse, and diseased tissues. Bacteria are also known as *germs* (**JURMS**) or *microbes* (**MEYE**-krohbs). Bacteria can exist almost anywhere: on the skin of the body, in water, air, decayed matter, secretions of body openings, on clothing, and beneath the nails.

Bacteria can be seen only with the aid of a *microscope* (**MEYE**-kroh-skohp). Fifteen hundred rod-shaped bacteria will barely cover the head of a pin.

TYPES OF BACTERIA

There are hundreds of different kinds of bacteria. However, bacteria are classified into two types, depending on whether they are beneficial or harmful.

1. Most bacteria are ***non-pathogenic*** (non-path-o-**JEN**-ik) organisms (helpful or harmless), which perform many useful functions, such as decomposing refuse and improving soil fertility. ***Saprophytes*** (sap-**RO**-fyts), non-pathogenic bacteria, live on dead matter and do not produce disease.
2. ***Pathogenic*** (path-o-**JEN**-ik) organisms (microbes or germs) are harmful, and although in the minority, produce disease when they invade plant or animal tissue. To this group belong the ***parasites*** (**PAR**-ah-syts), which require living matter for their growth.

It is because of pathogenic bacteria that beauty schools and salons must maintain certain sanitary and cleanliness standards.

Business Tips

Cosmetology is a field you grow into, and assistants and junior stylists who want to advance quickly will benefit from this advice from Jerry Gordon, owner of Gordon Designs in Chicago.

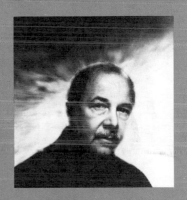

"Don't take the first job you're offered," advises Gordon. "Start by looking for a salon that offers advanced training, has a benefits package, and is willing to help you develop. Don't be disheartened by ads that read, 'Stylist with following wanted.' A salon that has to do this to generate new business is desperate and not the best place to be.

"When you find a salon you like, show a willingness to work hard. This isn't easy for young, eager stylists, but hair designing is a developed craft. You have to take orders, and learn the operation and culture of the salon, but a stylist who is trained in-house is the best asset a salon can have."

For those who dislike the idea of starting at the shampoo bowl, Gordon has this final advice: "Work on your patience," he says. "You've chosen a wonderful profession and you're embarking on a career that offers excitement, ego gratification, the opportunity to travel, and guaranteed on-the-job training. This is a very progressive field to be in, and you can go as far as you want."

PRONUNCIATIONS OF TERMS RELATING TO PATHOGENIC BACTERIA

Singular

coccus (**KOK**-us)

bacillus (bah-**SIL**-us)

spirillum (speye-**RIL**-um)

staphylococcus
   (staf-i-lo-**KOK**-us)

streptococcus
   (strep-to-**KOK**-us)

diplococcus
   (deye-ploh-**KOK**-us)

Plural

cocci (**KOK**-si)

bacilli (ba-**SIL**-i)

spirilla (spi-**RIL**-a)

staphylococci
   (staf-i-lo-**KOK**-si)

streptococci
   (strep-to-**KOK**-si)

diplococci (dip-lo-**KOK**-si)

CLASSIFICATIONS OF PATHOGENIC BACTERIA

Bacteria have distinct shapes that help to identify them. Pathogenic bacteria are classified as follows (Fig. 2.1):

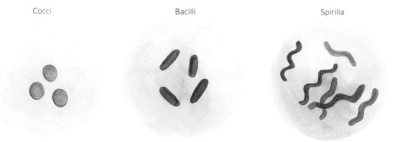

2.1—General forms of bacteria.

1. *Cocci* are round-shaped organisms that appear singly or in the following groups (Fig. 2.2):
   a) *Staphylococci:* Pus-forming organisms that grow in bunches or clusters. They cause abscesses, pustules, and boils.
   b) *Streptococci:* Pus-forming organisms that grow in chains. They cause infections such as strep throat.
   c) *Diplococci:* They grow in pairs and cause pneumonia.

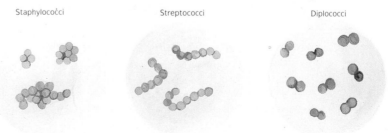

2.2—Groupings of bacteria.

2. *Bacilli* are short rod-shaped organisms. They are the most common bacteria and produce diseases such as tetanus (lockjaw), influenza, typhoid fever, tuberculosis, and diphtheria. (Fig. 2.3)
3. *Spirilla* are curved or corkscrew-shaped organisms. They are subdivided into several groups. Of chief importance to us is the *treponema pallida* (trep-o-**NE**-mah **PAL**-i-dah), which causes *syphilis* (**SIF**-i-lis).

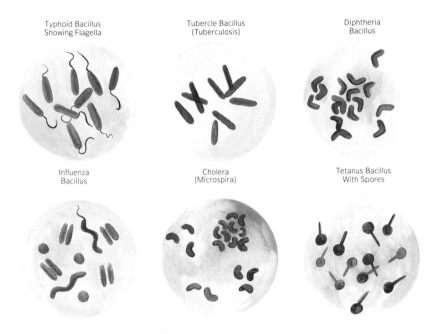

2.3 — Disease-producing bacteria.

Movement of Bacteria

Cocci rarely show active *motility* (self-movement). They are transmitted on the air, in dust, or in the substance in which they settle. Bacilli and spirilla are both motile and use hairlike projections, known as *flagella* (flah-**JEL**-ah) or *cilia* (**SIL**-ee-a), to move about. A whiplike motion of these hairs propels bacteria about in liquid.

BACTERIAL GROWTH AND REPRODUCTION

Bacteria generally consist of an outer cell wall and internal *protoplasm* (**PROH**-toh-plaz-em), material needed to sustain life. They manufacture their own food from the surrounding environment, give off waste products, and grow and reproduce. Bacteria have two distinct phases in their life cycle: the *active* or *vegetative stage*, and the *inactive* or *spore-forming stage*.

Active or Vegetative Stage

During the active stage, bacteria grow and reproduce. These micro-organisms multiply best in warm, dark, damp, or dirty places where sufficient food is available.

When conditions are favorable, bacteria grow and reproduce. When they reach their largest size, they divide into two new cells. This division is called *mitosis*. The cells formed are called *daughter cells*. When conditions are unfavorable, bacteria die or become inactive. (See chapter on cells, anatomy, and physiology.)

Inactive or Spore-Forming Stage

Certain bacteria, such as the anthrax and tetanus bacilli, form *spherical spores* with tough outer coverings during their inactive stage. The purpose is to be able to withstand periods of famine, dryness, and unsuitable temperatures. In this stage, spores can be blown about and are not harmed by disinfectants, heat, or cold.

When favorable conditions are restored, the spores change into the active or vegetative form, then grow and reproduce.

BACTERIAL INFECTIONS

There can be no infection without the presence of pathogenic bacteria. An infection occurs when the body is unable to cope with the bacteria and their harmful toxins. A *local infection* is indicated by a boil or pimple that contains pus. The presence of *pus* is a sign of infection. Bacteria, waste matter, decayed tissue, body cells, and living and dead blood cells are all found in pus. Staphylococci are the most common pus-forming bacteria. A *general infection* results when the bloodstream carries the bacteria and their toxins to all parts of the body, as in syphilis.

A disease becomes *contagious* (kon-**TAY**-jus) or *communicable* (ko-**MU**-ni-kah-bil) when it spreads from one person to another by contact. Some of the more common contagious diseases that prevent a cosmetologist from working are tuberculosis, common cold, ringworm, scabies, head lice, and virus infections.

The chief sources of contagion are unclean hands and implements, open sores, pus, mouth and nose discharges, and the common use of drinking cups and towels. Uncovered coughing or sneezing and spitting in public also spread germs.

Pathogenic bacteria can enter the body through:

1. A break in the skin, such as a cut, pimple, or scratch.
2. The mouth (breathing or swallowing air, water, or food).
3. The nose (air).
4. The eyes or ears (dirt).

The body fights infection by means of:

1. Unbroken skin, which is the body's first line of defense.
2. Body secretions, such as perspiration and digestive juices.
3. White cells within the blood that destroy bacteria.
4. Antitoxins that counteract the toxins produced by bacteria.

Infections can be prevented and controlled through personal hygiene and public sanitation.

OTHER INFECTIOUS AGENTS

Filterable viruses (fil-**TER**-a-bil **VI**-rus-es) are living organisms so small that they can pass through the pores of a porcelain filter. They cause the common cold and other respiratory (**RES**-pi-rah-torh-ee) and gastro-intestinal (digestive tract) (**GAS**-troh-in-**TES**-ti-nal) infections.

Parasites are organisms that live on other living organisms without giving anything in return.

Plant parasites or *fungi* (**FUN**-ji), such as molds, mildews, and yeasts, can produce contagious diseases, such as ringworm and *favus* (**FA**-vus), a skin disease of the scalp.

Animal parasites are responsible for contagious diseases. For example, the itch mite burrows under the skin, causing *scabies* (**SKAY**-beez), and infection of the scalp by lice is called *pediculosis* (pe-dik-yoo-**LOH**-sis).

Contagious diseases caused by parasites should never be treated in a beauty school or salon. Clients should be referred to a physician.

IMMUNITY

Immunity (i-**MYOO**-ni-tee) is the ability of the body to destroy bacteria that have gained entrance, and thus to resist infection. Immunity against disease can be natural or acquired and is a sign of good health. *Natural immunity* means natural resistance to disease. It is partly inherited and partly developed through hygienic living. *Acquired immunity* is something the body develops after it has overcome a disease, or through inoculation.

A human disease carrier is a person who is personally immune to a disease yet can transmit germs to other people. *Typhoid* (**TI** foid) *fever* and *diphtheria* (dif-**THEER**-i-a) can be transmitted in this manner.

Bacteria can be destroyed by disinfectants and by intense heat achieved by boiling, steaming, baking, or burning, and ultra violet rays. (This subject is covered in the chapter on sterilization and sanitation.)

Review Questions

BACTERIOLOGY

1. Why is bacteriology necessary?
2. Define bacteriology.
3. What are bacteria?
4. Where can bacteria exist? Give examples.
5. Define two types of bacteria.
6. What are parasites and saprophytes?
7. Name and define three forms of bacteria.
8. Name and define three types of cocci bacteria.
9. How do bacteria multiply?
10. Describe the active and inactive stages of bacteria.
11. How does bacteria move about?
12. Name two types of infection and define each.
13. What is a contagious or communicable disease?
14. How can infections be controlled or prevented?
15. Name two diseases produced by a) plant parasites and b) animal parasites.
16. Define immunity. Name two types.
17. How can bacteria be destroyed?

3

STERILIZATION AND SANITATION

LEARNING OBJECTIVES

After completing this chapter, you should be able to:

1. Describe the various methods of sterilization.
2. List the differences between sterilization and sanitation.
3. Describe how the spread of disease can be prevented.
4. Identify the methods of sanitation employed in the beauty salon.
5. Discuss why good sanitation practices in the beauty salon are necessary.

Sterilization

Sterilization is the process of making an environment germfree by destroying all bacteria, whether they are beneficial or harmful. Health departments and state boards of cosmetology recognize that it is impossible to completely sterilize all implements and equipment in the beauty school or salon. Therefore, it is generally recognized that the implements and equipment may be sanitized rather than sterilized. Throughout the entire text the term *sanitize* will be used to indicate all forms of sanitation.

Sterilization and sanitation are of practical importance to the cosmetologist because they deal with methods used either to prevent the growth of germs or to destroy them entirely when possible, particularly those responsible for infections and communicable diseases.

METHODS OF STERILIZATION AND SANITATION

Chemicals are the most effective sanitizing agents used in beauty salons to destroy or check the growth of bacteria. Chemical agents used for sanitizing are antiseptics and disinfectants.

1. An *antiseptic* (an-ti-**SEP**-tik) is a substance that may kill bacteria or retard their growth. As a general rule, antiseptics can be used safely on the skin.

2. A *disinfectant* (dis-in-**FEK**-tant) destroys most bacteria and is used to sanitize implements.

Several chemicals can be classified as both antiseptic and disinfectant. A strong solution such as *formalin* (**FOHR**-mah-lin) may be used as a disinfectant and a weak solution such as *quats* (**KWATS**) as an antiseptic.

Requirements of a good disinfectant:

1. Convenient to prepare
2. Quick acting
3. Practically odorless
4. Noncorrosive
5. Economical
6. Nonirritating to skin

There are many prepared and ready-to-use chemical disinfectant agents on the market. If these are used, select the ones that have been approved by your board of health or state board of cosmetology. Chemicals commonly used in the beauty salon are:

1. *Sodium hypochlorite* (**SOH**-di-um **HY**-po-chlor-it) to sanitize implements.
2. *Quaternary ammonium compounds* (quats) (**KWAH**-ter-nah-ree ah-**MOH**-nee-um **KOM**-pownds [**KWATS**]) to sanitize implements.
3. *Formaldehyde* (for-**MAL**-de-heyed) to sanitize implements.
4. *Alcohol* (**AL**-ko-hawl) to sanitize sharp cutting instruments and electrodes.
5. *Prepared commercial products* that clean floors, sinks, and toilet bowls.

A *wet sanitizer* is any covered receptacle large enough to hold a disinfectant solution in which the objects to be sanitized can be completely immersed. (Fig. 3.1) Wet sanitizers can be obtained in various sizes and shapes. Before immersing objects in a wet sanitizer containing a disinfectant solution, be sure to:

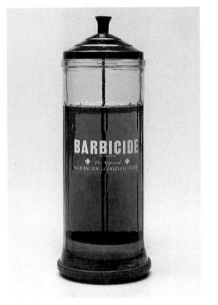

3.1 – Wet sanitizer.

1. Remove hair from combs and brushes.
2. Wash them thoroughly with hot water and soap.
3. Rinse them thoroughly.

This procedure prevents contamination of the solution. Further, soap and hot water remove most of the bacteria.

After the implements are removed from the disinfectant solution, they must be rinsed in clean water, wiped dry with a clean towel, and stored in a dry cabinet sanitizer until needed.

A *dry* or *cabinet sanitizer* is an airtight cabinet containing an active *fumigant.* A fumigant is a vapor that is used to keep clean objects sanitary. The sanitized implements are kept clean by storing them in the cabinet until they are needed.

How to prepare a fumigant. Place 1 tablespoonful (15 ml) of borax and 1 tablespoonful (15 ml) of formalin on a small tray on the bottom of the cabinet. This will form formaldehyde vapors. Replace chemicals regularly. They lose their strength, depending on how often the cabinet door is opened and closed.

Formalin is also available in tablet form. Follow the manufacturer's directions.

Ultra violet ray electrical sanitizers are effective for keeping combs, brushes, and implements clean until they are ready for use.

Combs, brushes, and implements must be sanitized before they are placed in the ultra violet sanitizer. Follow the manufacturer's directions for proper use.

CHEMICAL SANITIZING AGENTS

Sodium Hypochlorite
Sodium hypochlorite (common household bleach) compounds are frequently used to provide the sanitizing ability of chlorine.

One of the key advantages of chlorine is its ability to destroy viruses. A 10% solution is recommended with an immersion time of 10 minutes. Many prepared disinfectants contain sodium hypochlorite. Follow the manufacturer's directions for mixing and immersion time.

Quaternary Ammonium Compounds (QUATS)

These compounds are effective as disinfectants. They are available under different trade and chemical names. The advantages claimed for them are that they take a short time to disinfect; and they are odorless, colorless, nontoxic, and stable. A 1:1000 solution (1 part quats to 1,000 parts water) is commonly used to sanitize implements. Immersion time ranges from 1 to 5 minutes, depending on the strength of the solution used.

CAUTION

▶ *Before using any quats, read and follow the manufacturer's directions on the label as well as the accompanying literature.*

Formalin

Formalin is a sanitizing agent that can be used as either an antiseptic or a disinfectant, depending on its percentage strength. When purchased, formalin is approximately 37% to 40% formaldehyde gas in water. Because formaldehyde is a controversial substance, check with your state board of cosmetology before using.

Formalin is used in various strengths, for different purposes:

- 25% solution (equivalent to 10% formaldehyde gas) used to sanitize implements. Immerse implements in the solution for at least 10 minutes. (Preparation: 2 parts formalin, 5 parts water, 1 part glycerine)
- 10% solution (equivalent to 4% formaldehyde gas) used to sanitize combs and brushes. Immerse them for at least 20 minutes. (Preparation: 1 part formalin, 9 parts water)
- 5% solution (equivalent to 2% formaldehyde gas) used to cleanse the hands after they have been in contact with wounds, skin eruptions, etc. Also used to sanitize shampoo bowls and chairs. (Preparation: 1 part formalin, 19 parts water)

Sanitizing with Chemical Disinfectants

1. Wash implements thoroughly with soap and hot water.
2. Use a plain hot water rinse to remove all traces of soap.
3. Immerse implements in a wet sanitizer (containing approved disinfectant) for the required time.

▶ **NOTE:** Consult your state board of cosmetology or health department for a list of the approved disinfectants to be used in cosmetology schools and salons.

4. Remove implements from the wet sanitizer, rinse in water, and wipe dry with a clean towel.
5. Store sanitized implements in individually wrapped cellophane envelopes in a cabinet sanitizer or in an ultra violet ray cabinet until they are ready to be used.

Sanitizing with Alcohol

To sanitize electrodes and implements, use 70% alcohol or 99% isopropyl alcohol.

70% alcohol refers to ethyl or grain alcohol.
99% isopropyl alcohol is the same strength as 70% ethyl alcohol.

Implements with a fine cutting edge are best sanitized by rubbing the surface with a cotton pad dampened with 70% alcohol. This application prevents the cutting edges from becoming dull.

Electrodes (ee-**LEK**-trohds) can be safely sanitized by gently rubbing the exposed surface with a cotton pad dampened with 70% alcohol. Then place instruments in a dry sanitizer or an ultra violet ray sanitizer until ready for use.

PROPORTIONS FOR MAKING PERCENTAGE SOLUTIONS OF DISINFECTANTS

100% Active Liquid Concentrate	Strength
5 drops of liquid to 1 oz. (30 ml) water or 1 teaspoonful (5 ml) of liquid to 12 oz. (.36 l) water	1%
10 drops of liquid to 1 oz. (30 ml) water or 2 teaspoonfuls (10 ml) of liquid to 12 oz. (.36 l) water	2%
4 teaspoonfuls (20 ml) of liquid to 12 oz. (.36 l) water	4%
5 teaspoonfuls (25 ml) of liquid to 12 oz. (.36 l)water	5%
10 teaspoonfuls (50 ml) of liquid to 12 oz. (.36 l) water	10%

Table of Equivalents

Ordinary measured glass	8 oz. (.237 l)
1 pint	16 oz. (.475 l)
1 quart	32 oz. (.95 l)
½ gallon	64 oz. (1.9 l)

Business Tips

It's your first day in your new career. You've found the perfect salon and you can't wait to start doing hair. The only problem is, you don't have any appointments.

This is a scenario that every beginning stylist dreads. And, there is a way to overcome it that has proven effective and costs virtually nothing. Kenneth Anders, owner of five Kenneth's Designgroup salons in Columbus, Ohio, knows how to build a stylist's book. Anders's stylist promotion program accounts for 90% of his salon's business, and its implementation only requires time, not money.

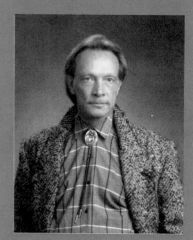

"The best advertising for any stylist, especially a beginner, is word-of-mouth," says Anders. "It quickly doubles and triples your income without a huge dollar investment.

"The program starts in the salon. Simply ask each client to tell three people to come to you. Hand them three of your business cards with his or her name written on the back. Then, tell that client that when those three cards are brought to you by *new* clients, he or she will earn a free haircut and style. After the appointment, follow up with a note that thanks the client for allowing you to do his or her hair, and includes a reminder to send you three clients to earn a free cut and style. Then, monitor the business cards as they come in."

As you develop your client base, don't be too concerned about giving away the free cuts. According to Anders, "Almost everyone will send you one client. The number who actually send in three, however, is quite small, so don't worry about giving away the farm."

Sanitizing Floors, Sinks, and Toilet Bowls

To sanitize floors, sinks, and toilet bowls in the beauty salon use a commercial product such as Lysol or pine oil. These contain the chemicals *cresol* (**KREE**-sohl) and *phenol* (**FEE**-nol) which are disinfectants. Deodorants can be used to offset offensive smells and add a refreshing scent.

Whichever disinfectant you use, make sure that it is properly diluted, as suggested by the manufacturer. (See chart on proportions for making percentage solutions of disinfectants on page 35.) Clients like to receive services in a beauty salon that is spotless. Get into the habit now. Keep everything clean and in order.

The use of chemical sanitizing agents involves certain dangers, unless safety measures are taken to prevent mistakes and accidents. Follow these safety rules:

1. Purchase chemicals in small quantities and store them in a cool, dry place; otherwise they could deteriorate when exposed to air, light, and heat.
2. Carefully weigh and measure chemicals.
3. Keep all containers labeled, covered, and under lock and key.
4. Do not smell chemicals or solutions because some of them have pungent odors and might irritate the membranes of your nose.
5. Avoid spilling when diluting chemicals.
6. Prevent skin burns by using forceps to insert or remove objects from the source of heat.
7. Keep a complete first aid kit on hand.

SANITIZING RULES

Chemical solutions in sanitizers should be changed regularly (according to state board of cosmetology regulations in your state).

Manicuring implements must be kept in a disinfectant solution (70% alcohol) during a manicure.

All articles must be clean and free from hair before being sanitized.

Sanitize electrical appliances by rubbing their surface with a cotton pad dampened with 70% alcohol.

All cups, finger bowls, or similar objects must be sanitized prior to being used for another client.

▶ NOTE: Immersing implements in a chemical solution must conform to state board of cosmetology regulations in your state.

COMMONLY USED DISINFECTANTS

Name	Form	Strength	How to Use
Quaternary Ammonium Compounds (Quats)	Liquid or tablet	1:1000 solution	Immerse implements in solution for 20 or more minutes.
Formalin	Liquid	25% solution	Immerse implements in solution for 10 or more minutes.
Formalin	Liquid	10% solution	Immerse implements in solution for 20 or more minutes.
Alcohol	Liquid	70% solution	Immerse implements or sanitize electrodes and sharp cutting edges 10 or more minutes.

COMMONLY USED ANTISEPTICS

Name	Form	Strength	Use
Boric Acid	White crystals	2-5% solution	Cleanse the eyes.
Tincture of Iodine	Liquid	2% solution	Cleanse cuts and wounds.
Hydrogen Peroxide	Liquid	3-5% solution	Cleanse skin and minor cuts.
Ethyl or Grain Alcohol	Liquid	60% solution	Cleanse hands, skin, and minute cuts. Not to be used if irritation is present.
Formalin	Liquid	5% solution	Cleanse shampoo bowl, cabinet, etc.
Chloramine-T (Chlorazene; Chlorozol)	White crystals	½% solution	Cleanse skin and hands, and for general use.
Sodium Hypochlorite (Javelle water; Zonite)	White crystals	½% solution	Rinse the hands.

Other approved disinfectants and antiseptics are being used in beauty salons. Consult your state board of cosmetology or your health department.

Public Sanitation

Public sanitation is the promotion of measures to protect public health and to prevent the spread of infectious diseases. The importance of sanitation cannot be overemphasized. Professional services bring the cosmetologist in direct contact with a client's skin, scalp, hair, and nails. By practicing the best sanitary measures you protect your client's health, as well as your own.

Various government agencies protect community health by providing for a wholesome food and water supply and the quick disposal of refuse. These steps are only a few of the ways in which the public health is safeguarded.

The air in a beauty salon should be kept fresh. It should not be dry or stagnant, nor should it have a stale, musty odor. Room temperature should be about 70 degrees Fahrenheit (21 degrees Celsius). The salon can be ventilated with the aid of an exhaust fan or an air-conditioning unit. Air-conditioning has the advantage of allowing you to regulate the quality and quantity of air brought into the salon. The temperature and moisture content of the air can be regulated by means of air-conditioning.

A person with an infectious disease is a source of contagion to others. Cosmetologists with colds or other communicable diseases must not be permitted to serve clients. Likewise, clients obviously suffering from an infectious disease must not be accommodated in a beauty salon. In this way, the best interests of other clients are served.

The state board of cosmetology and board of health in each state or locality have formulated sanitary regulations governing salons. Every cosmetologist must be familiar with these regulations and obey them.

Summary

Adherence to the following sanitary rules will result in cleaner and better service to the public:

1. Every salon must be well lighted, heated, and ventilated, and must be kept in a clean and sanitary condition.
2. The walls, curtains, and floor coverings in a salon also must be washed and kept clean.
3. All salons must be supplied with hot and cold running water. Drinking facilities (individual paper cups and/or fountain) should be provided.
4. All plumbing fixtures must be properly installed and work effectively.
5. The premises must be kept free from rodents, vermin, flies, or similar insects.
6. The salon should not be used for eating, sleeping, or living quarters.
7. All hair, cotton, or other waste material must be removed from the floor without delay and deposited in a closed container, then removed from the premises frequently.
8. Rest rooms must be kept sanitary and have a soap dispenser and individual paper towels.
9. Each cosmetologist must wear a clean uniform while working on clients.
10. The cosmetologist must cleanse his or her hands thoroughly before and after serving a client and after leaving the rest room.
11. A freshly laundered towel must be used for each client. Clean towels must be stored in a sanitized, closed cabinet. After use, soiled towels and linens must be placed immediately in containers provided for this purpose. Keep dirty towels away from clean towels.
12. Headrest coverings and neck strips must be changed for each client.
13. Do not permit the shampoo cape to come in contact with the client's skin.

14. The common use of powder puffs, lip color, cheek color, sponges, or styptic pencils is prohibited.

15. Keep lotions, ointments, creams, and powders in clean, closed containers. Use a clean spatula to remove creams or ointments from jars. Use sterile cotton pledgets to apply lotions and powders.
    Re-cover cosmetic containers after each use.

16. For manicuring, provide a sanitary container or finger bowl with an individual paper cup for each client.

17. Discard emery boards after use on a client.

18. Soiled combs, brushes, towels, or other used material must be removed from the tops of work stations immediately after use.

19. Clippies, hairpins, or bobby pins must not be placed in the mouth.

20. Combs or implements must not be carried in pockets of the uniform.

21. Hairnets must be washed after each use.

22. Clippies, curlers, bobby pins, or hairpins must be sanitized after each use.

23. All implements and articles used must first be sanitized and then placed in a dustproof or airtight container, or in a cabinet sanitizer.

24. Objects dropped on the floor are not to be used until they are sanitized.

25. Dogs, cats, birds, or other pets should not be permitted in a beauty school or salon.

▶ NOTE:

1. The responsibility for sanitation rests with each student in the cosmetology school and each cosmetologist in the salon. The manager must provide the necessities for school and salon sanitation.

2. You must obey the rules issued by the health department and the state board of cosmetology regarding acceptable methods of sanitation.

Review Questions

STERILIZATION AND SANITATION

1. What is sterilization?
2. What is the difference between sterilization and sanitation?
3. Name five methods of sterilization and sanitation.
4. What is the difference between an antiseptic and a disinfectant?
5. Name three chemical disinfectants.
6. Describe a wet sanitizer.
7. What is a fumigant?
8. What is a dry or cabinet sanitizer?
9. Why are good sanitation practices necessary in the salon?
10. Who formulates and governs sanitary regulations in beauty salons?

4

PROPERTIES OF THE SCALP AND HAIR

LEARNING OBJECTIVES

After completing this chapter, you should be able to:

1. Explain the purpose of hair.
2. Define what hair is.
3. Define the chief composition of hair.
4. Define the divisions of hair.
5. Discuss the facts relating to hair structure, growth, and distribution.
6. Describe the theories pertaining to the life and replacement of hair.
7. List the causes of changes in hair color.
8. Define basic scalp care.
9. Know how to perform scalp manipulation techniques.
10. Recognize the scalp and hair disorders commonly seen in the salon and school and know which can be treated there.

Introduction

As a hairstylist, it is important to have a technical knowledge of hair. This knowledge will be an asset to you as a professional cosmetologist.

Hair, like people, comes in a variety of colors, shapes, and sizes. To keep hair healthy and beautiful, proper attention must be given to its care and treatment. Applying a harsh cosmetic such as one that contains a lot of alcohol or providing improper hair services can cause the hair structure to become weakened or damaged. Knowledge and analysis of the client's hair, tactful suggestions for its improvement, and a sincere interest in maintaining its health and beauty should be primary concerns of every hairstylist.

Hair

The study of hair, technically called *trichology* (treye-**KOL**-o-jee), is important because stylists deal with hair on a daily basis. The chief purposes of hair are *adornment* and *protection* of the head from heat, cold, and injury.

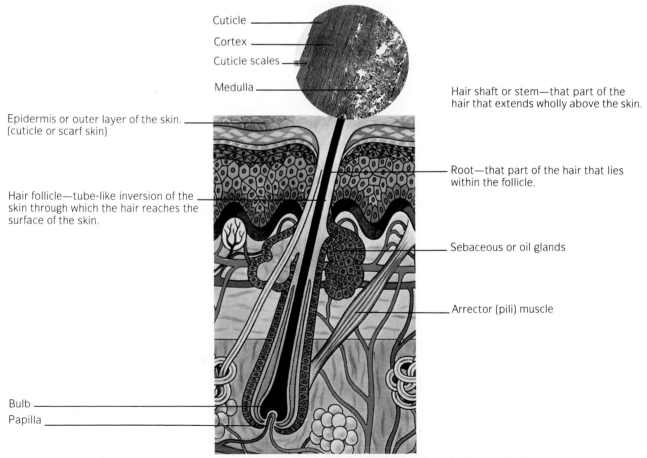

Cuticle

Cortex

Cuticle scales

Medulla

Hair shaft or stem—that part of the hair that extends wholly above the skin.

Epidermis or outer layer of the skin. (cuticle or scarf skin)

Root—that part of the hair that lies within the follicle.

Hair follicle—tube-like inversion of the skin through which the hair reaches the surface of the skin.

Sebaceous or oil glands

Arrector (pili) muscle

Bulb

Papilla

4.1—Cross section of skin and hair.

Hair is an *appendage* of the skin, a slender, threadlike outgrowth of the skin and scalp. (Fig. 4.1) There is no sense of feeling in hair, due to the absence of nerves.

COMPOSITION OF THE HAIR

Hair is composed chiefly of the protein *keratin* (**KER**-a-tin), which is found in all horny growths including the nails and skin. (Fig. 4.2) The chemical composition of hair varies with its color. Darker hair has more carbon and less oxygen; the reverse is true for lighter hair. Average hair is composed of 50.65% carbon, 6.36% hydrogen, 17.14% nitrogen, 5.0% sulfur, and 20.85% oxygen.

4.2 – Magnified view of hair cuticle, which is composed of keratin.

DIVISIONS OF THE HAIR

Full-grown human hair is divided into two principal parts: the root and the shaft.

1. The *hair root* is that portion of the hair structure located beneath the skin surface. This is the portion of the hair enclosed within the follicle.
2. The *hair shaft* is that portion of the hair structure extending above the skin surface.

Structures Associated with the Hair Root

The three main structures associated with the hair root are the follicle, bulb, and papilla.

The *follicle* (**FOL**-i-kel) is a tubelike depression, or pocket, in the skin or scalp that encases the hair root. (Fig. 4.3) Each hair has its own follicle, which varies in depth depending on the thickness and location of the skin. (We talk later in this chapter about the different types of hair.) One or more oil glands are attached to each hair follicle.

The follicle does not run straight down into the skin or scalp, but is set at an angle so that the hair above the surface flows

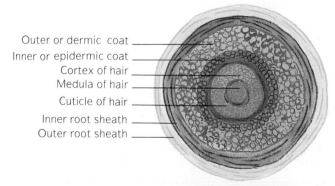

Outer or dermic coat
Inner or epidermic coat
Cortex of hair
Medula of hair
Cuticle of hair
Inner root sheath
Outer root sheath

4.3 – Cross section of the hair and follicle.

naturally to one side. This natural flow is sometimes called the *hair stream* of the scalp. It is fascinating that nature has allowed for hair to emerge from the scalp slanting in a given direction.

The *bulb* is a thickened, club-shaped structure which forms the lower part of the hair root. The lower part of the hair bulb is hollowed out to fit over and cover the hair papilla.

The *papilla* (pa-**PIL**-ah) is a small, cone-shaped elevation located at the bottom of the hair follicle and fits into the hair bulb. Within the hair papilla is a rich blood and nerve supply that contributes to the growth and regeneration of the hair. It is through the papilla that nourishment reaches the hair bulb. As long as the papilla is healthy and well nourished, it produces hair cells that enable new hair to grow.

Structures Associated with Hair Follicles

The *arrector pili* (a-**REK**-tohr **PIGH**-ligh) is a small involuntary muscle attached to the underside of a hair follicle. Fear or cold causes it to contract and the hair stands up straight, giving the skin the appearance of "gooseflesh." Eyelash and eyebrow hair do not have arrector pili muscles.

Sebaceous (si-**BAY**-shus), or oil, glands consist of little sac-like structures in the dermis. Their ducts are connected to hair follicles. Sebaceous glands frequently become troublemakers by overproducing and bringing on a common form of oily dandruff. Normal secretion of an oily substance from these glands, called **sebum** (**SEE**-bum), gives luster and pliability to the hair and keeps the skin surface soft and supple. The production of sebum is influenced by diet, blood circulation, emotional disturbances, stimulation of endocrine glands, and drugs.

Diet influences the general health of the hair. Eating too much sweet, starchy, and fatty foods can cause the sebaceous glands to become overactive and secrete too much sebum.

Blood circulation. The hair derives its nourishment from the blood supply, which, in turn, depends on the foods we eat for certain elements. In the absence of necessary foods, the health of the hair can be affected.

Emotional disturbances are linked with the health of the hair through the nervous system. Unhealthy hair can be an indication of an unhealthy emotional state.

Endocrine glands. The secretions of the endocrine glands influence the health of the body. Any disturbance of these glands can affect the health of the body and, ultimately, the health of the hair.

Drugs, such as hormones, can adversely affect the hair's ability to receive permanent waving and other chemical services.

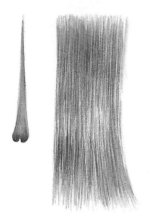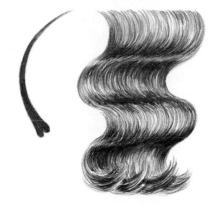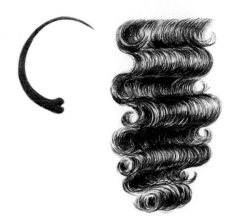

4.4a—Straight hair.   4.4b—Wavy hair.   4.4c—Curly hair.

HAIR SHAPES

Hair usually has one of three general shapes. (See Figs. 4.4a-c) As it grows out, hair assumes the shape, size, and curve of the follicle. A cross-sectional view of the hair under the microscope reveals that:

1. Straight hair is usually round.
2. Wavy hair is usually oval.
3. Curly or kinky hair is almost flat.

There is no strict rule regarding cross-sectional shapes of hair. Oval, straight, and curly hair have been found in all shapes. A myth exists that race or nationality determines the shape of hair—this is false. Anyone can have straight, wavy, or curly hair no matter what race or nationality. The direction of a hair as it projects out of the follicle determines each person's hair shape.

Direction of Hair Growth

Hair stream. Hair flowing in the same direction is known as the hair stream. It is the result of the follicles sloping in the same direction. Two such streams, sloping in opposite directions, form a natural parting of the hair.

Whorl. Hair that forms a circular pattern, as in the crown, is called a whorl. (Fig. 4.5)

Cowlick. A tuft of hair standing up is known as a cowlick. Cowlicks are more noticeable at the front hairline. However, they may be located on other parts of the scalp. When shaping or styling the hair, it is important to consider the direction of cowlicks. (Fig. 4.6)

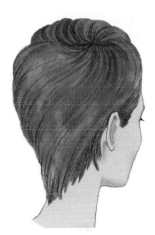

4.5—Whorl.

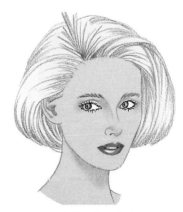

4.6—Cowlick.

LAYERS OF THE HAIR

The structure of the hair is composed of cells arranged in three layers (Also see Fig. 4.3 on page 45):

1. *Cuticle* (**KYOO**-ti-kel). The outside horny layer is composed of transparent, overlapping, protective scalelike cells, pointing away from the scalp toward the hair ends. Chemicals raise these scales so that solutions such as chemical relaxers, hair color, or permanent wave solutions can enter the hair cortex. The cuticle protects the inner structure of the hair.
2. *Cortex* (**KOR**-teks). The middle or inner layer, which gives strength and elasticity to the hair, is made up of a fibrous substance formed by elongated cells. This layer contains the pigment that gives the hair its color.
3. *Medulla* (mi-**DUL**-ah). The innermost layer is referred to as the pith, or marrow, of the hair shaft and is composed of round cells. The medulla may be absent in fine and very fine hair.

HAIR DISTRIBUTION

Hair is distributed all over the body, except on the palms of the hands, soles of the feet, lips, and eyelids. There are three types of hair on the body:

1. *Long hair* protects the scalp against the sun's rays and injury, gives adornment to the head, and forms a pleasing frame for the face. Soft, long hair also grows in the armpits of both sexes and on the faces of men. Male hormones, however, make a man's facial hair coarser than a woman's.
2. *Short or bristly hair*, such as the eyebrows and eyelashes, adds beauty and color to the face. Eyebrows divert sweat from the eyes. The eyelashes help protect the eyes from dust particles and light glare.
3. *Lanugo* (lah-**NOO**-goh) hair is the fine, soft, downy hair on the cheeks, forehead, and nearly all other areas of the body. It helps in the efficient evaporation of perspiration.

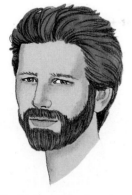

4.7—Hair on the head and face.

Technical Terms Given to Hair on the Head and Face

Barba (**BAR**-ba)—the face
Capilli (kah-**PIL**-i)—the head
Cilia (**SIL**-ee-a)—the eyelashes
Supercilia (soo-per-**SIL**-ee-a)—the eyebrows (Fig. 4.7)

HAIR GROWTH

If the hair is normal and healthy, each individual hair goes through a steady *cycle* of events: *growth, fall,* and *replacement*. You will notice that the average growth of healthy hair on the scalp is about ½" (1.25 cm) per month. The rate of growth of human hair differs on specific parts of the body, between sexes, among races, and with age. Scalp hair also differs among individuals in strength, elasticity, and waviness.

The growth of scalp hair occurs more rapidly between the ages of 15 to 30, but declines sharply between 50 to 60. Scalp hair grows faster on women than on men. Hair growth also is influenced by seasons of the year, nutrition, health, and hormones.

Climatic conditions and *seasonal changes* affect hair in the following ways:

1. Humidity and moisture deepen the natural wave.
2. Cold air causes the hair to contract.
3. Heat causes the hair to swell or expand and absorb moisture.

Here are some myths about hair growth:

1. Close clipping, shaving, trimming, cutting, or singeing have an effect on the rate of hair growth. This is *not* true.
2. The application of ointments and oils increases hair growth. This is *not* true. Ointments and oils lubricate the hair shaft, but they *do not* feed the hair.
3. Hair grows after death. This is *not* true. The flesh and skin contract, thus there is the appearance of hair growth.
4. Singeing the hair seals in the natural oil. This is *not* true.

Normal Hair Shedding

A certain amount of hair is shed daily. This is nature's method of making way for new hair. The average daily shedding is estimated at 50 to 80 hairs. Hair loss beyond this estimated average indicates some scalp or hair abnormality.

LIFE AND DENSITY OF THE HAIR

The exact life span of hair has not been agreed upon. The average life of hair ranges from 2 to 4 years. Factors such as sex, age, type of hair, heredity, and health have a bearing on the duration of hair life.

The area of an average head is about 120 square inches (780 cm²). There is an average of 1,000 hairs to a square inch (6.5 cm²). The number of hairs on the head varies with the color of the hair: blonde, 140,000; brown, 110,000; black, 108,000; red, 90,000.

NATURAL REPLACEMENT OF THE HAIR

Hair depends on the papilla for its growth. As long as the papilla is not destroyed, the hair will grow. If the hair is pulled out from the roots, it will grow again. But should the papilla be destroyed, the hair will never grow again. In humans, new hair replaces old hair in the following manner:

1.   The bulb loosens and separates from the papilla. (Fig. 4.8a)
2.   The bulb moves upward in the follicle.
3.   The hair moves slowly to the surface where it is shed.
4.   The new hair is formed by cell division, which takes place at the root of the hair around the papilla. (Fig. 4.8b)

Eyebrows and eyelashes are replaced every 4 to 5 months.

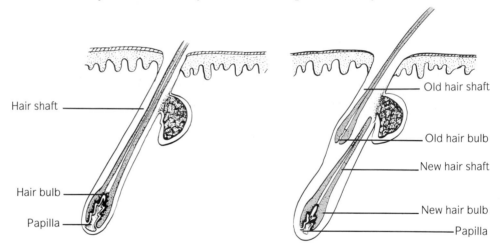

4.8a—At an early stage of shedding, the hair shows its separation from the papilla.

4.8b—At a later stage of the hair shedding, you will note a new hair growing from the same papilla.

COLOR OF THE HAIR

The natural color of hair, its strength, and its texture depend mainly on heredity. The cortex contains coloring matter, minute grains of *melanin* (**MEL**-a-nin), or pigment. Although there is no definite scientific proof, it appears that pigment is derived from the color-forming substances in the blood, as is all pigment of the human body. The color of a person's hair, how light or dark it is, depends on the number of grains of pigment in each strand.

An *albino* (al-**BEYE**-no) is a person born with white hair, the result of an absence of coloring matter in the hair shaft, accompanied by no marked pigment coloring in the skin or irises of the eyes.

To give successful hair lightening and tinting services, you need to know about natural hair color and distribution of hair pigment.

Graying of Hair

Gray hair is caused by the absence of color pigment in the cortical layer. It is really *mottled* hair—spots of white or whitish yellow scattered about in the hair shafts. Gray hair is just that—it grows that way from the hair bulb. It does not begin to grow as another color that turns gray.

In most cases, the graying of hair is a result of the natural aging process in humans, although graying also can occur as a result of some serious illness or nervous shock. An early diminishing of pigment brought on by emotional tensions can also cause the hair to turn gray.

Premature graying of hair in a young person is usually the result of a defect in pigment formation occurring at birth. Often it will be found that several members of a family are affected with premature grayness.

Business Tips

Shampoo technicians and assistants can build their bank accounts and their credibility with clients when they learn to prescribe hair and scalp treatments. At Salon Gianni, Montclair, New Jersey, these treatments bring in substantial amounts of money each week for technicians.

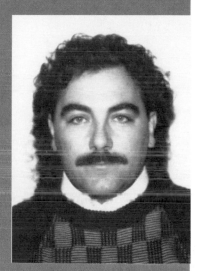

Says Gianni, "Learn all you can about trichology and hair conditions so that you can immediately recognize porosity, over-bleaching, thermal damage, or other hair and scalp problems. As soon as the client is seated at the shampoo bowl, look at her hair and begin to talk about its condition in a professional way." Gianni's salon offers half-hour aromatherapy scalp massages, hair shaft treatments, and customized problem-solving treatments. Also popular is a color-refreshing "hair cocktail," which is done at the shampoo bowl. The client's color formula is mixed with equal parts peroxide and shampoo and left on for 5 to 10 minutes to brighten faded color.

According to Gianni, all it takes to sell services is to suggest them, and along with each service sale is an opportunity for a retail sale.

"Just remember that the home care product cannot replace regular salon treatments," says Gianni. "Treatments are not simply conditioners. They are in-depth problem solvers, and they represent the easiest sale that you can make because you are truly doing the client a favor."

While beautiful, healthy hair is a woman's crowning glory, don't neglect the male client. According to Gianni, men are particularly concerned about hair loss, and the key to success with them is to always discuss such sensitive matters in private.

Hair Analysis

Much of the cosmetologist's time is taken up with servicing and styling clients' hair. For this reason, you should be able to recognize the condition and type of a client's hair and be able to analyze it.

CONDITION OF THE HAIR

Knowledge of hair and skill in determining its condition can be acquired by constant observation using the senses available to you: sight, touch, hearing, and smell.

1. *Sight*. Observing the hair will immediately give you some knowledge about its condition. Being able to look at hair contributes approximately 15% to its analysis, and touching the hair is the final determining factor.
2. *Touch*. Cosmetologists are guided by the touch or feel of the hair in making a professional hair analysis. When the sense of touch is fully developed, fewer mistakes will be made in judging the hair.
3. *Hearing*. Listen to what clients tell you about their hair, health problems, reactions to cosmetics and medications they might be taking. You will be in a better position to analyze the condition of hair more accurately.
4. *Smell*. Unclean hair and certain scalp disorders create an odor. If the client generally has good health, you might suggest regular shampooing and proper rinsing.

QUALITIES OF THE HAIR

Qualities by which human hair is analyzed are *texture*, *porosity*, and *elasticity*.

Texture

Hair texture refers to the degree of coarseness or fineness of the hair, which may vary on different parts of the head. Variations in hair texture are due to:

1. *Diameter of the hair*, whether coarse, medium, fine, or very fine. Coarse hair has the greatest diameter; very fine hair has the smallest.
2. *Feel of the hair*, whether harsh, soft, or wiry.

Types of Hair

Medium hair is the normal type most commonly seen in the salon or school. This type of hair does not present any special problem. *Fine* or *very fine hair* requires special care. Its microscopic structure usually reveals that only two layers, the cortex and cuticle, are present. *Wiry hair*, whether coarse, medium, or fine, has a hard, glassy finish caused by the cuticle scales lying flat against the hair shaft. It takes longer for chemicals such as permanent wave solutions, tints, or lighteners to penetrate this type of hair.

Porosity

Hair porosity is the ability of all types of hair to absorb moisture *(hygroscopic quality)*. Hair has *good porosity* when the cuticle layer is raised from the hair shaft and can absorb a fair or normal amount of moisture or chemicals. *Moderate porosity* (normal hair) is most often seen in the salon or school. It is less porous than hair with good porosity. Usually hair with good or moderate porosity presents no problem when receiving hair services, whether permanent waving, hair tinting, or lightening. *Poor porosity* (resistant hair) exists when the cuticle layer is lying close to the hair shaft and absorbs the least amount of moisture. Hair with poor porosity requires thorough analysis and strand tests before the application of hair cosmetics. *Extreme porosity* is seen in hair in poor condition. It may be due to tinting, lightening, or damage from continuous or faulty treatments.

Elasticity

Hair elasticity is the ability of hair to stretch and return to its original form without breaking. Hair can be classified as having good elasticity, normal elasticity, or poor elasticity. (Refer to the chapter on permanent waving for more information.) Hair with normal elasticity is springy and has a lively and lustrous appearance. Normal dry hair is capable of being stretched about one-fifth of its length; it springs back when released. Wet hair can be stretched 40% to 50% of its length. Porous hair stretches more than hair with poor porosity.

CAUTION

▶ *You should see by now that hair is hair and you must analyze each client individually. Never make a snap judgment based on race or nationality that a client will have a particular hair type.*

Disorders of the Hair

CANITIES

Canities (ka-**NIT**-eez) is the technical term for gray hair. Its immediate cause is the loss of natural pigment in the hair. There are two types:

1. Congenital canities exists at or before birth. It occurs in albinos and occasionally in persons with normal hair. A patchy type of congenital canities may develop either slowly or rapidly, depending upon the cause of the condition.
2. Acquired canities may be due to old age, or onset may occur prematurely in early adult life. Causes of acquired canities may be worry, anxiety, nervous strain, prolonged illness, or heredity.

RINGED HAIR

Ringed hair is alternate bands of gray and dark hair.

HYPERTRICHOSIS

Hypertrichosis (hi-per-tri-**KOH**-sis), or *hirsuties*, means superfluous hair, an abnormal development of hair on areas of the body normally bearing only downy hair.

TRICHOPTILOSIS

Trichoptilosis (tri-kop-ti-**LOH**-sis) is the technical term for *split hair ends*. (Fig. 4.9a)

TRICHORRHEXIS NODOSA

Trichorrhexis nodosa (**TRIK**-o-rek-sis no-**DO**-sa), or *knotted hair*, is a dry, brittle condition including formation of nodular swellings along the hair shaft. (Fig. 4.9b) The hair breaks easily and there is a brushlike spreading out of the fibers of the broken-off hair along the hair shaft. Softening the hair with conditioners may prove beneficial.

MONILETHRIX

Monilethrix (moh-**NIL**-e-thriks) is the technical term for *beaded hair.* (Fig. 4.9c) The hair breaks between the beads or nodes. Scalp and hair treatments may improve the hair condition.

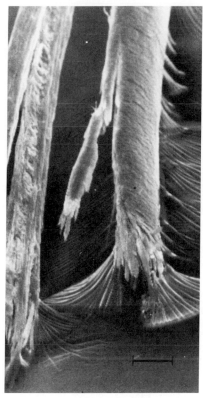
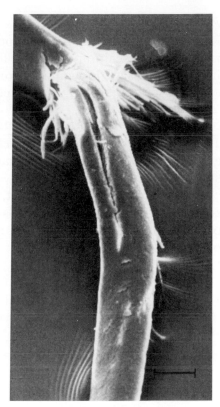
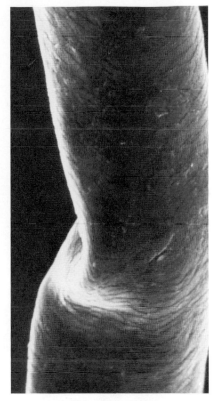

4.9a—Split hair ends.   4.9b—Knotted hair.   4.9c—Beaded hair.

FRAGILITAS CRINIUM

Fragilitas crinium (frah-**JIL**-i-tas **KRI**-nee-um) is the technical term for *brittle hair* or split ends. The hairs may split at any part of their length. Conditioning hair treatments may be recommended.

Scalp Care

A basic requisite for a healthy scalp is cleanliness and stimulation. The scalp and hair should be kept clean by frequent treatment and shampooing. A healthy, clean scalp will resist a variety of disorders.

SCALP MANIPULATIONS

Since the same manipulations are given with all scalp treatments, you should learn to give them with a continuous, even motion, which will stimulate the scalp and/or soothe the client's tension. Scalp massage is most effectively applied as a series of treatments, once a week for normal scalp and more frequently for scalp disorders, under the direction of a dermatologist.

Anatomy

Knowing the muscles, the location of blood vessels, and the nerve points of the scalp and neck will help guide you to those areas in which massage movements are to be directed for the most beneficial results. (See chapter on cells, anatomy, and physiology.)

Scalp Manipulation Technique

There are several ways in which scalp manipulations may be given. The following routine may be changed to meet your instructor's requirements.

With each massage movement, place the hands under the hair so the length of the fingers, balls of the fingertips, and cushions of the palms can stimulate the muscles, nerves, and blood vessels of the scalp area.

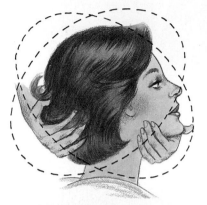

4.10—Relaxing movement.

1. RELAXING MOVEMENT. Cup the client's chin in your left hand; place your right hand at the base of her skull, and rotate head gently. Reverse positions of your hands and repeat. (See Fig. 4.10)

2. SLIDING MOVEMENT. Place your fingertips on each side of the client's head; slide your hands firmly upward, spreading the fingertips until they meet at the top of the head. Repeat four times. (See Fig. 4.11)

3. SLIDING AND ROTATING MOVEMENT. Same as movement No. 2, except that after sliding the fingertips 1" (2.5 cm), you rotate and move the client's scalp. Repeat four times. (See Fig. 4.12)

4. FOREHEAD MOVEMENT. Hold the back of the client's head with your left hand. Place stretched thumb and fingers of your right hand on the client's forehead. Move your hand slowly and firmly upward to 1" (2.5 cm) past the hairline. Repeat four times. (See Fig. 4.13)

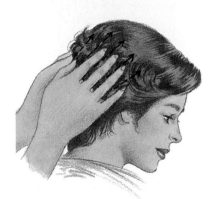

4.11—Sliding movement.

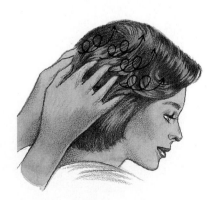

4.12—Sliding and rotating movement.

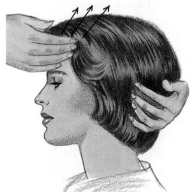

4.13—Forehead movement.

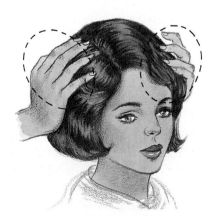

4.14—Scalp movement.

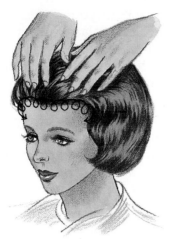

4.15—Hairline movement.

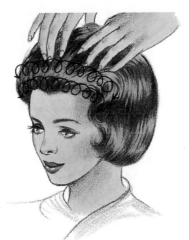

4.16—Front scalp movement.

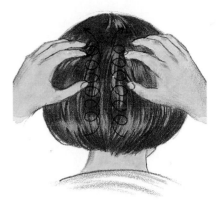

4.17—Back scalp movement.

5. SCALP MOVEMENT. Place the palms of your hands firmly against the client's scalp. Lift the scalp in a rotary movement, first with your hands placed above her ears, and second with your hands placed at the front and back of her head. (See Fig. 4.14)

6. HAIRLINE MOVEMENT. Place the fingers of both hands at the client's forehead. Massage around her hairline by lifting and rotating. (See Fig. 4.15)

7. FRONT SCALP MOVEMENT. Dropping back 1" (2.5 cm), repeat preceding movement over entire front and top of the scalp. (See Fig. 4.16)

8. BACK SCALP MOVEMENT. Place the fingers of each hand on the sides of the client's head. Starting below her ears, manipulate the scalp with your thumbs, working upward to the crown. Repeat four times. Repeat thumb manipulations, working toward the center back of the head. (See Fig. 4.17)

9. EAR-TO-EAR MOVEMENT. Place your left hand on the client's forehead. Massage from the right ear to the left ear along the base of her skull with the heel of your hand, using a rotary movement. (See Fig. 4.18)

10. BACK MOVEMENT. Place your left hand on the client's forehead and stand to the left of her. Using your right hand, rotate from the base of the client's neck, along the shoulder, and back across the shoulder blade to the spine. Slide your hand up the client's spine to the base of her neck. Repeat on the opposite side. (See Fig. 4.19)

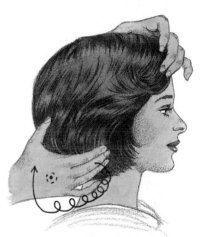

4.18—Ear-to-ear movement.

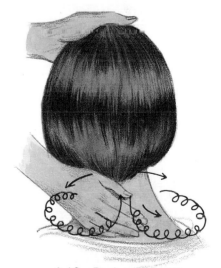

4.19—Back movement.

11. SHOULDER MOVEMENT. Place both your palms together at the base of the client's neck. With rotary movement, catch muscles in the palms and massage along the shoulder blades to the point of her shoulders, and then back again. Then massage from the shoulders to the spine and back again. (See Fig. 4.20)

12. SPINE MOVEMENT. Massage from the base of the client's skull down the spine with a rotary movement. Using a firm finger pressure, bring your hand slowly to the base of the client's skull. (See Fig. 4.21)

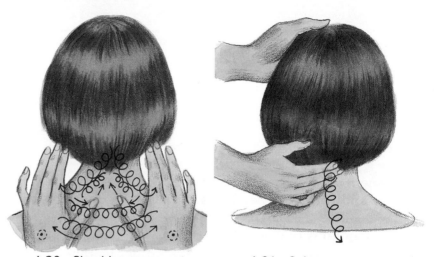

4.20 — Shoulder movement.   4.21 — Spine movement.

Disorders of the Scalp

Just as the skin is continually being shed and replaced, the uppermost layer of the scalp is also being cast off all the time. Ordinarily, these *horny scales* loosen and fall off freely. The natural shedding of these horny scales should not be mistaken for dandruff.

DANDRUFF

Dandruff consists of small, white scales that usually appear on the scalp and hair. The medical term for dandruff is *pityriasis* (pit-i-**REYE**-ah-sis). Long neglected, excessive dandruff can lead to baldness. The nature of dandruff is not clearly defined by medical authorities although it is generally believed to be of infectious origin. Some authorities hold that it is due to a specific microbe.

A direct cause of dandruff is the excessive shedding of the *epithelial*, or surface, *cells.* Instead of growing to the surface and falling off, these horny scales accumulate on the scalp.

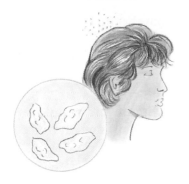
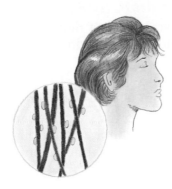
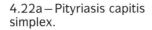

4.22a—Pityriasis capitis simplex.

4.22b—Pityriasis steatoides.

Indirect or associated causes of dandruff are a sluggish condition of the scalp, possibly due to poor circulation, infection, injury, lack of nerve stimulation, improper diet, and uncleanliness. Contributing causes are the use of strong shampoos and insufficient rinsing of the hair after a shampoo. The two principal types of dandruff are:

1. *Pityriasis capitis simplex* (**CAH**-pit-is **SIM**-pleks)—dry type. (Fig. 4.22a)
2. *Pityriasis steatoides* (ste-a-**TOY**-dez)—a greasy or waxy type. (Fig. 4.22b)

Pityriasis capitis simplex (dry dandruff) is characterized by an itchy scalp and small white scales, which are usually attached to the scalp in masses, or scattered loosely in the hair. Occasionally, they are so profuse that they fall to the shoulders. Dry dandruff is often the result of a sluggish scalp caused by poor circulation, lack of nerve stimulation, improper diet, emotional and glandular disturbances, or uncleanliness. *Treatment:* Frequent scalp treatments, use of mild shampoos, regular scalp massage, daily use of antiseptic scalp lotions, and applications of scalp ointments.

Pityriasis steatoides (greasy or waxy type of dandruff) is a scaly condition of the epidermis (surface skin). The scales become mixed with sebum, causing them to stick to the scalp in patches. There may be itchiness, causing the person to scratch the scalp. If the greasy scales are torn off, bleeding or oozing of sebum may follow. Medical treatment is advisable.

Both forms of dandruff are considered to be contagious and can be spread by the common use of brushes, combs, and other articles. Therefore, the cosmetologist must take the necessary precautions to sanitize everything that comes into contact with the client.

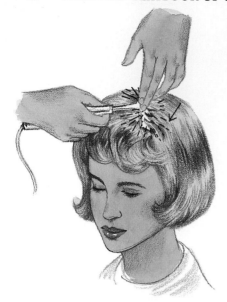

4.23a—Applying high-frequency current with glass rake electrode.

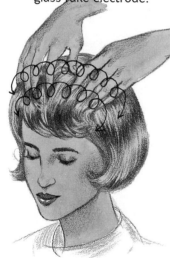

4.23b—Applying indirect high-frequency current, cosmetologist manipulates the scalp.

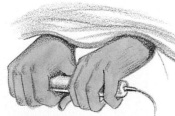

4.23c—While cosmetologist manipulates the scalp, the client holds metal electrode.

Dandruff Treatment

A scalp with a dandruff condition may be treated by using the following procedure:

1. Drape client. (See chapter on draping.)
2. Brush the client's hair for 5 minutes.
3. Apply a scalp preparation according to the scalp's condition (dry or oily). (See sections on dry and oily hair scalp treatments on pages 64 and 65.)
4. Apply infrared lamp for about 5 minutes. (See chapter on electricity and light therapy.)
5. Give scalp manipulations, using indirect high-frequency current. (Fig. 4.23a) (See chapter on electricity and light therapy.)
6. Shampoo with corrective anti-dandruff lotion.
7. Thoroughly towel-dry the hair.
8. Use direct high-frequency current for 3 to 5 minutes. (Figs. 4.23b, 4.23c) (See chapter on electricity and light therapy.)
9. Apply scalp preparation suitable for the condition.
10. Set, dry, and style the hair.
11. Clean up your work station.

ALOPECIA

Alopecia (al-oh-**PEE**-shee-ah) is the technical term for any abnormal hair loss. The natural falling out of the hair should not be confused with alopecia. As we learned earlier, when hair has grown to its full length, it falls out and is replaced by a new hair. The natural shedding of hair occurs most frequently in spring and fall. Hair loss due to alopecia is not replaced unless special treatments are given to encourage hair growth. Hairstyles such as ponytails and tight braids cause tension on the hair and can contribute to constant hair loss or baldness.

Alopecia senilis (se-**NIL**-is) is the form of baldness that occurs in old age. This loss of hair is permanent.

Alopecia prematura (pre-mah-**CHUR**-ah) is the form of baldness that begins any time before middle age with a slow, thinning process. This condition is caused when hairs fall out and are replaced by weaker ones.

Alopecia areata (air-ee-**AH**-tah) is the sudden falling out of hair in round patches, or baldness in spots, sometimes caused by anemia, scarlet fever, typhoid fever, or syphilis. Patches are round or irregular in shape and can vary in size from ½″ to 2″ or 3″ (1.3 to 5.1 or 7.6 cm) in diameter. Affected areas are slightly depressed, smooth, and very pale, due to a decreased blood supply. In most conditions of alopecia areata, the nervous system has been subjected to some injury. Since the flow of blood is influenced by the nervous system, the affected area also is poorly nourished. (Fig. 4.24)

Treatment for Alopecia

Alopecia appears in a variety of different forms, caused by many abnormal conditions. Sometimes an alopecia condition can be improved by proper scalp treatments.

Procedure for Alopecia Treatment

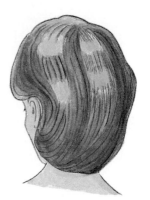

4.24—Alopecia areata.

1. Drape client.
2. Brush the client's hair for about 5 minutes.
3. Apply a medicated scalp ointment as directed by a physician.
4. Apply infrared light for about 5 minutes.
5. Give scalp manipulations. You may use the faradic or indirect high-frequency current.
6. Use a mild shampoo.
7. Towel-dry the hair.
8. Apply direct high-frequency current for about 5 minutes.
9. Apply medicated scalp lotion.
10. Repeat scalp manipulations; include neck, shoulders, and upper back.
11. Set hair; dry with warm or cool air, and style hair.
12. Clean up your work station.

Procedure for Alopecia Areata Treatment

1. Drape client.
2. Give regular scalp manipulations.
3. Shampoo the hair according to its condition; if scalp is very tender, use a mild shampoo.
4. Dry the hair and scalp thoroughly.
5. Expose the scalp to ultra violet rays for 5 to 10 minutes, especially the bald spots. (Fig. 4.25)
6. Apply ointment or lotion with light manipulations on the bald spots.
7. Apply high-frequency current for about 5 minutes. If an ointment is used, apply direct current; if a lotion is used, apply indirect current.
8. Style the hair, using a comb only.
9. Clean up your work station.

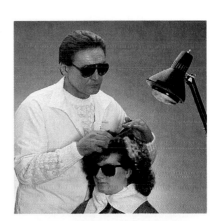

4.25—Applying ultra violet rays.

VEGETABLE PARASITIC INFECTIONS

Tinea (**TIN**-ee-ah) is the medical term for ringworm. Ringworm is caused by vegetable parasites. All forms are contagious and can be transmitted from one person to another. The disease is commonly carried by scales or hairs containing fungi. Bath tubs, swimming pools, and unsanitized articles are also sources of transmission.

Ringworm starts with a small, reddened patch of little blisters. Several such patches may be present. Any ringworm condition should be referred to a physician.

Tinea capitis (**KAP**-i-tis), ringworm of the scalp, is characterized by red papules, or spots, at the opening of the hair follicles. (Fig. 4.26) The patches spread and the hair becomes brittle and lifeless. It breaks off, leaving a stump, or falls from the enlarged open follicles.

Tinea favosa (fa-**VO**-sah), also **favus** (**FA**-vus) or *honeycomb ringworm,* is characterized by dry, sulfur-yellow, cuplike crusts on the scalp, called *scutula* (**SKUT**-u-la), which have a peculiar odor. (Fig. 4.27) Scars from favus are bald patches that may be pink or white and shiny. It is *very contagious* and should be referred to a physician.

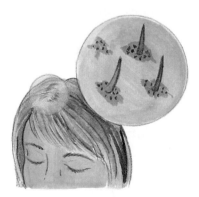 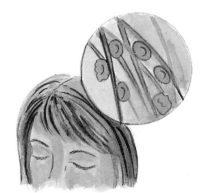

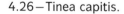

4.26—Tinea capitis.   4.27—Favus.

ANIMAL PARASITIC INFECTIONS

Scabies "itch" is a highly contagious, animal parasitic skin disease, caused by the itch mite. Vesicles and pustules can form from the irritation of the parasites or from scratching the affected areas.

Pediculosis (pe-dik-yoo-**LOH**-sis) *capitis* is a contagious condition caused by the **head louse** (animal parasite) infesting the hair of the scalp. (Fig. 4.28) As the parasites feed on the scalp, itching occurs and the resultant scratching can cause an infection.

The head louse is transmitted from one person to another by contact with infested hats, combs, brushes, or other personal articles. To kill head lice, advise the client to apply larkspur tincture, or other similar medication, to the entire head before retiring. The next morning, the client should shampoo with germicidal soap. Treatment should be repeated as necessary. Never treat a head lice condition in the salon or school.

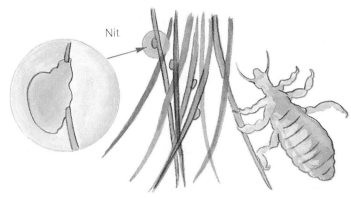

4.28—Head louse.

STAPHYLOCOCCI INFECTIONS

Furuncle (fu-**RUN**-kel), or boil, is an acute staphylococci infection of a hair follicle that produces constant pain. (Fig. 4.29) It is limited to a specific area and produces a pustule perforated by a hair.

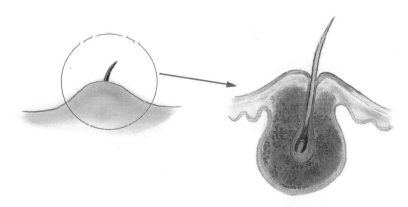

4.29—Furuncle (boil).

Carbuncle (**KAHR**-bun-kul) is the result of an acute staphylococci infection and is larger than a furuncle. Refer the client to a physician.

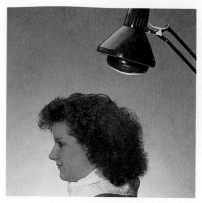

4.30—Applying heat with infrared lamp.

GENERAL HAIR TREATMENTS

The purpose of a general scalp treatment is to keep the scalp and hair in a clean and healthy condition. Regular scalp treatments also are beneficial in preventing baldness.

Procedure for Normal Hair and Scalp

1. Drape client.
2. Brush hair for about 5 minutes.
3. Apply scalp cream.
4. Apply infrared lamp for about 5 minutes. (Fig. 4.30)
5. Give scalp manipulations for 10 to 20 minutes.
6. Shampoo the hair.
7. Towel-dry the hair to remove excess moisture.
8. Apply suitable scalp lotion.
9. Set, dry, and style hair.
10. Clean up your work station.

Dry Hair and Scalp Treatments

This treatment should be used when there is a deficiency of natural oil on the scalp and hair. Select scalp preparations containing moisturizing and emollient materials. Avoid the use of strong soaps, preparations containing a mineral oil or sulfonated oil base, greasy preparations, and lotions with a high alcohol content.

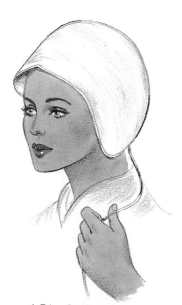

4.31—Scalp steamer.

1. Drape client.
2. Brush client's hair for about 5 minutes.
3. Apply the scalp preparation for this condition.
4. Apply the scalp steamer for 7 to 10 minutes, or wrap the head in warm steam towels for 7 to 10 minutes. (Fig. 4.31)
5. Give a mild shampoo.
6. Towel dry the hair and scalp thoroughly.
7. Apply moisturizing scalp cream sparingly with a rotary, frictional motion.
8. Stimulate the scalp with direct high-frequency current, using the glass rake electrode, for about 5 minutes.
9. Set, dry, and style the hair.
10. Clean up your work station.

Oily Hair and Scalp Treatments

Excessive oiliness is caused by the over-activity of the sebaceous (oil) glands. Manipulate the scalp and knead it to increase the blood circulation to the scalp. Any hardened sebum in the pores of the scalp will be removed with the correct degree of pressing and squeezing. To normalize the function of these glands, excess sebum should be flushed out with each treatment.

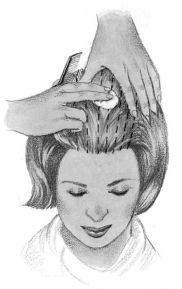

4.32 – Applying scalp lotion with cotton pledget.

1. Drape client.
2. Brush client's hair for about 5 minutes.
3. Apply a medicated scalp lotion to the scalp only with a cotton pledget. (Fig. 4.32)
4. Apply infrared lamp for about 5 minutes.
5. Give scalp manipulations. (Optional: Faradic or sinusoidal current may be used.) (Figs. 4.33a, 4.33b)
6. Shampoo with a corrective shampoo for oily scalp.
7. Towel dry the hair.
8. Apply direct high-frequency current for 3 to 5 minutes.
9. Apply a scalp astringent.
10. Set, dry, and style the hair.
11. Clean up your work station.

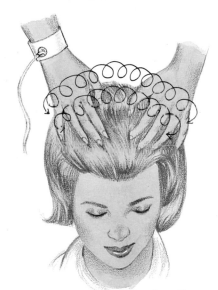

4.33a – Applying faradic current, cosmetologist manipulates the scalp.

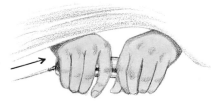

4.33b – While cosmetologist manipulates scalp, client holds the electrode.

CAUTION

▶ *Do not use high-frequency current on hair treated with tonics or lotions having alcohol content.*

Corrective Hair Treatment

A corrective hair treatment deals with the hair shaft, not the scalp. Dry and damaged hair can be greatly improved by conditioners. Hair treatments are especially beneficial and extremely important when given approximately a week or 10 days before, and a week or 10 days after, a permanent wave, tint, lightener, toner, or chemical hair straightening treatment.

Dry hair may be softened quickly with a conditioning preparation applied directly on the hair shaft. The product used for this purpose is usually an emulsion containing cholesterol and related compounds.

Some conditioners function more effectively when heat is applied to induce penetration into the cortex. The heat applied to the hair opens the cuticle's imbrications, and permits significantly more corrective agents to enter the hair shaft. This provides more conditioning benefits.

1. Drape client.
2. Brush the client's hair for about 5 minutes.
3. Apply a mild shampoo.
4. Towel dry the hair.
5. Apply a conditioner according to the manufacturer's directions.
6. Set, dry, and style hair.
7. Clean up your workstation.

Review Questions

PROPERTIES OF THE SCALP AND HAIR

1. What is the purpose of hair?
2. What is hair?
3. What is hair composed of?
4. What are the two principal parts of hair?
5. What factors influence hair growth?
6. What are the theories relating to the life and density of hair?
7. What determines the color of a person's hair?
8. What is the basic requisite for a healthy scalp?

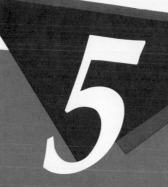

5

DRAPING

LEARNING OBJECTIVES

After completing this chapter, you should be able to:

1. List the methods of draping and preparing the client for cosmetology services.

2. Demonstrate draping for wet hair services.

3. Demonstrate draping for chemical services.

4. Demonstrate draping for dry hair services.

Introduction

The comfort and protection of the client must always be considered during cosmetology services. Protection of the skin and clothing assures clients that the cosmetologist is personally and professionally concerned about their comfort and safety.

Methods of draping depend on the service being performed. Several procedures are presented in this text, although those taught by your instructor are also acceptable. Consideration for the client is one of your most important responsibilities as a cosmetologist.

The following instructions are important before draping a client for any type of service:

1. Prepare materials and supplies for the service.
2. Sanitize hands.
3. Ask the client to remove all neck and hair jewelry and store it away.
4. Remove objects from the client's hair.
5. Turn the client's collar to the inside. (See Fig. 5.1)
6. Proceed with the appropriate draping method.

In the following procedures the purpose of the towel or neck strip is for sanitary reasons, to prevent contact of the cape with the client's skin.

DRAPING FOR WET HAIR SERVICES

Shampooing, Scalp and Hair Care, and Haircutting

1. Place a towel lengthwise across the client's shoulders, crossing the ends beneath the chin.
2. Place the cape over the towel and fasten in the back so that the cape does not touch the client's skin.
3. Place another towel over the cape and secure in front.

For haircutting, the towel should be removed after shampooing and replaced with a neck strip. This allows the hair to fall naturally without obstruction.

DRAPING FOR CHEMICAL SERVICES

Hair Color, Perms, and Relaxers

1. Slide towel down from back of client's head and place lengthwise across the client's shoulders. (See Fig. 5.2)

2. Cross the ends of the towel beneath the chin and place the cape over the towel. Fasten in the back and adjust the towel over the cape. (See Fig. 5.3)

3. Fold the towel over the top of the cape and secure in front. (See Fig. 5.4)

4. It is advisable to apply a protective cream around the hairline immediately prior to the application of chemicals to the hair. This prevents possible skin irritation.

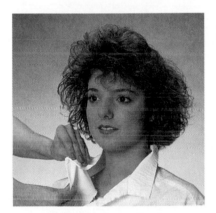

5.1   Turning collar in.

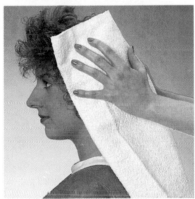

5.2—Sliding towel down around client's neck.

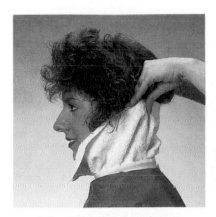

5.3—Adjusting towel over cape.

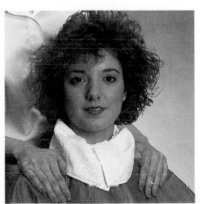

5.4—Folding towel over.

DRAPING FOR DRY HAIR SERVICES

Brushing or Thermal Design

1. Secure a neck strip around the client's neck. (See Fig. 5.5)
2. Place the cape over the neck strip and fasten so that the cape does not touch the client's skin. (See Fig. 5.6)
3. Fold the uncovered portion of the neck strip down over the cape. Make sure that no part of the cape touches the client's neck. (See Fig. 5.7)

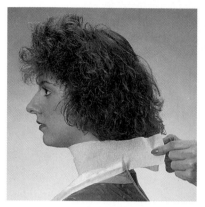

5.5—Placing neck strip.

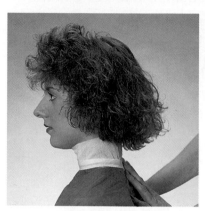

5.6—Placing cape over neck strip.

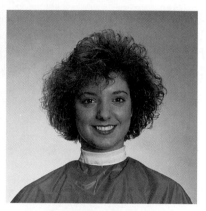

5.7—Folding neck strip down over cape.

Comb-Out

1. Secure a neck strip around the client's neck.
2. Place the cape over the neck strip and fasten so that the cape does not touch the client's skin. (See Fig. 5.8) Capes especially designed for this service can be used.

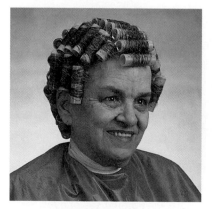

5.8—Draping for a comb-out.

People Skills

As you look forward to your career in the salon, you'll face the constant challenge of effective client communication. Be prepared for anything to happen!

Van Council, co-owner of Van Michael Salon in Atlanta and internationally renowned platform artist for Joico, encounters his fair share of sticky situations as he services thirty clients a day. Because Van Michael Salon has a reputation for excellent service, Council often deals with clients who have had a hair nightmare at another salon. How does he handle this situation?

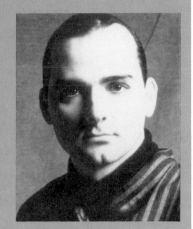

By being honest about what can and can't be done with fragile or damaged hair. Council recalls one client whose hair was irreparably damaged by over bleaching. Her hair was dry, brittle, and broken, and her request, of course, was to immediately transform her hair into beautifully conditioned locks with subtle highlights.

Council's first step was to listen, without interrupting, to her list of requests. Then, he explained the realistic options and outcomes. Once the client understood and agreed upon a corrective service that would eliminate her severest streaks and condition her hair, Council asked her to repeat her expectations to him. When he was certain that she accurately understood what to expect, he proceeded with the service.

Good communication takes time, but it is vital to client satisfaction. When you're honest with clients about what to expect, they'll appreciate it.

Review Questions

DRAPING

1. What must a cosmetologist take into consideration when performing any service?
2. What is draping?
3. Why is draping so important?
4. Why is a towel or neck strip used in draping?
5. What are the four preliminary steps before draping a client?
6. What are the differences when draping for wet hair services, dry hair services, and chemical services?

6

SHAMPOOING, RINSING, AND CONDITIONING

LEARNING OBJECTIVES

After completing this chapter, you should be able to:

1. List the reasons for good hygienic care of the hair and scalp.

2. Identify the various types of shampoos.

3. Demonstrate the procedure for shampoo manipulations.

4. List the professional methods of cleansing the hair and scalp with and without water.

5. Identify the various types of rinses.

6. Demonstrate the proper use of various types of rinses.

Introduction

Shampooing is the first step of a great many salon services, and a good shampoo sets the stage for a successful salon visit. In salons where the stylist gives the shampoo, the client may use this initial experience to evaluate the professional expertise of the stylist. Clients assume that the stylist who shampoos with a high level of professionalism will perform all additional services at that same level of competency and concern. In salons where there is a separate shampoo person, the client may use the experience to judge the professionalism of the salon. Therefore, the client who enjoys the shampoo service is more likely to request additional services and recommend the stylist and the salon to potential clients.

Shampooing is an important preliminary step for a variety of hair services and is given primarily to cleanse the hair and scalp. However, the psychological effects of a pleasurable and relaxing experience at the shampoo bowl will help to ensure that the client visits the salon on a regular basis.

To be effective, a shampoo must remove all dirt, oils, cosmetics, and skin debris without adversely affecting either the scalp or hair. It is important to analyze the condition of the client's hair and scalp and to check for disease or disorders. A client with an infectious disease should not be treated in the salon and should be referred to a physician.

Unless the scalp and hair are cleansed regularly, the accumulations of oil and perspiration, which mix with the natural scales and dirt, offer a breeding place for disease-producing bacteria. This can lead to scalp disorders.

Hair should be shampooed as often as necessary, depending on how quickly the scalp and hair become soiled. As a general rule, oily hair should be shampooed more often than normal or dry hair.

WATER

Chemically, water is composed of hydrogen and oxygen (H_2O). Depending on the kinds and quantities of other minerals present, it can be classified as either hard or soft water. You will be able to make a more professional shampoo selection if you know whether the salon water is hard or soft.

Soft water is rain water or water that has been chemically softened. It contains small amounts of minerals and, therefore, allows shampoos to lather freely. For this reason, it may be preferred for shampooing.

Hard water contains certain minerals that lessen the ability of shampoo to lather. However, it can be softened by a chemical process.

SELECTING THE CORRECT SHAMPOO

Many types of shampoos are available. As a professional cosmetologist, you should learn the composition and action of a shampoo to determine whether or not it will serve your intended purpose. Read the label and accompanying literature carefully so that you can make an informed decision.

Select the shampoo according to the condition of the hair. Hair is not considered normal if it has been:

Lightened   Abused by the use of harsh shampoos
Toned or tinted   Damaged by improper care
Permanent waved   Damaged by exposure to the elements
Chemically relaxed   such as sun, cold, heat, wind

REQUIRED MATERIALS AND IMPLEMENTS

Prior to giving a shampoo, gather all necessary materials and implements. Don't forget that the client should be properly draped. The relaxing mood and the professional quality of the shampoo is destroyed if you dash off to get a forgotten item, leaving the client wet and dripping in the shampoo bowl. Required materials and implements are:

Towels   Hair rinse (optional)
Shampoo cape   Neck strip
Shampoo   Comb and hairbrush

BRUSHING

Hairbrushes made of natural bristles are recommended for hair brushing. Natural bristles have many tiny overlapping layers, or scales, which clean and add luster to the hair, while nylon bristles are shiny and smooth and recommended for hairstyling.

You should include a thorough hair brushing as a part of every shampoo and scalp treatment, with the following exceptions:

1. Do not brush before giving a chemical service.
2. Do not brush if the scalp is irritated.

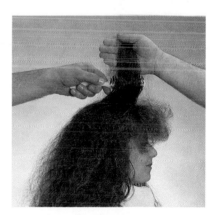

6.1 — Brushing the hair.

Brushing stimulates the blood circulation to the scalp, helps remove dust, dirt, and hair spray buildup from the hair, and gives hair added sheen. (Fig. 6.1) Therefore, you should brush the hair whether the scalp and hair are in a dry or oily condition. Do not use the comb to loosen scales from the scalp.

To brush the hair, first part it through the center from front to nape. Then part a section about ½″ (1.25 cm) off the center parting to the crown of the head. Holding this strand of hair in the left hand between the thumb and fingers, lay the brush (held in the right hand) with the bristles well down on the hair close to the scalp; rotate the brush by turning the wrist slightly, and sweep the bristles the full length of the hair shaft. Repeat three times. Then part the hair again ½″ (1.25 cm) from the first parting and continue until the entire head has been brushed.

SHAMPOO PROCEDURE

Preparation

1. Seat your client comfortably at your work station.
2. Select and arrange the required materials.
3. Wash your hands.
4. Place a neck strip and shampoo cape around the client's neck. (Be sure that the client's collar lies smoothly under the garment before the neck strip is adjusted.)
5. Remove all hairpins and combs from the hair.
6. Ask client to remove earrings and glasses and to put them in a safe place.
7. Examine the condition of the client's hair and scalp.
8. Brush the hair thoroughly.
9. Re-drape with shampoo cape and towel.
10. Seat the client comfortably at the shampoo sink.
11. Adjust the shampoo cape over the back of the shampoo chair. (Fig. 6.2)
12. Adjust the volume and temperature of the water spray.

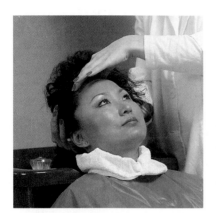

6.2—Support client's head with your right hand and place the cape over the back of the chair.

Consider the client's preference in adjusting the water temperature. Turn on the cold water first and gradually add warm water until you obtain a comfortably warm temperature. Test the temperature of the water by spraying it on the inner side of your wrist. The temperature of the water must be constantly monitored by keeping one finger over the edge of the spray nozzle and in contact with the water.

Procedure

1. *Saturate, wet hair thoroughly,* with warm water spray. Lift the hair and work it with your free hand to saturate the scalp. Shift your hand to protect the client's face, ears, and neck from the spray when working around the hairline. (Figs. 6.3–6.5)
2. *Apply small quantities of shampoo to the hair,* beginning at the hairline and working back. Work into a lather using the pads or cushions of the fingers.

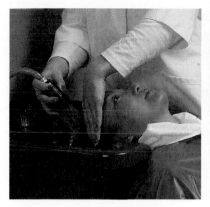

6.3—Protecting the face.

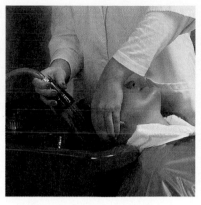

6.4—Protecting the ears.

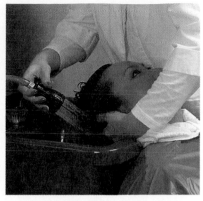

6.5—Protecting the neck.

Reminders

In massaging the scalp, do not use firm pressure if:

- You will be giving the client a chemical service after the shampoo.
- The client's scalp is tender or sensitive.
- The client requests less pressure.

3. *Manipulate scalp.*

   a) Begin at the front hairline and work in a back-and-forth movement until the top of the head is reached. (See Fig. 6.6)

   b) Continue in this manner to the back of the head, shifting your fingers back 1" (2.5 cm) at a time.

   c) Lift the client's head, with your left hand controlling the movement of the head. With your right hand, start at the top of the right ear and, using the same movement, work to the back of the head. (See Fig. 6.7)

   d) Drop your fingers down 1" (2.5 cm) and repeat the process until the right side of the head is covered.

   e) Beginning at the left ear, repeat steps c and d.

   f) Allow the client's head to relax and work around the hairline with your thumbs in a rotary movement.

   g) Repeat these movements until the scalp has been thoroughly massaged.

   h) Remove excess shampoo and lather by squeezing the hair.

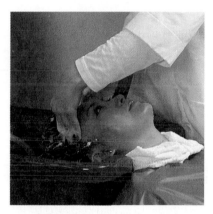

6.6—Manipulating scalp.

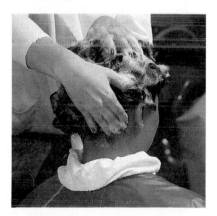

6.7—Lifting client's head.

4. *Rinse hair thoroughly* with a strong spray.
   a) Lift the hair at the crown and back with the fingers of your left hand to permit the spray to rinse the hair thoroughly.
   b) Cup your left hand along the napeline and pat the hair, forcing the spray of water against the base scalp area.

5. *If required, apply shampoo again.*
   a) Repeat the procedure using steps 2, 3, and 4 as outlined above. You will need less shampoo because partially clean hair lathers more easily.

6. *Partially towel dry.*
   a) Remove excess moisture from the hair at the shampoo bowl.
   b) Wipe excess moisture from around the client's face and ears with the ends of the towel.
   c) Lift the towel over the back of the client's head and drape the head with the towel.
   d) Place your hands on top of the towel and massage until the hair is partially dry. (Fig. 6.8)

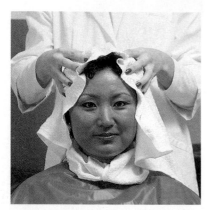

6.8–Towel drying the hair.

Completion

1. Comb the hair, beginning with the ends at the nape of the client's neck.
2. Change the drape if necessary.
3. Style the hair as desired.

Cleanup

1. Discard used materials, and place unused supplies in their proper place.
2. Place used towels in the towel hamper.
3. Remove hair from combs and brushes; wash with hot, soapy water; rinse; and place in wet disinfectant for the required time.
4. Sanitize the shampoo bowl.
5. Cleanse your hands.

SHAMPOOING CHEMICALLY TREATED HAIR

Chemically treated hair tends to be drier and more fragile than non-chemically treated hair. Therefore, a mild shampoo formulated for chemically treated hair is recommended. Chemically treated hair also tends to tangle. To remove tangles, comb gently from the bottom of the head and hair strand. Do not force the comb through the hair. Use a conditioner if necessary.

TYPES OF SHAMPOOS

Shampoo accounts for the highest dollar expenditure in hair care products. Consumer studies show the current growth pattern in the shampoo market to be in the direction of the professional salon. You will have to be more knowledgeable and sophisticated about the products used, more proficient in using them, and able to sell these products to your clients.

Thousands of good shampoos exist, one for every conceivable type of hair or scalp condition a client could have: dry, oily, fine, coarse, limp, lightened, permed, relaxed, or chemically un-treated. There are shampoos that add highlights and others that remove them. There are shampoos that deposit a coating on the hair, and there are shampoos to strip coating off the hair.

The ingredients list is the key to determining which shampoo will leave a client's hair lustrous and manageable, treat a scalp or hair condition, or prepare hair for chemical treatment. Most shampoos have many common ingredients, and it is your responsibility as a professional cosmetologist to understand the chemical composition in order to select the best shampoo for each particular service and client.

General descriptions of different types of shampoos are listed below. The section entitled "Chemistry of Shampoos" in the chapter on chemistry has detailed information about the chemical ingredients that make up the different types of shampoos.

Explaining pH

Before discussing acid-balanced shampoos, you should know something about pH (potential hydrogen) levels in shampoo. This will help you to select the proper shampoo for your client. The amount of hydrogen in a solution is measured on a pH scale that has a range from 0 to 14. The amount of hydrogen in a solution determines whether it is more alkaline or more acid. A shampoo that is more acid can have a pH rating from 0 to 6.9; a shampoo that is more alkaline can have a pH rating from 7 to 14. The higher the pH rating (more alkaline), the stronger and harsher the shampoo is to the hair. A high pH shampoo can leave the hair dry and brittle. (Also see pH scale in the chapter on chemistry.)

Acid-balanced Shampoos

An acid-balanced shampoo is one that falls within the 4.5 to 6.6 range, an acceptable pH range. Any shampoo can become acid balanced by the addition of citric, lactic, or phosphoric acid.

Proponents of acid-balanced shampoo state that an acid pH of 4.5 to 5.5 is essential to prevent excessive dryness and hair damage during the cleansing process, while the Consumer's Union's chemists consider the difference between a pH of 5 and a pH of 8 too small to affect the hair and scalp in the limited time of an average application.

Business Tips

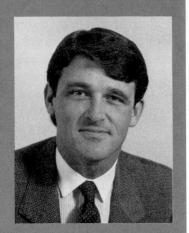

"If you want to be successful, start off as a true assistant to a master, not a shampoo slave." That's the advice from Gary Ahlquist, a consultative educator from San Diego, who trains and lectures all across the country. "In Europe, the master/associate relationship produces new masters," says Ahlquist. "Here, 19-year-olds with nine months of education think that they should command large commissions right away.

"If you want to do it right, find the greatest master stylist you can and offer to act as his or her assistant. An assistant does not just shampoo. He or she does all the manual labor, such as wrapping perms, checking curls, and applying color. The master consults with the client, performs the design cut, and does 25% of the finishing. He or she steps in when the assistant has dried the hair to the damp stage.

"In the ideal relationship, the assistant has the respect of the master designer and anticipates what's needed instead of waiting to be told everything. Many master/assistant relationships don't work because clients only get to see the assistant taking orders, and never learn to respect him or her. He or she has to go to another salon to become a master in his or her own right.

"Working with assistants is the only way salons and stylists can make great money. With a full-time assistant and a part-time assistant, a master designer can work as many as four chairs in a salon, and if one person can work that many chairs, he or she can pay the assistant well."

Ahlquist's additional advice: Specialize, learn to sell retail, develop your client consulting skills, and learn all that you can about supply and demand. Says Ahlquist of the latter, "If you're booked three months in advance, raise your prices; work smarter, not harder."

Conditioning Shampoos

Virtually every shampoo available on the professional market contains one or more conditioning agents designed to make the hair smooth and shiny, to avoid damage to chemically treated hair, and to improve the manageability of the hair. Protein, dimethicone, biotin, hydantoin, oleyl alcohol, and cocoamphocarboxyglycinate are just a few examples of conditioning agents that are used to assist shampoos in meeting current grooming needs.

Medicated Shampoos

Medicated shampoos contain special chemicals or drugs that are very effective in reducing excessive dandruff or other scalp conditions. These are prescribed by a physician. They generally are quite strong and will affect the color of tinted or lightened hair.

Dry Shampoos

A dry shampoo is usually given when the client's health does not permit a wet shampoo. Only a few of these products are available on the market today. Follow the manufacturer's recommended directions when giving a dry shampoo. Do not give a dry shampoo before performing a chemical service. (Fig. 6.9)

Color or Highlighting Shampoos

(See chapters on hair coloring and chemistry.)

Shampoos for Hairpieces and Wigs

Prepared wig cleaning solutions are now available. (See chapter on the artistry of artificial hair.)

HAIR RINSES

A hair rinse consists of a mixture of water with a mild acid, coloring agent, or ingredients designed to serve a particular purpose. (Fig. 6.10)

Acid Rinses

Acid rinses are used to restore the pH balance to the hair and to remove soap scum. The fatty acids found in soap combine with the minerals in water to form a soap scum that cannot be completely removed from the hair with plain water. Therefore, the hair tends to become coated, dull, and difficult to comb. Because soap is not currently used in the manufacture of professional shampoos, you will not find acid rinses in many salons.

The types of acids used in prepared acid hair rinses are:

Citric acid from the juice of a lime, orange, or lemon.

Tartaric acid, which is obtained from residues in wine making.

Acetic acid, which is present in vinegar.

Lactic acid, which is lactose or sugar of milk.

Conditioners and Cream Rinses

A conditioner or cream rinse is a commercial product with a creamy appearance that is used after shampooing. It is intended to soften hair, add luster, and make tangled hair easier to comb. Conditioners and cream rinses coat the hair shaft to make it slick and smooth. This temporary coating allows the comb to glide easily through the hair and often gives the false impression that the hair has been restored to its original healthy condition.

Used occasionally, conditioners and cream rinses are useful to remove tangles. However, habitual use can lead to future hair care problems. The coating ingredients can build up on the hair, making it prematurely heavy and oily. This can lead the client to shampoo more frequently, causing further damage to the hair.

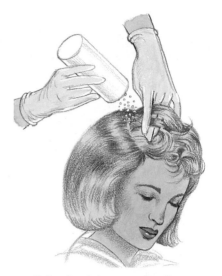

6.9—Applying powder dry shampoo.

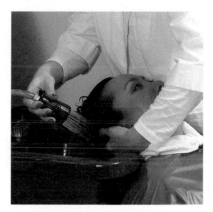

6.10—Rinsing the hair

An endless cycle is created because conditioners and cream rinses give the illusion of curing a problem that they are actually compounding. Professional conditioning treatments are an effective solution to the problem.

Acid-balanced Rinses

Acid-balanced rinses are commercially formulated to prevent the fading of color after a tint or toner application. This rinse is acid balanced to close the cuticle and trap within it the color molecules. This helps to prevent fading. Citric acid is probably the most commonly used ingredient in an after-rinse, but most also contain a mild moisturizer to leave the hair soft, pliable, and easy to comb.

Medicated Rinses

Medicated rinses are formulated to control minor dandruff conditions. Follow the manufacturer's instructions.

Color Rinses

Color rinses highlight or add temporary color to the hair. These rinses remain on the hair until the next shampoo. (For additional information, see the chapter on hair coloring.)

Review Questions

SHAMPOOING, RINSING, AND CONDITIONING

1. Why is a professional shampoo important?
2. What is the purpose of a shampoo?
3. Why and how often should the hair be shampooed?
4. How do you determine the proper shampoo to use?
5. Name two types of water.
6. Why is brushing important prior to shampooing?
7. When is it not appropriate to brush before shampooing?
8. What does pH mean?
9. How is pH measured?
10. Why is pH in shampoo important?
11. What is a hair rinse?
12. What is the function of an acid rinse?
13. What type of rinse is intended to soften the hair, add luster, and remove tangles?
14. What type of rinse prevents fading of color after a tint or toner application?
15. How does an acid-balanced rinse prevent fading?
16. What is a medicated rinse?
17. What is the purpose of a color rinse?

7

HAIRCUTTING

LEARNING OBJECTIVES

After completing this chapter, you should be able to:

1. Describe why professional haircutting is a foundation for hairstyling and permanent waving.

2. Explain the correct use of the basic haircutting implements.

3. Demonstrate proper hair sectioning and its relationship to professional haircutting.

4. Demonstrate how to cut and use a guideline in haircutting.

5. List the various techniques used in hair thinning.

6. List the basic techniques for cutting with scissors or with a razor.

7. Define the terms related to professional haircutting.

Introduction

As a cosmetology student, you will learn to master the art and techniques of *haircutting.* Your haircutting skills will increase your professional qualifications in the salon. Thorough instruction is required in the proper way to cut and shape the hair, using a regular scissors, thinning shears, or a razor. Instruction must be followed by continual practice under the guidance of an instructor. A good haircut serves as a foundation for attractive hairstyles and for other services performed in the salon. A cosmetology education is not complete until you have acquired the artistic skill and judgment necessary for successful haircutting.

Hairstyles should accentuate the client's good points while minimizing his or her poor features. In selecting a suitable hairstyle, take into consideration the client's head shape, facial contour, neckline, and hair texture. However, you should also be guided by the client's wishes, personality, and lifestyle.

IMPLEMENTS USED IN HAIRCUTTING

The quality and selection of implements is important in order to accomplish a good haircut. To do your best work, the cosmetology student should buy and use only superior implements from a reliable manufacturer. However, improper use will quickly destroy the efficiency of any implement, no matter how perfectly it might be made at the factory.

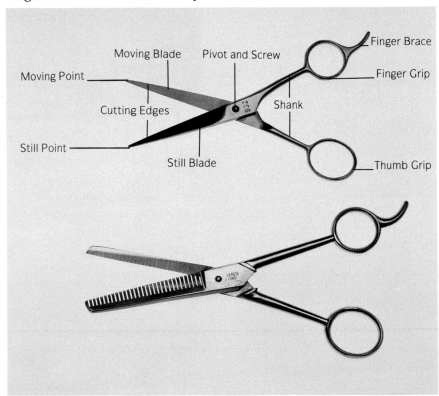

7.1 — Haircutting scissors (top); thinning shears, one blade notched (bottom).

The following are the implements used in haircutting (Figs. 7.1, 7.2):

Regular haircutting scissors
Thinning shears (single- or double-notched blades)

Razors with safety guards
Hair clippers (See Fig. 7.33)
Combs and clippies (See Fig. 9.1 for illustrations of clippies)

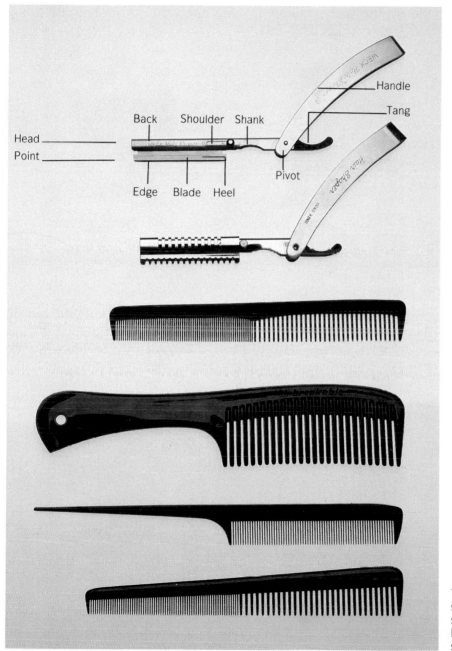

7.2—From top to bottom: straight razor; straight razor with safety guards; all-purpose comb; large-tooth comb; tail comb; hair shaping comb.

SECTIONING FOR HAIRCUTTING

By following a practical step-by-step procedure, you will soon learn how to give a professional haircut. The first step is to section the hair properly. The following illustrations cover the practical and accepted methods for dividing the hair into either four or five sections. In any case, follow your instructor's methods for dry or wet haircutting.

Four-Section Parting

Part hair down the center from the forehead to the *nape* (the back of the neck) and also across the top of the head from ear to ear. Pin up the four sections, leaving hair around the hairline to use as a guide. (Figs. 7.3, 7.4)

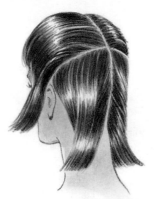

7.3 — Four-section parting.

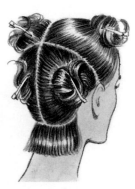

7.4 — Four-section with guideline.

Five-Section Parting

Five-section parting with subparting panels: section and pin up hair in the order shown in the illustrations.

The back section (No. 5) can be divided into sections No. 5a and No. 5b for easier handling. (Figs. 7.5–7.7)

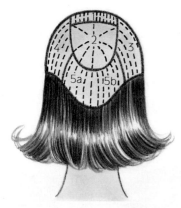

7.5 — Back view.

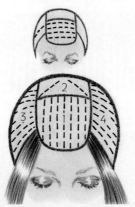

7.6 — Top section No. 1 may be subparted either in a horizontal or vertical direction.

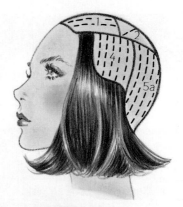

7.7 — Side view.

Alternative Five-Section Method

Another way to divide the hair into five sections is to part the hair across the *crown* (the top part of the head) from ear to ear, then subdivide the hair in the same order as shown in the illustration. (Fig. 7.8)

HOLDING HAIR SHAPING IMPLEMENTS

Scissors (Shears)

Haircutting scissors are handled correctly by inserting the third (ring) finger into the ring of the still blade and placing the little finger on the finger brace. The thumb is inserted into the ring of the movable blade. The tip of the index finger is braced near the pivot of the scissors in order to have better control. (Fig. 7.9)

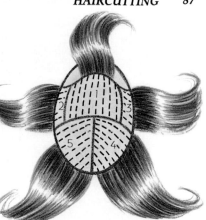

7.8 — Hair divided into five sections with center back parting.

Thinning Shears

Excess bulk is easily removed from the hair with a thinning shear. As can be seen in Fig. 7.1, thinning shears are quite similar to haircutting scissors, except that they have one or both blades *notched* or *serrated.* The single-notched edge cuts more hair. Which one is used depends on the preference of the cosmetologist. The notches provide a way to thin the hair in a uniform manner. Both thinning shears and cutting scissors are held in the same way. (Figs. 7.10, 7.11)

Holding Comb and Scissors

During the haircutting process, you will be holding both comb and scissors. Practice by closing the blades of the scissors, removing the thumb from the ring, and resting the scissors in the palm. Hold the scissors securely with the ring finger. The comb is held between the thumb and fingers. (Fig. 7.12)

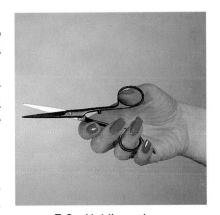

7.9 — Holding scissors (shears).

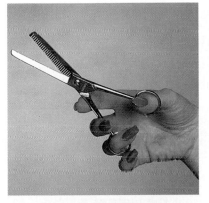

7.10 — Holding thinning shears with one blade notched.

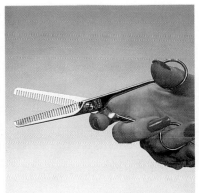

7.11 — Holding thinning shears with both blades notched.

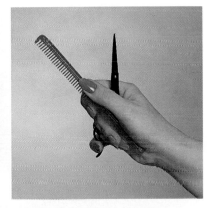

7.12 — Holding comb and scissors.

▶ NOTE: When combing the hair, hold the comb and scissors in the right hand, as shown. When shaping (cutting) the hair, hold the comb in the left hand. To save time, do not put down the comb or scissors during shaping.

HAIR THINNING

The purpose of *thinning* or *texturizing* hair is to remove excess bulk without shortening its length. For best results, use the following suggestions:

1. When using a razor for thinning or shaping, first dampen the hair.
2. When using thinning shears or regular scissors, the hair may be either dry or damp.

Hair texture determines the point where thinning should start on the hair strand. As a rule, fine hair may be thinned closer to the scalp than coarse hair. Fine hair is softer and more pliable, and when cut very short will lie flatter on the head. On the other hand, if coarse hair is thinned too close to the scalp, the short, stubby ends will protrude through the top layer.

The amount of hair you thin depends on the particular hairstyle. As a guide, start thinning different textures of hair as follows:

1. *Fine hair:* ½" to 1" (1.25 to 2.5 cm) from the scalp
2. *Medium hair:* 1" to 1½" (2.5 to 3.75 cm) from the scalp
3. *Coarse hair:* 1½" to 2" (3.75 to 5 cm) from the scalp

Hair Thinning Areas

There are several areas where it is *not* advisable to thin the hair (Fig. 7.13):

1. At the nape of the neck (ear to ear).
2. At the side of the head, above ears.
3. Around the facial hairline. Usually hair is not heavy at the hairline.
4. In the hair part. The cut ends will be seen in the finished hairstyle.

▶ NOTE: Never thin the hair near the ends of a strand; to do so will render the hair shapeless.

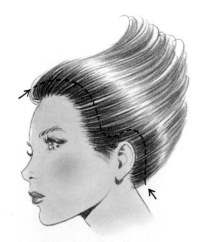

7.13—Dotted line shows hair that does not require thinning.

CAUTION

▶ *During the thinning process, remember that you can always go back and remove more hair if necessary. However, once the hair has been cut, it is impossible to replace and you might have difficulty in achieving the desired hairstyle.*

Thinning with Thinning Shears

When using the thinning shears, grip the hair firmly and evenly by overlapping the middle finger slightly over the index finger.

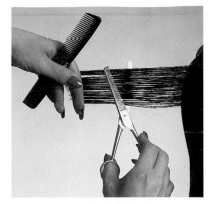

7.14—Thinning with thinning shears.

Procedure

1. Pick up a section of hair from ½" to 1" (1.25 to 2.5 cm) wide by 2" to 3" (5 to 7.5 cm) long, depending on the hair's texture.
2. Hold the section straight out from the scalp between the middle and index fingers.
3. Place thinning shears 1" to 2" (2.5 to 5 cm) from the scalp.
4. Cut the section by partly closing the thinning shears three-quarters through the strand. (Fig. 7.14)
5. Move out another 1½" (3.75 cm) and cut again.
6. Repeat if necessary.

▶ **NOTE:** It is advisable to avoid thinning the top part of the section.

Thinning with Haircutting Scissors (Shears)

When using regular haircutting scissors to thin the hair, pick up smaller sections of hair than when using the thinning shears. This process of thinning with scissors is known as *slithering* or *effilating*, and requires a different technique. (Fig. 7.15)

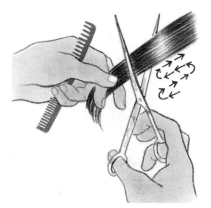

7.15—Thinning with haircutting scissors (shears).

Procedure

1. Hold a section of hair straight out between the middle and index fingers.
2. Place the hair in the scissors so that only the underneath hair will be cut.
3. Slide the scissors about 1" to 1½" (2.5 to 3.75 cm) down the section, closing them slightly each time the scissors are moved toward the scalp.
4. Repeat this procedure twice on each section.

Alternate method: Hold the hair with the thumb and index finger. (Fig. 7.16)

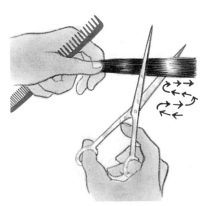

7.16—Holding the hair with thumb and index finger.

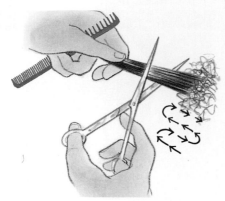

7.17—Slithering the hair after back-combing.

Back-combing method: The short hair may be back-combed and then slithered. (Fig. 7.17)

HAIRCUTTING WITH SCISSORS

Scissor shaping can be done either on dry or wet hair.

Dry shaping. If hair is shaped while dry, it is recommended that you first shampoo and completely dry the hair prior to shaping.

Wet shaping. The hair can be shaped immediately after it has been shampooed.

Preparation

1. Seat the client; adjust the neck strip and plastic cape.
2. Analyze the head shape, facial features, and hair texture.
3. Decide on a suitable haircut with the client.
4. Comb and brush the hair free of tangles.

Procedure

1. Divide the hair into five sections.
2. Determine the length of the *nape guideline hair,* the section that will serve as a length guide while you cut the hair.
3. *Blunt cut* (cutting hair straight without slithering) the guideline strand of nape hair. (See Fig. 7.18)
   a) Blunt cut the strand on the left side, using the strand closest to the earlobe and using the earlobe as a guide. (See Fig. 7.19)
   b) Blunt cut the strand on the right side to match the left side.
   c) Blunt cut from back center to left front. (See Fig. 7.20)
   d) Blunt cut from back center to right front for completed guideline. (See Fig. 7.21)

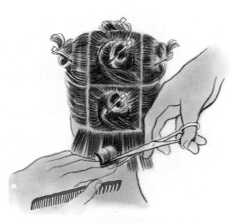

7.18—Blunt cutting strand at center nape to desired length.

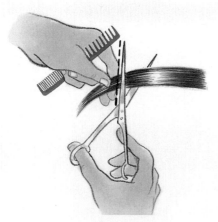

7.19—Blunt cutting.

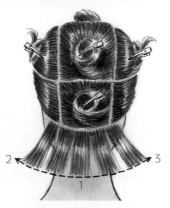

7.20—Following up by cutting all remaining guideline hair.

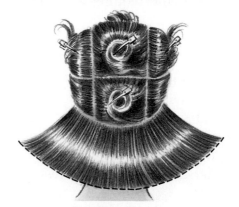

7.21—Properly cut guideline hair.

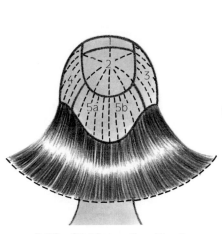
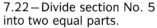

7.22—Divide section No. 5 into two equal parts.

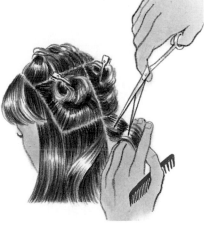

7.23—Blunt cutting section No. 5b.

7.24—Crown section.

4. Let down section No. 5 and divide into two equal parts (No. 5a and No. 5b). Match length with guideline hair. (See Fig. 7.22) Either the left side or the right side may be done first. Hold hair panels out from the head while blunt cutting. (See Fig. 7.23) Continue cutting sections No. 3 and No. 4 in the same manner.

Crown Section

Crown section No. 2. Hold the pie-shaped strands out from the head; match length by picking up strands from the section already cut. Continue around the head, matching the length with sides and back hair. (See Figs. 7.24, 7.25)

Top Front Section

Divide section No. 1 into two parts. Pick up hair in the middle section using a few strands of previously cut hair from the crown as a guide. Maintain the hand movement in a 45° (.785 rad) arc. Proceed to cut both parts of section No. 1 in the prescribed manner. (See Figs. 7.26, 7.27)

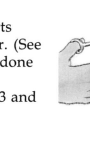

7.25—Shaping crown section.

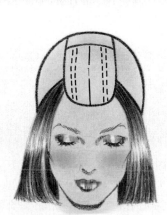

7.26—Top view section No. 1 with vertical partings.

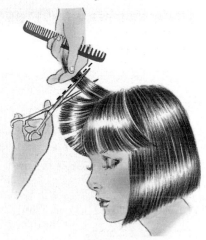

7.27—Shaping top section.

If bangs are to be cut, work directly in front of the client for even cutting. Test hair for bounce (elasticity), then determine the desired length. If the bangs are to be short, use the bridge of the nose as a guide. If the style is to be long, shape strands to blend into the length of the sides. (See Figs. 7.28–7.30)

Reducing bulk. To complete cutting the hair, remove excess bulk by thinning with a razor, thinning shears, or scissors. It is recommended that all hair be checked for proper length.

People Skills

There's a saying that the only good business is repeat business. But how do you build a following in a salon? According to Geri Mataya, owner of Uptown Hair Design in Pittsburgh, developing a personal sales technique ensures repeat clients.

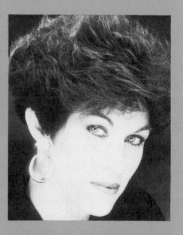

Says Mataya, whose staff members' client retention ranges from 50% to 90%, "The difference between the stylist who has a high retention rate and the one who isn't getting repeat business is that the successful stylist knows how to service clients."

Her easy tips for service are: Listen to the client and give her your full attention so you can do what she wants, not what you want. Then, always give an extra she doesn't expect, such as a scalp massage during a shampoo, coffee while she waits, or a compliment about how she looks. Lastly, give her a reason to return by suggesting a service to think about for next time and booking that next appointment before she leaves.

Adds Mataya, "Take sales and psychology classes so that you can determine something about your client and what she wants. The 'know-it-all' is easy because she'll tell you exactly what she likes. The hardest client to service is the undecided one. For her, think minimal, because she isn't ready for a major change. Gain her trust by trimming her hair and styling it differently. Then suggest a change for her to think about until her next appointment.

"If you're getting a lot of clients but not retaining them, you can't blame the salon or the owner. Learn to identify with your client's needs, even if she's very different from you, and you can't help but succeed."

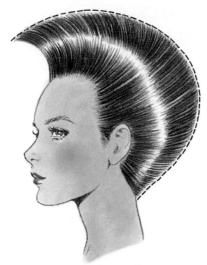

7.28—Correct uniform shaping.

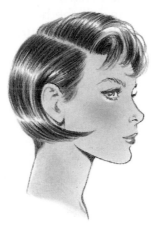

7.29—Completed shaping with bang effect and/or off-face style.

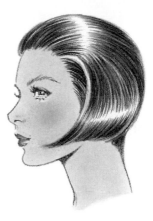

7.30—Hair shaping for straight back style.

Completion

Remove the neck strip and plastic cape. Thoroughly clean all hair clippings from the cape, client's clothing, and the work area. You may then proceed with the next professional service desired by the client.

SHINGLING

Shingling is cutting the hair close to the nape and gradually longer toward the crown, without showing a definite line.

Regardless of the current hair fashions, there will always be clients who prefer to have their hair cut short. To satisfy these clients, you must know how to shingle the hair. The accompanying illustrations show how to accomplish shingling with the use of shears and comb. (See Figs. 7.31, 7.32)

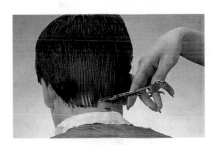

7.31—Outlining neckline.

Procedure

Shingling should be done at eye level. Start by outlining neckline. Hold the hair in the comb and cut upward in a graduated effect. When you reach the top of the section being shingled, turn the comb downward and comb the hair. Proceed, section by section, until the entire back of the head is shingled in a smooth, uniform manner.

▶ NOTE: In shingling, the blades of the scissors are held parallel with the comb; only the top blade moves and does the cutting.

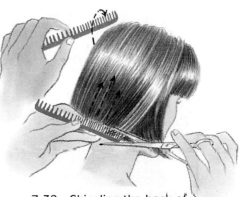

7.32—Shingling the back of the head.

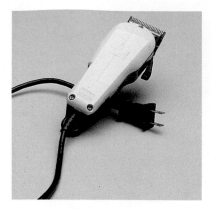

7.33—Electric haircutting clippers.

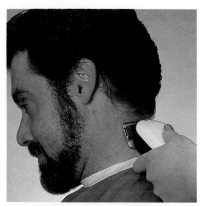

7.34—Cleaning the neck with clippers.

USE OF CLIPPERS ON THE NECKLINE

There is a mistaken notion that using clippers to "clean" the neckline makes the hair grow in thicker on the neck. This is not true, because the amount of human hair can only be as great as the number of follicles in the area. Use of clippers or any other implement does not increase the number of follicles. (Figs. 7.33, 7.34)

USING THE RAZOR

The successful cosmetologist must be versatile in handling all haircutting implements efficiently, including the straight razor.

How to Hold the Razor

Finger wrap hold. Place the thumb in the groove part of the *shank* and fold the fingers over the handle of the razor. The *guard* faces the cosmetologist while working. (See Fig. 7.35)

Three-finger hold. Place three fingers over the shank, the thumb in the groove of the shank, and the little finger in the hollow part of the tang. (See Fig. 7.36)

▶ NOTE: When combing the hair, hold the razor and comb in the right hand. (See Fig. 7.37) When cutting the hair with a razor, hold the comb in the left hand. Do not put down the comb or razor.

When using the razor, keep the hair damp to avoid pulling the hair and to prevent dulling the razor.

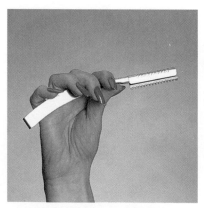

7.35—Finger wrap hold.

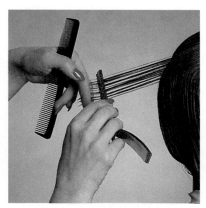

7.36—Blunt razor cutting.

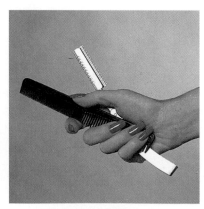

7.37—Holding razor and comb.

Changing Blades

Removing an old blade. Remove the guard. With the left hand, hold the shaper firmly above the joint. Catch the blade in the teeth of the upper part of the guard and push out the blade. (See Fig. 7.38)

Inserting a new blade. Slide the blade into the groove, pushing the end carefully with your fingers. Place the tooth end of the guard into the blade notch and slide the blade in until it clicks into position. Slide the guard over the blade, making sure the free or open end is over the cutting edge of the blade.

Thinning with a Razor

Hold a strand of wet hair straight out between the middle and index fingers. Place the razor flat, not erect, about ½" (1.25 cm) from the scalp (depending on the hair texture), and use short, steady strokes toward the hair ends. (See Figs. 7.39–7.41)

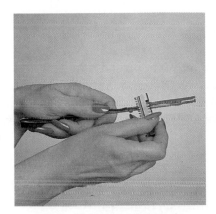

7.38—Removing old blade.

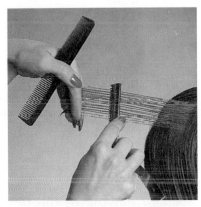

7.39—Thinning with razor.

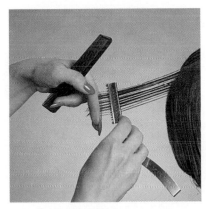

7.40—Tapering hair ends with razor.

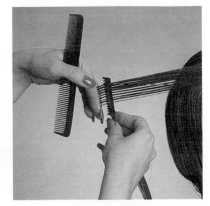

7.41 Razor under-cutting with upward stroke.

Haircutting with a Razor

Preparation

1. Seat the client; adjust the neck strip and plastic cape.
2. Analyze the head shape, facial features, and hair texture.
3. Decide on a suitable haircut with the client.
4. Comb and brush the hair free of tangles.
5. Shampoo and cut the hair while it is wet.

Procedure

1. Divide the hair into five sections.
2. Determine the length of the nape guideline hair.
3. Blunt cut a guideline strand of nape hair. (See Fig. 7.42)
   a) Blunt cut a strand on the left side; use the earlobe as a guide.
   b) Blunt cut a strand on the right side to match the left side.
   c) Use guideline hair to cut from the back center to the left front and back center to the right front. (See Fig. 7.43)
   d) Complete guideline. (See Fig. 7.44)

Cutting back sections No. 5a and No. 5b. Divide section No. 5 into two parts (sections No. 5a and No. 5b). From the center of section No. 5a, pick horizontal strands. Pick up a guideline strand for length. When guideline hair falls away, cut the hair, moving hands out and upward into a 45° (.785 rad) arc. (See Fig. 7.45)

Cutting section No. 4. Proceed to cut to the left into section No. 4 in the same manner.

Cutting section No. 3. Return to section No. 5b and cut this section, moving to the right into section No. 3, always lifting hands in an upward 45° (.785 rad) arc as the hair is cut. Measure carefully with guideline hair.

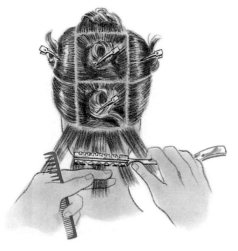

7.42 — Blunt cutting a strand at center nape for desired hair length.

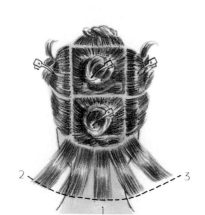

7.43 — Following up by cutting all remaining guideline hair.

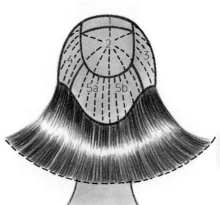

7.44 — Completed guideline.

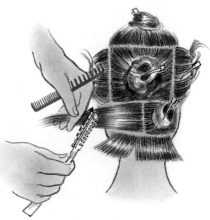

7.45 — Shaping section No. 5a.

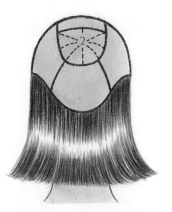

7.46—Section No. 2.

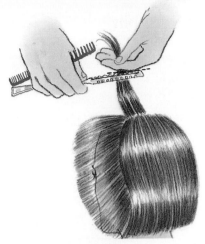

7.47—Shaping section No. 2.

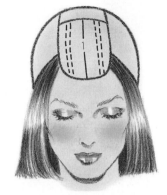

7.48—Section No. 1 shown with vertical parting.

Cutting section No. 2. Next, proceed to cut section No. 2 (crown), using the previously cut hair as a guide. (See Figs. 7.46, 7.47)

Cutting section 1. Divide section No. 1 into two parts. Pick up hair in the middle of the section using a few strands of previously cut hair from the crown as a guide. Maintain the hand movement in a 45° (.785 rad) arc. Proceed to cut both parts of section No. 1 in the prescribed manner. (See Figs. 7.48, 7.49)

Bangs. To cut bangs evenly, work directly in front of the client. Test hair for bounce (elasticity), then determine the desired length. If the bangs are to be short, use the bridge of the nose as a guide. If the style is to be long, shape strands to blend into the length of the sides.

Reducing bulk. To complete cutting the hair, remove excess bulk by thinning with a razor, thinning shears, or scissors. Be sure to check hair for proper length. (See Figs. 7.50, 7.51)

Completion. Remove the neck strip and plastic cape. Thoroughly clean all hair clippings from the cape, client's clothing, and the work area. You may then proceed with the next professional service desired by the client.

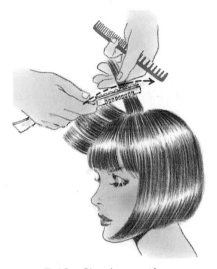

7.49—Shaping section No. 1.

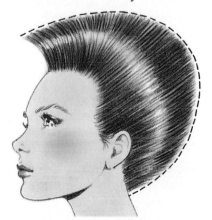

7.50—Correct uniform shaping.

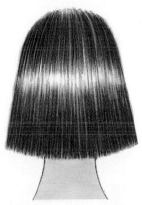

7.51—Back view—uniform shaping.

People Skills

One of the biggest challenges you'll face as a working stylist is dealing successfully with human dynamics. Maintaining good relationships with your co-workers is as vital as having great client relationships, because co-workers are your daily support system.

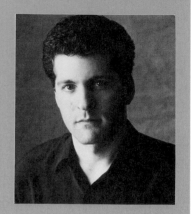

Carmine Minardi, a salon owner who started with 250 clients and now boasts 4,000 for his entire salon, offers this advice for getting off on the right foot: "The most successful stylists reach that point by having the support and help of their co-workers. As you gain their respect and get them to share ideas, hints, and tips, you'll learn more from them than you will from any educational seminar.

"When you interview for a job, tell the owner that at some point you'd like to be introduced to the entire staff. When you begin working, always offer to help your colleagues, even if it means staying late. To become a great stylist, you have to be a fantastic assistant first. By helping others and creating a feeling of positive energy, it's inevitable that you'll become sensitive enough to tune in to the needs and feelings of others, which is the biggest key to success.

"Under these circumstances, the hardest thing might be to be able to take criticism well, but a sensitive person is always open to criticism and ready to learn from it. Showing you're flexible is the strongest statement you can make about yourself."

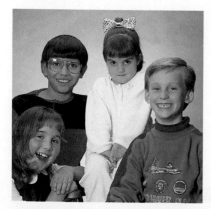

7.52—Popular hairstyles for children.

LEARN TO HANDLE CHILDREN

Special consideration should be given to children and teenagers. Hairstylists who are patient and know how to handle children will attract the parents to their salons for their own hairstyling. (Fig. 7.52)

CUTTING OVERLY CURLY HAIR

Overly curly hair has special characteristics, as have other types of hair, that require certain techniques for styling. Most important to you is the ability to visualize and create a hairstyle that will enhance the appearance of the client. Knowing the correct cutting and styling techniques and using common sense in their application are basic to the success of the hairstylist. One method for shaping and styling overly curly hair is outlined below. Your instructor may also have alternate methods for you to use.

Procedure

1. Drape the client for hair shaping.

2. Shampoo and thoroughly dry the hair.

3. Apply an *emollient* (i-**MOL**-yent) (softening) product lightly to the scalp and hair to replace lost oil.

4. Begin in the crown. Using a wide-tooth comb or a hair lifter, comb the hair upward and slightly forward, extending the hair length as long as possible. Continue until all hair has been combed out from the scalp and evenly distributed around the head. Combing in a circular pattern will usually help avoid splits.

5. Cut the hair. Visualize the style and length of hair desired. Start by tapering the sides, and cut in the direction the hair will be combed.

6. Taper the back part of the head to blend with the sides.

7. Trim the extreme hair ends in the crown and top areas to the desired length.

8. For an off-the-face hairstyle, comb hair up and backward. For a forward movement, comb hair up and forward.

9. Blend side hair with the top, crown, and back hair.

10. Outline the hairstyle at the sides, around the ears, and in the nape area, using either scissors or a trimmer (clipper).

11. Check silhouette of shaping, making sure it is blended.

12. Give a finishing touch. Fluff the hair slightly with a hair lifter, wherever needed. Spray the hair lightly to give it a natural, lustrous sheen. (See Fig. 7.53)

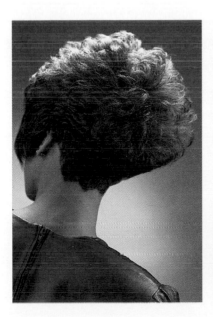
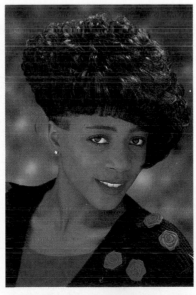
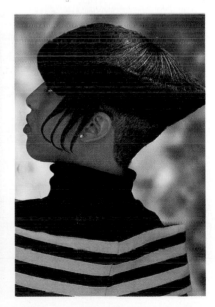

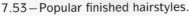
7.53—Popular finished hairstyles.

Review Questions

HAIRCUTTING

1. Why is the mastery of haircutting so important to the student?
2. What four factors should be taken into consideration when choosing a hairstyle for your client?
3. What are the tools used in haircutting?
4. What is the first step in haircutting?
5. What is the purpose of thinning the hair?
6. How close to the scalp should you thin: a) fine hair; b) medium hair; c) coarse hair?
7. In which areas is it advisable not to thin the hair?
8. Define slithering.
9. What is the purpose of a guideline?
10. What is shingling?
11. For what purpose is the clipper used?
12. Why is a razor used on damp hair?
13. What is tapering?
14. Overly curly hair is cut wet or dry?

8

FINGER WAVING

LEARNING OBJECTIVES

After completing this chapter, you should be able to:

1. Explain the purpose of finger waving.
2. Demonstrate the different types of finger waves.
3. List the steps in the finger waving procedure.

Introduction

Finger waving is the art of shaping and directing the hair into alternate parallel waves and designs using the fingers, comb, waving lotion, and hairpins or clippies.

You may wonder why you are learning a technique that is not frequently requested by many clients anymore. Training in finger waving is important because it teaches you the technique of moving and directing hair. It also helps you develop the dexterity, coordination, and finger strength required for professional hairstyling. In addition, it provides valuable training in creating hairstyles and in molding hair to the curved surface of the head. It is an excellent introduction to hairstyling.

PREPARATION

Always wash your hands before giving your client any salon service. Make sure all necessary implements have been sanitized and towels and other supplies are clean and fresh. Prepare the client in the same manner as you would for a shampoo.

Shampoo the client's hair at the shampoo bowl, towel-blot the hair, and seat the client comfortably at your station.

More natural soft-looking waves are obtained with hair that has a natural wave or has been permanently waved than with straight hair. A finger wave correctly done complements the client's head as well as her facial features.

FINGER WAVING LOTION

Waving lotion makes the hair pliable and keeps it in place during the finger waving procedure.

Waving lotion is made from Karaya gum, which is found in trees of Africa and India. This gum can be diluted to a thin, watery consistency, generally for use on fine hair, or its consistency can be more concentrated for use on regular or coarse hair. A good waving lotion is harmless to the hair and does not flake when it dries.

APPLICATION OF LOTION

Part the hair down to the scalp, comb smooth, and arrange it to conform to the planned style. The hair will move more easily if you use the coarse teeth of the comb. Follow the natural growth pattern when combing and parting the hair. You will find the hair easier to mold, and it will not buckle or separate in the crown area.

Waving lotion is applied to the hair while it is damp. This permits the lotion to be distributed smoothly and evenly. Use an applicator to apply the waving lotion and a comb to distribute it through the hair. Do not use an excessive amount of waving lotion.

▶ **NOTE:** Apply lotion to one side of the head at a time; this prevents it from drying and requiring additional applications.

To determine the natural hair growth, comb the hair away from the face, and push hair forward gently with the palm of your hand. As you will learn in the chapter on hairstyling, the hair will fall in its natural growth pattern.

The finger wave may be started on either side of the head. However, in this presentation, the hair is parted on the left side of the head and the wave is started on the right (heavy) side of the head.

Horizontal Finger Waving

SHAPING THE TOP AREA

Using the index finger of your left hand as a guide, shape the top hair with a comb, using a circular movement. Starting at the hairline, work toward the crown in 1½" to 2" (3.7 to 5 cm) sections at a time until the crown has been reached. (See Fig. 8.1)

Forming the First Ridge

Place the index finger of the left hand directly above the position for the first ridge. With the teeth of the comb pointing slightly upward, insert the comb directly under the index finger. Draw the comb forward about 1" (2.5 cm) along the fingertip. (See Fig. 8.2)

With the teeth still inserted in the ridge, flatten the comb against the head in order to hold the ridge in place. (See Fig. 8.3)

Remove the left hand from the head and place the middle finger above the ridge and the index finger on the teeth of the comb.

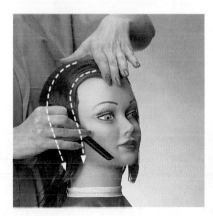

8.1—Shape top area.

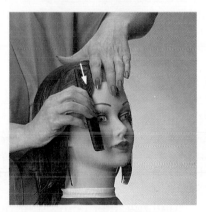

8.2—Draw hair about 1" (2.5 cm) toward fingertip.

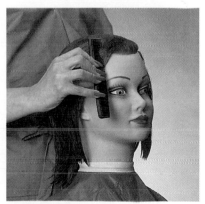

8.3—Flatten comb against head.

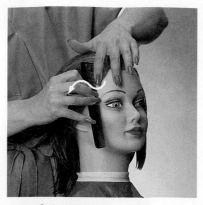

8.4—Emphasize ridge.

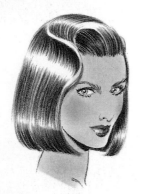

8.5—Comb hair in semi-
circular direction.

Emphasize the ridge by closing the two fingers and applying pressure to the head. (See Fig. 8.4)

▶ NOTE: Do not try to increase the height or depth of a ridge by pinching or pushing with fingers; such movements will create over-direction of the ridge.

Without removing the comb, turn the teeth downward, and comb the hair in a right semicircular direction to form a dip in the hollow part of the wave. (See Fig. 8.5)

Follow this procedure, section by section, until the crown has been reached, where the ridge phases out. (See Fig. 8.6)

The ridge and wave of each section should match evenly, without showing separations in the ridge and hollow part of the wave.

Forming the Second Ridge

Begin at the crown area. (See Fig. 8.7) The movements are the reverse of those followed in forming the first ridge. The comb is drawn from the tip of the index finger toward the base of the index finger, thus directing formation of the second ridge. All movements are followed in a reverse pattern until the hairline is reached, thus completing the second ridge. (See Fig. 8.8)

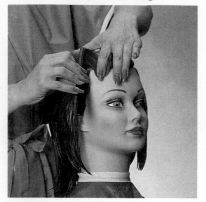

8.6—Complete first ridge at the crown.

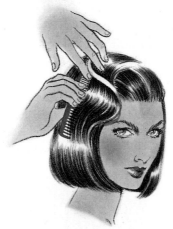

8.7—Start the second ridge.

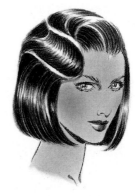

8.8—Complete second ridge.

Forming the Third Ridge

Movements for the third ridge closely follow those used in creating the first ridge. However, the third ridge is started at the hairline and extended back toward the back of the head. (See Fig. 8.9)

Continue alternating directions until the side of the head has been completed. (See Fig. 8.10)

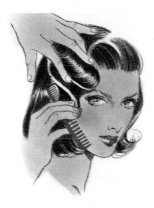

8.9—Start the third ridge.

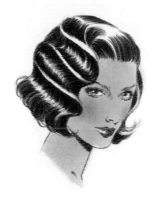

8.10—Complete right side.

LEFT SIDE OF THE HEAD

Use the same procedure for the left (light) side of the head as you used for finger waving the right (heavy) side of the head.

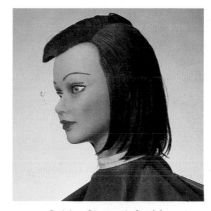

8.11—Shape left side.

Procedure

1. Shape the hair. (See Fig. 8.11)
2. Starting at the hairline, form the first ridge, section by section, until the second ridge of the opposite side is reached. (See Fig. 8.12)
3. Both the ridge and the wave must blend without splits or breaks, with the ridge and wave on the right side of the head. (See Fig. 8.13)
4. Start with the ridge and wave in the back of the head and proceed, section by section, toward the left side of the face.
5. Continue working back and forth until the entire side is completed. (See Fig. 8.14)

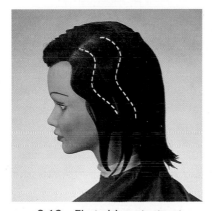

8.12—First ridge starts at hairline.

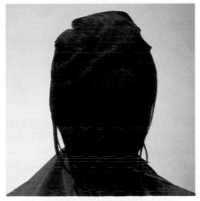

8.13—Ridge and wave matched in the crown area.

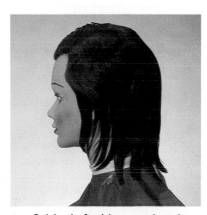

8.14—Left side completed.

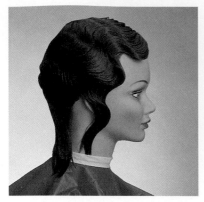

8.15—Completed hairstyle, right side.

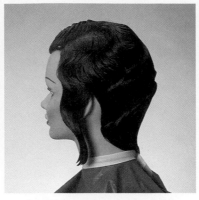

8.16—Completed hairstyle, left side.

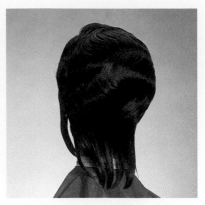

8.17—Completed hairstyle, back view.

6.   Figures 8.15–8.17 illustrate the completed hairstyles.

Completion

1.   Place net over hair, secure with hairpins or clippies if needed, and safeguard the client's forehead and ears while under the dryer with cotton, gauze, or paper protectors.
2.   Adjust the dryer to medium heat and allow hair to dry thoroughly.
3.   Remove client from under dryer.
4.   Remove clippies or pins and hairnet from hair.
5.   Comb out and reset waves into a soft coiffure.
6.   Clean up work station.
7.   Sanitize combs, hairpins, clippies, and hairnet after each use.

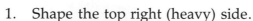

Alternate Method of Finger Waving

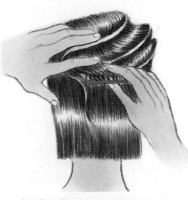

8.18—Finger waving around the head.

Hair parted on left side. The following is an alternate method to perform finger waving:

1.   Shape the top right (heavy) side.
2.   Phase out the first ridge starting at the front ***right*** side, and working around to the crown.
3.   Start a ridge on the ***left*** front side and go all around the head, finishing on the front right hairline. (Fig. 8.18)
4.   Start another ridge on the front right hairline and finish on the left front side. Continue, left to right and right to left, until the entire head is completed.

     This method eliminates the need to match ridges and waves at the back of the head. (Completion is the same as it is for the horizontal method of finger waving.)

Vertical Finger Waving

In vertical finger waving, the ridges and waves run up and down the head, while in horizontal finger waving they go parallel around the head.

The procedure for making vertical ridges and waves is the same as it is for horizontal finger waving.

1. Make side part, extending from forehead to crown.
2. Form shaping in a semicircular effect. (See Figs. 8.19, 8.20)

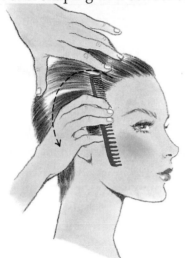
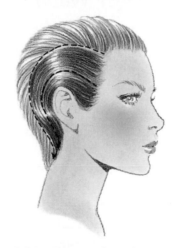

8.19—Form shaping.   8.20—First section of wave.

3. Make first section of ridge and wave. (See Fig. 8.21)
4. Continue with additional sections until the part is reached.

Start the second ridge at the hair part. Start the third ridge at the hairline. Complete side. (See Fig. 8.22) (Completion is the same as it is for horizontal finger waving.)

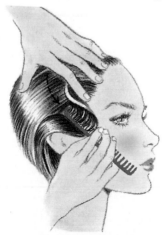
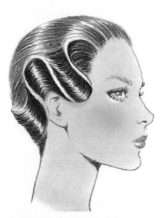

8.21—Start first wave.   8.22—Completed finger wave.

Shadow Wave

A shadow wave is a shallow wave with low ridges that are not very sharp. The waves are formed in the regular manner, but the comb does not penetrate to the scalp. The hair layers underneath are not waved. This type of wave is sometimes desirable for a client who wishes to dress her hair very close to the head.

Reminders and Hints on Finger Waving

1. Wash hands and have available sanitized implements and supplies.
2. Avoid the use of an excessive amount of waving lotion.
3. Use hard rubber combs with both fine and coarse teeth.
4. Before finger waving, locate the natural or permanent wave in the hair.
5. To emphasize the ridges of a finger wave, press the ridge between the fingers, holding the fingers against the head.
6. To wave the underneath hair, insert the comb through the hair to the scalp.
7. For a longer-lasting finger wave, mold the waves in the direction of the natural growth.
8. To safeguard the client's forehead and ears from intense heat while under dryer, use cotton, gauze, or paper protectors.
9. Place a net over the hair to protect the setting while it is being dried.
10. Thoroughly dry the hair before combing it out.
11. Prolonged drying under heat will dry the natural oils of the hair and scalp.
12. Finger waves will not remain in place if the hair is combed out before it has been completely dried.
13. Lightened or tinted hair that tangles is easier to comb if a cream rinse is used.
14. Lightly spraying the hair with lacquer will hold the finger wave longer and give the hair a sheen.

Success Spotlight

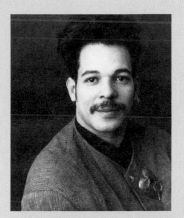

As a Puerto Rican immigrant who studied chemical engineering, Balmer Galindez could not continue his studies in the United States until he learned English. Once he did, he chose a beauty career over science because, "While struggling with a language barrier, I discovered it was easy to express my concepts in fashion in my own way. I became a hair designer because I liked hands-on learning and the fact that there are no set rules to creativity, except that every style from the past is reborn in a new way."

Galindez, who worked behind the chair for 8 years before opening his own salon in New York City offers this advice to would-be success stories: "Seek knowledge. Even Picasso had to learn the basics before he could go beyond them to be creative. Execute what you learn and always strive to improve on it. Help others and grow with them because one mind makes for a knowledgeable person, but three minds together make a genius."

According to Galindez, the influence of the Hispanic market in the United States is growing so fast that opportunities for bilingual cosmetologists are boundless. Proving this, he recently moved from salon owner to platform artist, teaching in the first all-Spanish language cosmetology seminar held in the Bronx.

Review Questions

FINGER WAVING

1. What is the purpose of finger waving?
2. What is the purpose of finger waving lotion?
3. Name the different types of finger waves.
4. List five reminders or hints for better finger waving.

9

WET HAIRSTYLING

LEARNING OBJECTIVES

After completing this chapter, you should be able to:

1. Define hairstyling.
2. List the basic elements of hairstyling.
3. Demonstrate the proper use and care of implements employed in hairstyling.
4. List and analyze the characteristics of a client's appearance prior to a hairstyling service.

Introduction

Before you can become a proficient stylist you must first understand hair structure, permanent waving, hair straightening, thermal waving and curling, hair coloring, hair chemistry, the action of conditioners, and the overall importance of hair shaping.

Hairstyling is creating wearable art. To be a successful stylist you must be able to apply basic art principles to hairstyling in order to change along with fashion trends.

The elementary rules of art that you use to style hair are weight and balance, form, rhythm, shape, composition, contrast, elevation, texture, structure, and the use of space. The accomplishments of styling, decoration, and incorporating new ideas become easier as you gain experience.

As you gain experience you will become adept at using art principles and applying them appropriately to each client. It is advisable for you to take note of your client's physical form so that you will be better able to balance the hairstyle to the individual.

Examine your client's hair before starting the shampoo. This gives you the opportunity to take note of hair growth direction and texture and helps you visualize a becoming and personalized hairstyle. (Fig. 9.1)

Hairstyling Basics

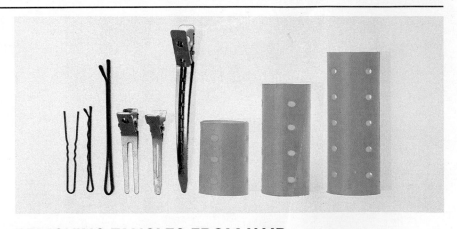

9.1—Implements and materials used in hairstyling—left to right: hairpin; bobby pin; roller pin; double prong clip; single prong clip; duckbill clamp; short roller; medium roller; long roller.

REMOVING TANGLES FROM HAIR

It is necessary to remove tangles from your client's hair before you shampoo, cut, or style it. This will prevent damage and matting. To remove tangles, follow this procedure:

1. Begin at the nape with a coarse-toothed comb or cushioned brush.
2. Separate a small section and brush across and down each strand.
3. Work across the back, in small sections, gradually progressing to the crown.
4. The size of the sections you use will depend on the thickness, length, curliness, condition, and elasticity of the hair.

5. Once the tangles are removed, proceed with the service. (Figs. 9.2–9.4)

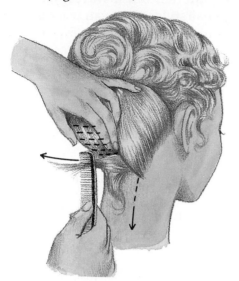

9.2—Removing tangles in nape area.

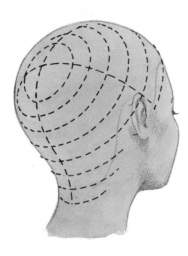

9.3—Combing pattern for removing tangles.

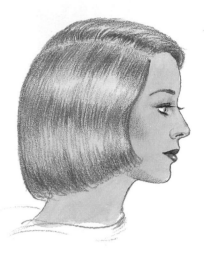

9.4—Tangles removed.

MAKING A PART

Clean partings make hairstyles look professional. Use any one of these common methods.

1. Comb hair straight and tightly back from the face. Draw your comb toward the back of the head in an even line. Hold the light side firm while combing the heavy side away from the parting. (Figs. 9.5–9.7)

2. Using the end of a tail comb, draw a clean, clear line.

3. To make use of a *natural part,* comb wet hair straight back. Place the palm of the left hand on the head and push forward. You will notice the hair split apart into sections. These sections are the natural partings.

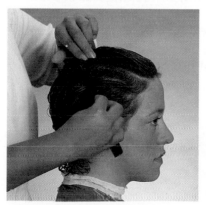

9.5—Drawing comb back full length.

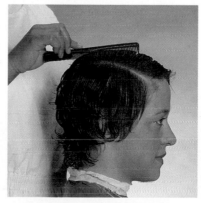

9.6—Combing hair above and below part.

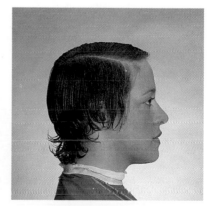

9.7—Hair combed with straight part.

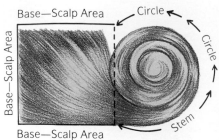

9.8—Parts of a curl.

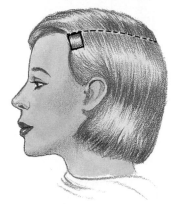

9.9—Pin curl base.

PIN CURLS

Pin curls provide the bases for all patterns, lines, waves, curls, and rolls that you use as you create hairstyles. You can use them on straight, permanent-waved, and naturally curly hair. Pin curls work best if the hair is properly tapered and wound smoothly. This makes springy and long-lasting curls with good direction and definition.

Parts of a Curl

Pin curls are constructed of three principal parts: *base, stem,* and *circle.* (Fig. 9.8)

1. The *base* is the stationary, or immovable, foundation of the curl, which is attached to the scalp. (Fig. 9.9)
2. The *stem* is the section of the pin curl, between the base and first arc (turn) of the circle, which gives the circle its direction, action, and mobility.
3. The *circle* is the part of the pin curl that forms a complete circle. The size of the curl governs the width of the wave and its strength.

Mobility of a Curl

The amount of movement (mobility) of a section of hair is determined by the *stem* and *circle*. Curl mobility is classified as *no-stem, half-stem,* and *full-stem.*

1. The *no-stem curl* is placed directly on the base of the curl. It produces a tight, firm, long-lasting curl.
2. The *half-stem curl* permits more freedom, since the curl (circle) is placed one-half off the base. It gives good *control* to the hair and produces *softness* in the finished wave pattern.
3. The *full-stem curl* allows for the greatest mobility. The curl is placed completely off the base. The base may be a square, triangular, half-moon, or rectangular section depending on the area of the head in which the full-stem curls are used. It gives as much freedom as the length of the stem will permit. If it is exaggerated, the hair near the scalp will be flat and almost straight. It is used for a *strong direction* of the hair and a *weaker wave pattern.* (Figs. 9.10–9.12)

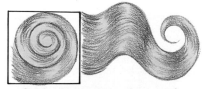

9.10—No-stem curl opened out.

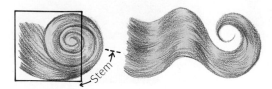

9.11—Half-stem curl opened out.

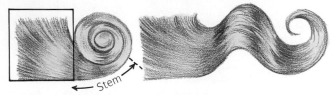

9.12—Full-stem curl opened out.

Open and Closed Center Curls

Open center curls produce even, smooth waves and uniform curls. *Closed center curls* produce waves that decrease in size toward the end. They are good for fine hair or if a fluffy curl is desired. Notice the difference in the waves produced by pin curls with open centers and those with closed centers. The size of the curl determines the size of the wave. If you make pin curls with the ends outside the curl, the resulting wave will be narrower near the scalp and wider toward the ends. (Figs. 9.13, 9.14)

Curl and Stem Direction

Curls may be turned toward the face, away from the face, upward, downward, or diagonally. You determine what the finished result will be by the direction in which you place the stem of the curl. Curl and stem direction is referred to as:

1. *Forward movement*—toward the face.
2. *Reverse movement*—backward or away from the face. (Figs. 9.15–9.18)

These illustrations are intended to show stem directions and curl placements and are not illustrations of pin curl patterns.

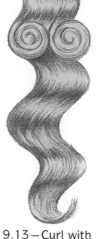
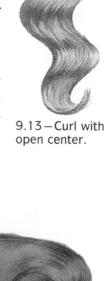

9.13—Curl with open center. 9.14—Curl with closed center.

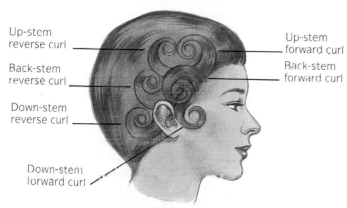

Up-stem reverse curl
Back-stem reverse curl
Down-stem reverse curl
Down-stem forward curl
Up-stem forward curl
Back-stem forward curl

9.15—Forward movement.

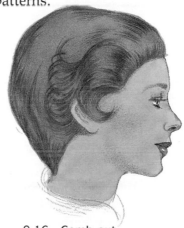

9.16—Comb-out.

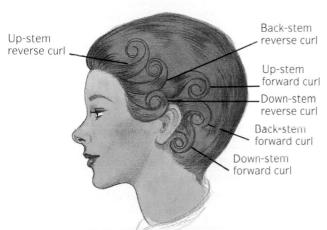

Up-stem reverse curl
Back-stem reverse curl
Up-stem forward curl
Down-stem reverse curl
Back-stem forward curl
Down-stem forward curl

9.17—Backward movement.

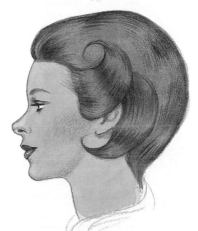

9.18—Comb-out.

Clockwise and Counterclockwise Curls

The terms *clockwise curls* and *counterclockwise curls* are used to describe the direction of pin curls. Curls formed in the same direction as the movement of the hands of a clock are known as clockwise curls. Curls formed in the opposite direction of the movement of the hands of a clock are known as counterclockwise curls. (Figs. 9.19, 9.20)

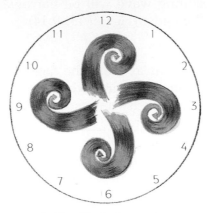

9.19 — Clockwise curls.

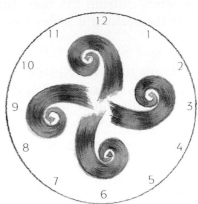

9.20 — Counter-clockwise curls.

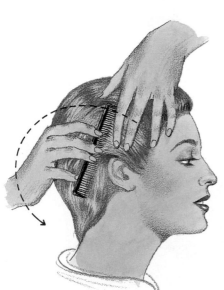

9.21 — Forming side forward vertical shaping.

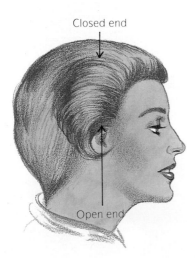

9.22 — Finished side forward vertical shaping.

Shaping for Pin Curl Placements

A *shaping* is a section of hair that you mold into a design to serve as a base for a curl or wave pattern.

Shapings are classified as forward and reverse; diagonal, vertical, or horizontal; oblong or circular.

Circular shapings are pie-shaped with the open end smaller than the closed end. They work well as the first forward shaping in a hairstyle that moves away from the face. In a wave pattern, the forward circular shaping would be followed by a reverse circular curl.

Oblong shapings are waves that remain the same width throughout the shaping.

Forward shapings are directed toward the face. This type of shaping is *oval* (larger in size at its closed end).

Procedure

To make a forward, vertical shaping on the side of the head, direct the hair in a circular motion, moving back from the face, upward, then downward and toward the face. The size of the shaping determines the resulting hairstyle. (Figs. 9.21, 9.22)

2. To make a top forward shaping, comb-direct the hair in a circular motion, away from the forehead, pivoting the comb to create a circular effect toward the face. (Figs. 9.23, 9.24)

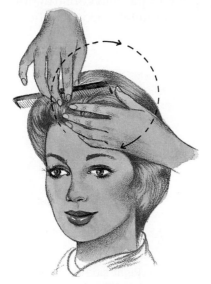

9.23—Forming oval shaping for top forward movement.

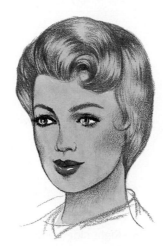

9.24—Finished oval shaping for top forward movement.

Reverse shapings are comb-directed downward, then immediately upward in a circular motion, away from the face. (Figs. 9.25, 9.26)

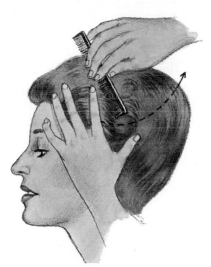

9.25—Forming left side reverse vertical shaping.

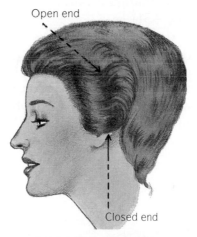

Open end

Closed end

9.26—Finished left side reverse vertical shaping.

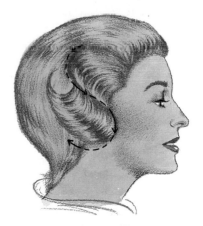

9.27—Diagonal shaping.

Diagonal shapings are variations of the forward shaping with the exception that the shaping is formed diagonally to the side of the head. (Fig. 9.27)

Vertical side shapings are directed in a way that places the open and closed ends in a vertical fashion.

Horizontal shapings are comb-directed parallel with the parting. They are recommended for pin curl parallel construction and where a wave design is carried completely around the head. (Figs. 9.28, 9.29)

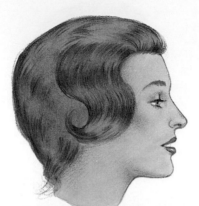

9.28—Right side horizontal shaping.

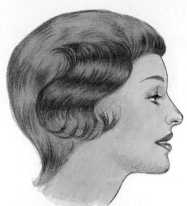

9.29—Right side reverse horizontal shaping.

PIN CURL FOUNDATIONS OR BASES

Before you begin to make your pin curls, divide the hair into sections or panels. Then you are ready to subdivide the sections into the type of foundations or bases required for the various curls. The most commonly shaped bases you will use are rectangular, triangular, arc (half-moon or C-shape), and square. (Figs. 9.30, 9.31)

To avoid splits in the finished hairstyle, you must use care when selecting and forming the curl base. Further uniformity of curl development can only be achieved if the sections of hair are as equal as possible. Each curl must lie flat and smooth on its base. If extended too far off the base you will get just direction with a loose curl away from the scalp. The finished curl, however, is not affected by the shape of the base.

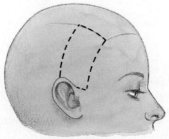

9.30—Panel.

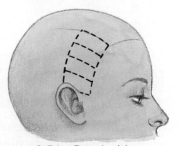

9.31—Panel with rectangular bases.

Rectangular base pin curls are usually recommended at the side front hairline for a smooth upsweep effect. To avoid splits in the comb-out, the pin curls must overlap. (Fig. 9.32)

Triangular base pin curls are recommended along the front or facial hairline to prevent breaks or splits in the finished hairstyle. The triangular base allows a portion of the hair from each curl to overlap the next and comb into a uniform wave without splits. (Figs. 9.33, 9.34)

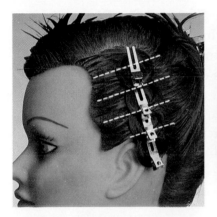

9.32—Rectangular base.

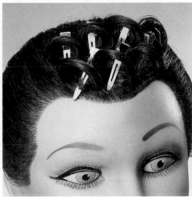

9.33—Triangular base.

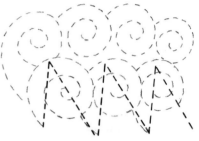

9.34—Detail of triangular base.

Arc base, also known as half-moon or C-shape base, pin curls are carved out of a shaping. Arc base pin curls give good direction and may be used for an upsweep effect or a French twist at the lower back of the head. (Figs. 9.35, 9.36)

Square base pin curls are used for even construction suitable for curly hairstyles without much volume or lift. They can be used on any part of the head and will comb out with lasting results. To avoid splits in the comb-out, stagger the sectioning as shown in the illustration (square base, brick-lay fashion). (Fig. 9.37)

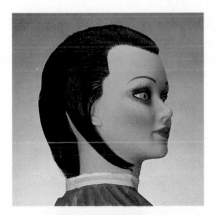

9.35 Arc base side.

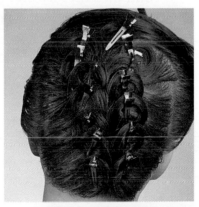

9.36—Arc base—back of head.

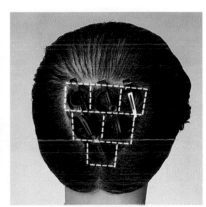

9.37—Square base.

PIN CURL TECHNIQUES

You will learn to make pin curls several ways. We illustrate several methods of forming pin curls. Your instructor might demonstrate other methods that are equally correct.

Carved Curls or Sculptured Curls

Pin curls, carved out of a shaping without disturbing the shaping, are usually referred to as *carved curls.* You can form these curls on either the right side or the left side of the head.

Procedure for Forming Pin Curls on the Right Side

1. Wet hair thoroughly with water or setting lotion.
2. Comb smoothly and form shaping. (See Fig. 9.38)
3. Start making curls at the open end of the shaping.
4. Slice strand for first curl. (See Fig. 9.39) Use your finger to hold the curl in place.
5. *Ribbon* the strand by forcing it through the comb while applying pressure with the thumb on the back of comb to create tension. (See Figs. 9.40, 9.41)

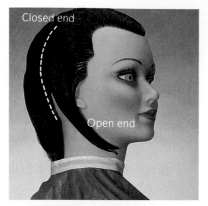

9.38 — Shaping.

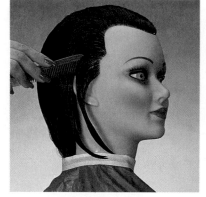

9.39 — Slicing.

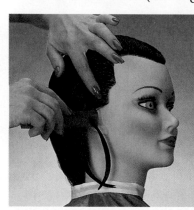

9.40 — Holding base with finger.

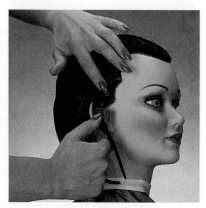

9.41 — Ribboning.

6. Form the curl forward. (See Fig. 9.42)
7. Wind the curl around your index finger. (See Fig. 9.43)

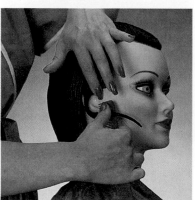

9.42 — Forming.

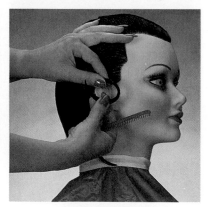

9.43 — Winding.

8. Slide the curl off your finger, keeping the hair ends inside the center of the curl. (See Fig. 9.44)
9. Mold the curl into the shaping. (See Fig. 9.45)
10. Hold the curl in shaping. (See Fig. 9.46)
11. Anchor the curl with clip. (See Fig. 9.47)

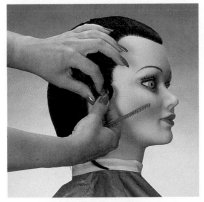

9.44—Sliding off finger.

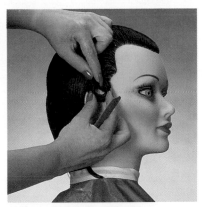

9.45—Molding.

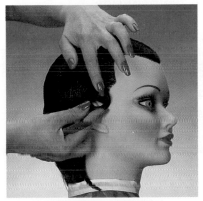

9.46—Holding curl.

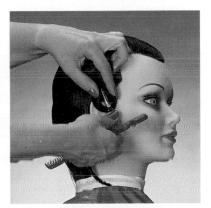

9.47—Anchoring.

CAUTION

▶ *Be very careful not to destroy your shaping as you comb or pin the curl.*

Whenever a longer-lasting curl movement is desired, stretch the hair strand and apply tension. You can accomplish this by ribboning and stretching the strand. Firmly comb it between the spine of the comb and the thumb in the direction of the curl movement.

Sculptured curl arrangements backed up with a second row of pin curls comb out into strong ridge waves. (Figs. 9.48–9.50)

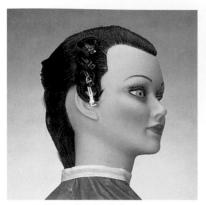

9.48—Finished first row.

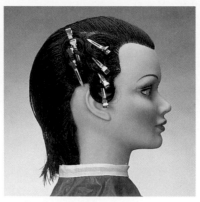

9.49—Sculpture curl arrangement backed up with a second row of curls.

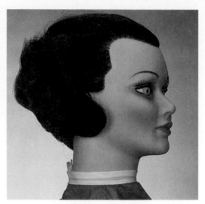

9.50—Curls combed into waves with a strong ridge.

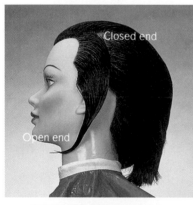

9.51—Shaping.

Procedure for Forming Pin Curls on the Left Side

Making pin curls on the left side of the head requires a different technique from making them on the right side.

1. Wet hair thoroughly with water or setting lotion. Comb smooth and form the shaping. (See Fig. 9.51) Note open and closed ends of shaping.
2. Slice a strand out of shaping. (See Fig. 9.52)
3. Stretch a strand by ribboning it through the comb. (See Figs. 9.53, 9.54)

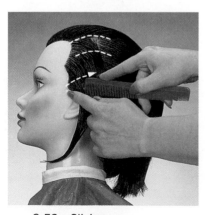

9.52—Slicing.

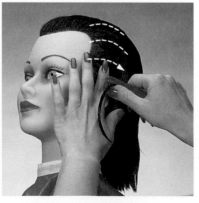

9.53—Holding base with finger and stretching strand by pulling through the comb.

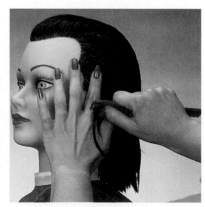

9.54—Ribboning.

4. Form a forward curl.
5. Wind the strand around your index finger. (See Fig. 9.55)
6. Slide the curl off tip of your finger and mold into shaping. (See Fig. 9.56)
7. Hold the curl in shaping. (See Fig. 9.57)
8. Anchor with a clip. (See Fig. 9.58)

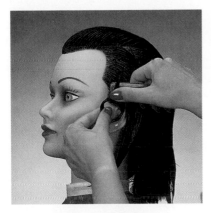

9.55—Winding.

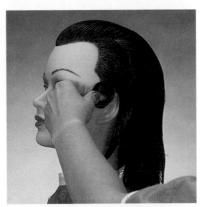

9.56—Sliding off finger.

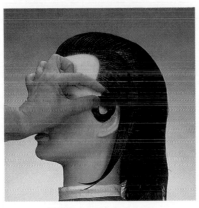

9.57—Holding curl.

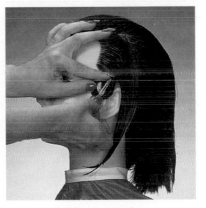

9.58—Anchoring.

What You Should Know about Pin Curls

1. Pin curls must fit within the curvature of a shaping. (See Fig. 9.59)
2. Curls should overlap one another.
3. The size of the curls graduates from small at the open end to large at the closed end.

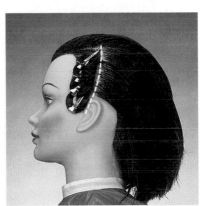

9.59—Finished first row.

4. Reverse shaping for backup curls. (See Fig. 9.60)
5. To slice a strand, the tip of your comb should touch the tip of your finger halfway through shaping. (See Fig. 9.61)
6. To ribbon hair you will use the coarse or fine teeth of the comb depending on the hair texture. (See Fig. 9.62)

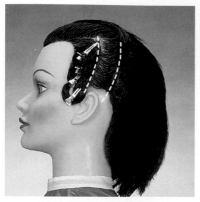
9.60 – Reverse shaping.

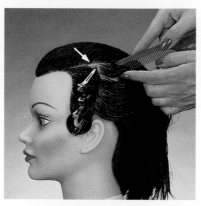
9.61 – Slicing.

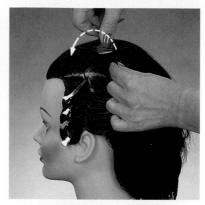
9.62 – Ribboning.

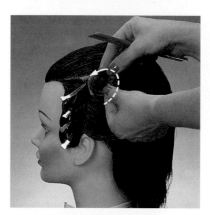
9.63 – Placing curl.

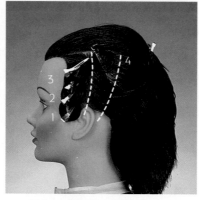
9.64 – Completed first curl.

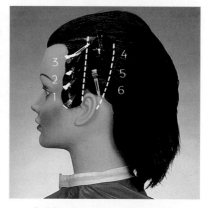
9.65 – Completed reverse shaping.

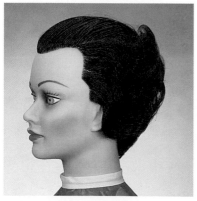
9.66 – Comb-out.

7. Ribbon the tip of the strand with fine teeth for a neat closing of the curl and place on base. (See Fig. 9.63)
8. Complete top reverse curl and divide shaping into strands for the next two curls. (See Fig. 9.64)
9. Complete the second row of curls within the curve of the shaping. (See Fig. 9.65)
10. Comb out the forward and reverse pin curl setting into a full, wide wave. (See Fig. 9.66)

ANCHORING PIN CURLS

Anchoring pin curls correctly ensures that curls hold firmly where you have placed them, so that the hairstyle you have planned develops properly.

There are several methods for inserting clips or clippies, but they are always inserted from the *open* end of the shaping. Whichever way you choose, keep in mind that it is essential not to disturb the base or sculpture as you insert the clip.

Procedure

To anchor the pin curl correctly, gently slide the clip or clippie through part of the base and/or stem at an angle and across the ends of the curl. This will hold the curl securely without it unfurling, sagging, or flipping over.

1. Clips should be anchored in such a manner that they do not interfere with the formation or placement of other curls or with any other step in setting the hair.
2. To avoid indentation or impressions across the hair, it is advisable not to pin across the center of the entire curl.
3. The size of the clips used should be governed by the size of the curl. Curls made with small strands or fine hair cannot support the weight of a double-prong clip, but perform better if pinned in place with a single-prong clip (clippie) or hairpin. However, a clippie or hairpin might not be able to support the weight of coarse or thick hair. Use your own judgment.
4. Clips that are placed against the skin, ear, or scalp can become very hot during the drying process. If clips must touch the skin, simply place cotton under the part of the clips touching these areas. (Figs. 9.67–9.70)

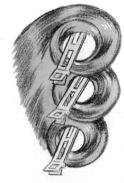

9.67—Hairline forward pin curls (clockwise curl).

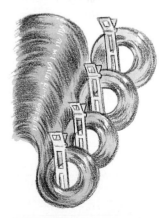

9.70—Ridge reverse pin curls (counter-clockwise curls).

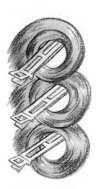

9.68—Forward pin curls equal in size. Any place on the head.

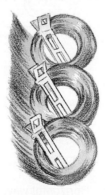

9.69—Reverse pin curls (counter-clockwise curls). Equal in size. Any place on the head.

EFFECTS OF PIN CURLS

Pin curl patterns have been designed to achieve specific style effects. Always take care to ensure that pin curls lie evenly and are placed in the direction in which they will be combed; otherwise, you will find yourself fighting uneven wave or curl design.

1. A *vertical wave* produces the best result when it begins with a reverse shaping, followed by a pin curl pattern. (Figs. 9.71, 9.72)

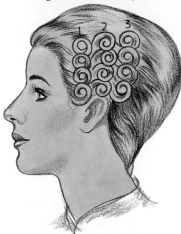 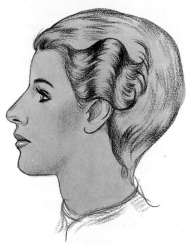

9.71—Vertical wave pin curl pattern.

9.72—Vertical wave comb-out.

2. A *horizontal wave* is first shaped in a forward semicircular fashion, from the hair part downward. The pin curls are then set. (Figs. 9.73, 9.74)

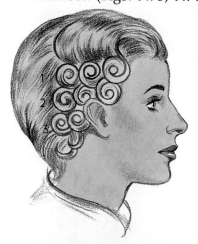 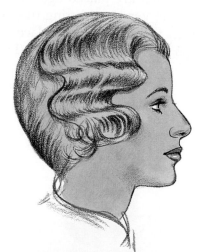

9.73—Horizontal wave pin curl pattern.

9.74—Horizontal wave comb-out.

3. *Interlocking movement* involves two directional rows of pin curls and produces clash (an area where two wave patterns are placed back to back to build volume). First row—back stem with forward curls. Second row—forward stem with

reverse curls. Comb-out—the clash area is interlocked. (Figs. 9.75, 9.76)

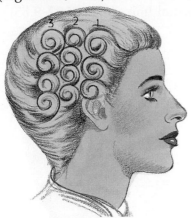

9.75—Setting pattern.

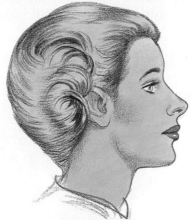

9.76—Comb-out.

4. **Waved top.** (Figs. 9.77–9.79)

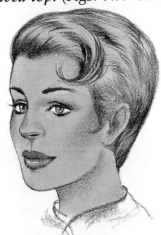

9.77 Shaping.

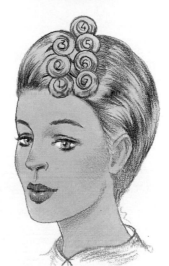

9.78—Setting pattern.

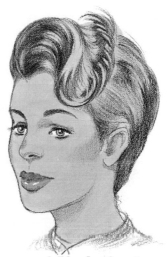

9.79—Comb-out.

5. **Diagonal waves** are made by shaping hair in an oval forward. Then start the pin curls at the open end. (Figs. 9.80, 9.81)

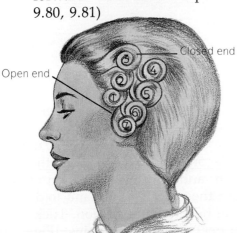

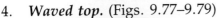

9.80—Setting pattern

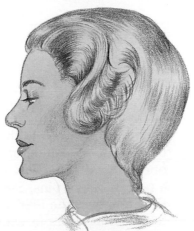

9.81—Comb-out.

6. For *waved bangs,* shape the hair and set the pin curls into waves starting at the open end. For fine hair use more pin curls than you would for normal hair. (Figs. 9.82–9.85)

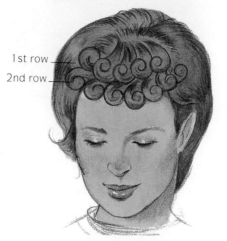

1st row
2nd row

9.82 — Setting pattern for fine hair.

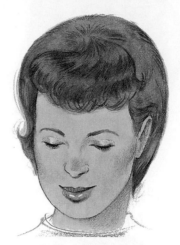

9.83 — Comb-out.

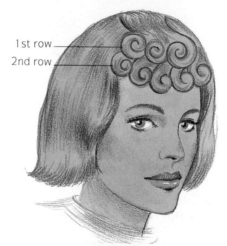

1st row
2nd row

9.84 — Setting pattern for normal hair.

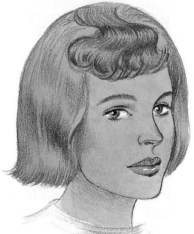

9.85 — Comb-out.

7. A *French twist* is set by parting off the back area and making a vertical center part. Comb both sections together, as they will be in the finished comb-out. Shape large, smooth pin curls into the two long vertical shapings. Comb out by back-brushing or back-combing the area. Smooth one side with a narrow brush, and pin the ends down with a row of bobby pins. Smooth the other section, and fold the ends over the first hair in herringbone fashion. Tuck the ends in, and pin with a neat row of bobby pins. (Figs. 9.86, 9.87)

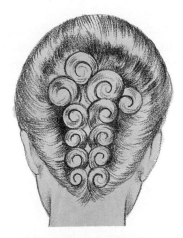

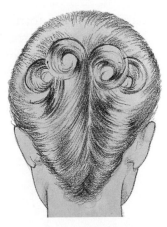

9.86—Setting pattern for normal hair.

9.87—Comb-out and pinning.

8. *Ridge curls* are pin curls placed behind the ridge of a shaping or finger wave. They are useful when a loose wave with good definition is desired. You must be careful not to disturb the ridge when slicing out the strands for the curls. (Figs. 9.88–9.91)

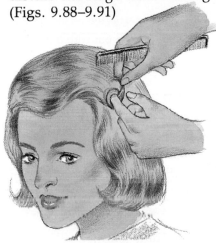

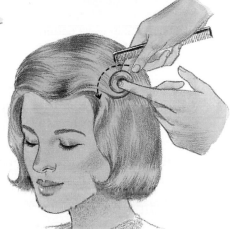

9.88—Wind hair around fingertip.

9.89—Slide strand off finger and roll it to base of ridge.

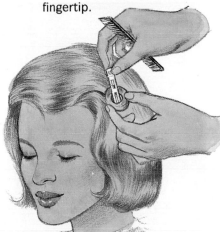

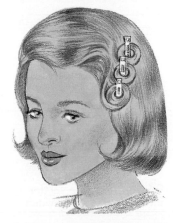

9.90—Anchor curl with clippie.

9.91—Completed ridge curl.

9. *Skip waves* are formed by a combination of finger waves and pin curl patterns. The pin curls are placed in *alternate* finger wave formations. This technique is recommended when side, smooth-flowing vertical waves are desired. For best results the hair should be 3″ to 5″ (7.5 to 12.5 cm) in length. It is not suitable for very curly or fine hair. (Figs. 9.92–9.94)

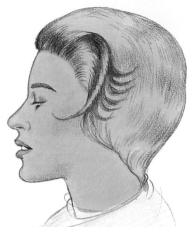

9.92 – Shaping and ridge for vertical finger wave.

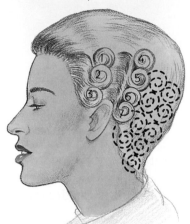

9.93 – Skip wave pattern for fluff ends.

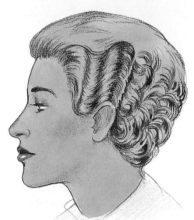

9.94 – Comb-out with fluff ends.

CASCADE OR STAND UP CURLS

The *cascade or stand up curl* is the forerunner of the roller. It provides for height in the finished hairstyle and may be used with rollers or alone. It is wound from the ends to the scalp, as a roller is. The center opening is made large, and the curl is pinned in a standing position. (Figs. 9.95–9.102)

Procedure
Wet hair thoroughly with water or setting lotion.

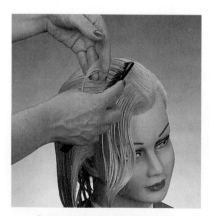

9.95 – Comb, divide, and smooth strand.

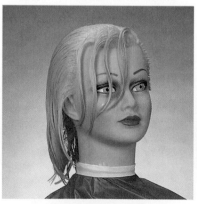

9.96 – Divide the section into strands for individual curls.

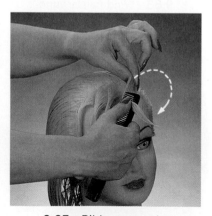

9.97 – Ribbon strand.

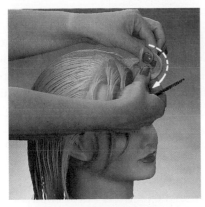

9.98—Direct strand.

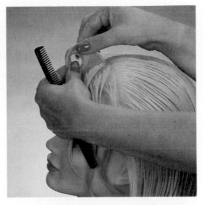

9.99—Wind the strand, being sure to keep the curl round.

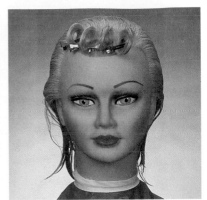

9.100—Anchor the curl securely at the base.

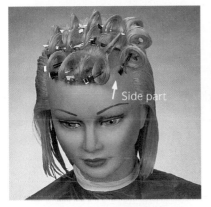

9.101—Top setting.

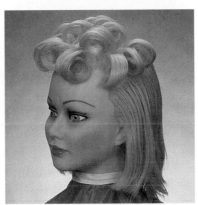

9.102—Comb out as you would a roller set.

SEMI-STAND UP CURLS

Semi-stand up curls are stand up curls that have been carved out of a shaping and pinned in a semi-standing position. A top wave effect can be achieved with semi-stand up curls. After the shaping is in place, make three counterclockwise curls, and back them up with four clockwise curls. (Figs. 9.103–9.105)

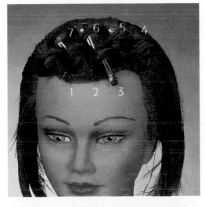

9.103—Semi-stand up curl setting.

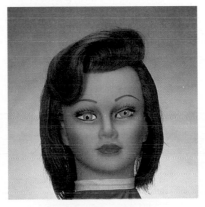

9.104—Comb-out.

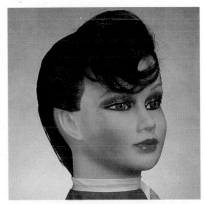

9.105—(Alternate) Comb-out.

ROLLER CURLS

You can use rollers to create the same effects as stand up curls. They are simply molds for stand up curls, which allow you to have more control over the hair. Like stand up curls, they create a great deal of lift and volume. There are advantages to using roller curls rather than pin curl methods.

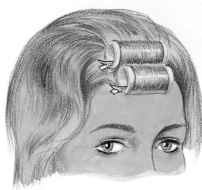

9.106—Roller curls.

1. One roller can accommodate the equivalent of two to four stand up curls.
2. Rollers give more security to hair when it is wet, so there is no chance of having your finely executed curls collapse.
3. The tension with which hair can be placed on a roller gives the finished curl a bounce and life that a pin curl cannot provide.
4. Rollers come in various sizes, lengths, and shapes to fulfill most hairstyling needs. (Fig. 9.106)

Roller Technique

1. Section hair into panels, then subdivide each panel into roller bases.
2. The size of the base should be almost the same size as the roller. If a roller is 3″ (7.5 cm) long and 1″ (2.5 cm) wide, the base for it should be 2½″ (6.25 cm) long and 1″ (2.5 cm) wide. The size of the base will be guided by the size of the roller.
3. Hair must be wet so that it will be flexible, stretchable, and adhere to plastic rollers.
4. Prepare a roller section by combing the strand firmly and smoothly at a 45° (.785 rad.) angle. (See Figs. 9.107, 9.108a–b)
5. Wrap ends of the hair smoothly against the roller.

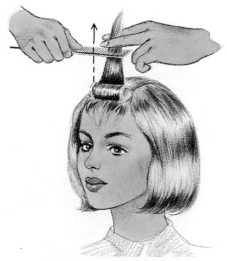

9.107—Strand preparation.

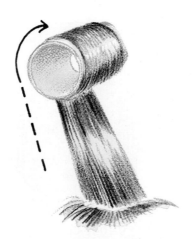

9.108a—45° angle.

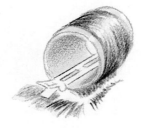

9.108b—Anchor with clip.

6. Place both thumbs over the hair ends and roll the roller firmly toward the scalp. (See Figs. 9.109, 9.110)

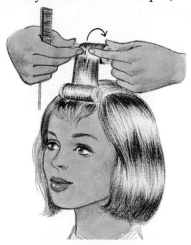 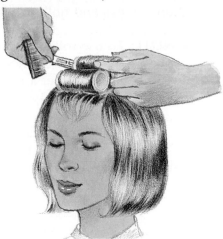

9.109—Winding roller.   9.110—Pinning roller.

7. Hold the roller in position while clipping. (See Figs. 9.111–9.114)

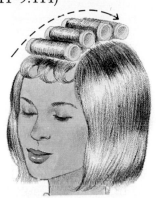 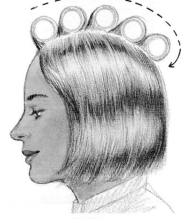

9.111—Complete panel of roller curls from hairline to crown with strands left out for bang effect.

9.112—Roller setting for off-the-face effect.

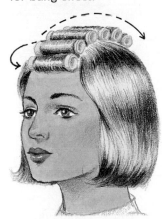 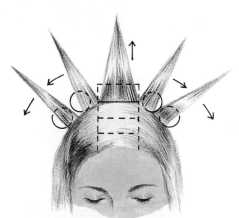

9.113—Roller curl pattern for bang effect.

9.114—The angle at which hair should be held from the head for roller placement.

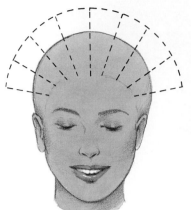

9.115—Sectioning of different lengths of hair for rollers.

Roller Size

Rollers are most effective in creating lift and volume, and indentation (valleys and hollows) in hairstyles.

▶ **NOTE:** To use rollers to their best advantage, it is important for the hair length to be more than three times the rollers' diameter. For example, a roller with a 1½″ (3.75 cm) diameter is for use on hair that is 4½″ (11.25 cm) long. (Fig. 9.115)

A strand of hair that is 4½″ (11.25 cm) long will wrap around a 1″ (2.5 cm) roller one full turn. The result will be a soft puff with minimum curl on the ends. (Figs. 9.116, 9.117)

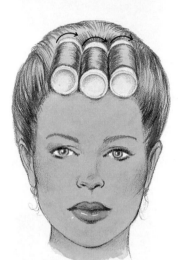
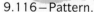
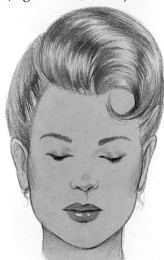

9.116—Pattern.   9.117—Comb-out.

When using a ¾″ (1.85 cm) roller on hair that is 4½″ (11.25 cm) long, the strand will wrap around 1½ times. The result will be a curlier set. (Figs. 9.118, 9.119)

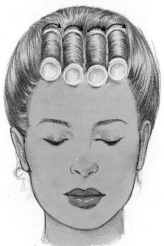
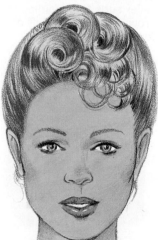

9.118—Pattern.   9.119—Comb-out.

One-half-inch (1.25 cm) rollers permit the hair to wrap around two or more times, resulting in a deep, soft wave with clash. (The hair ends turn in the opposite direction from the movement.) Notice that you need more rollers to cover the same area. (Figs. 9.120, 9.121)

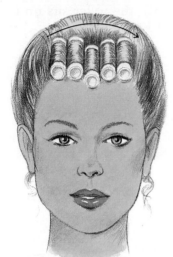

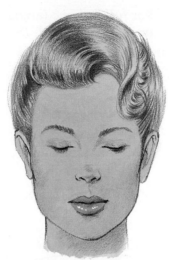

9.120—Pattern.

9.121—Comb-out.

▶ **NOTE:** The length of the hair and size of the roller affect the finished hairstyle. If you use a roller that is 1½" (3.75 cm) in diameter on hair that is 6" to 7" (15 to 17.5 cm) long, you will get different results than you would with hair that is 3" to 5" (7.5 to 12.5 cm) in length.

BARREL CURLS

A barrel curl serves as a substitute for a curl formed around a roller. It may be used where there is insufficient room to place a roller. However, it does not provide the tension that is present in roller wrapping.

The barrel curl is made in a similar manner as the stand up curl, with a flat base and containing much more hair. (Fig. 9.122)

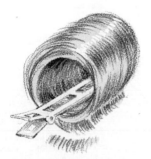

9.122—Barrel curl.

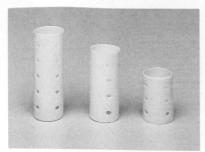

9.123—Rollers of similar width and various lengths.

Volume and Indentation

Volume is created by the base of the curl (the direction of the hair up from the head) and the size of roller. (Fig. 9.123)

1. For *full volume* (angle of strand), the roller sits on its base, or is overdirected. (See Figs. 9.124, 9.125)

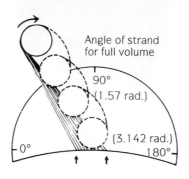

9.124—Full volume.

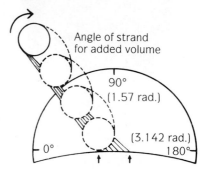

9.125—Added volume.

2. For *medium volume,* the roller rests ½" (1.25 cm) off the base. (It is slightly underdirected.) (See Fig. 9.126)

3. *For a small amount of lift,* the roller sits off the base. (It is underdirected.) (See Fig. 9.127)

4. To create *indentation or hollowness,* keep the hair close to the head and roll to ½" (1.25 cm) off the base. (See Fig. 9.128)

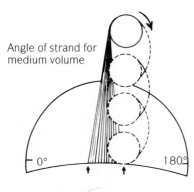

9.126—Medium volume.

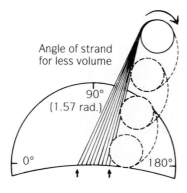

9.127—Less volume.

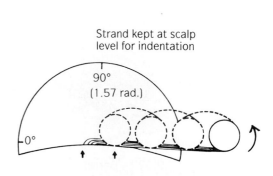

9.128—Indentation.

5. Figs. 9.129 to 9.132 demonstrate how a finished style can be created by setting for volume and indentation.

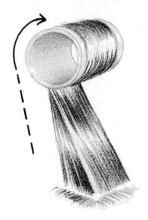
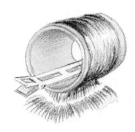

9.129a—Creates volume.

9.129b—Anchor with clip.

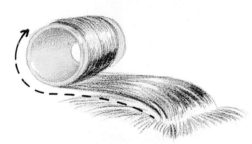
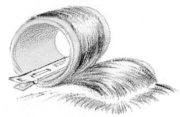

9.130a—Creates indentation or hollowness.

9.130b—Anchor with clip.

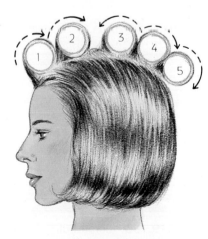
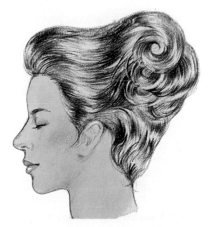

9.131—Setting pattern: 1st two rollers—volume; 3rd roller—indentation; 4th and 5th rollers—volume.

9.132—Comb-out.

Cylinder Circular Roller Action

Hair that is directed in a circular fashion is referred to by various names, such as radial motion, circular movement, curvature movement, curvature roller action, rotary motion or movement, spotmatic movement, contour movement, and so on.

The spot or area from which the hair is directed to form a circular movement is also referred to by any of the following terms: balance point, swing point, terminal point, pivot point, pendulum point, radial point, fulcrum point, radiation point, rotary point, and spotmatic point.

Roller action is created by the way the hair is molded around the roller. This roller action can be varied by using different size rollers and setting patterns. (Figs. 9.133–9.146)

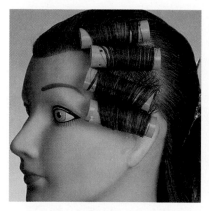

9.133 — Short hair (slender rollers).

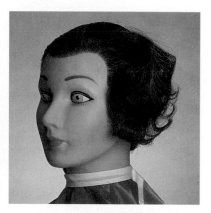

9.134 — Comb-out.

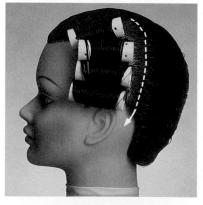

9.135 — Medium length hair (medium size rollers).

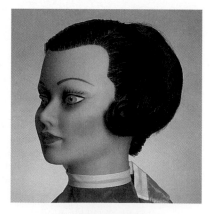

9.136 — Comb-out.

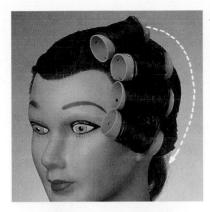

9.137—Long hair (large rollers).

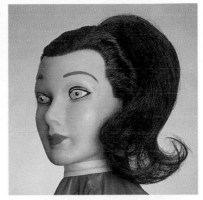

9.138—Comb-out.

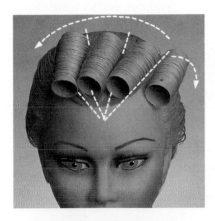

9.139—Top—cylinder rollers set in wedge-shaped partings in a circular manner.

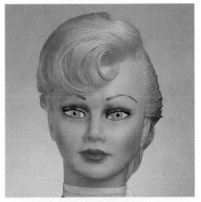

9.140—Comb-out in a forward shell effect with bangs.

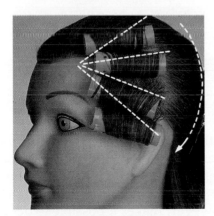

9.141—Side—cylinder rollers set in wedge-shaped partings.

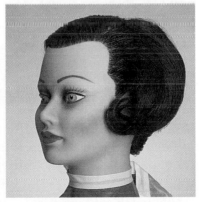

9.142—The comb-out gives a circular movement toward the face.

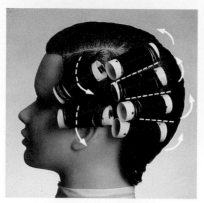

9.143—Special side effects—side roller setting with sculpture curl in front of ear.

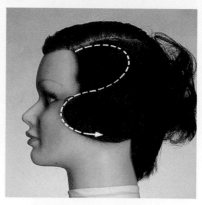

9.144—The comb-out produces an "S" wave formation effect.

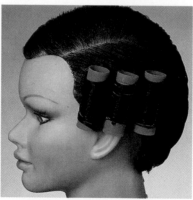

9.145—To create a ridge line and indentation (hollowness), set the hair on rollers at an angle.

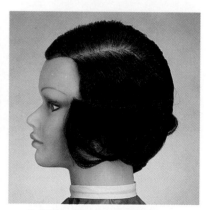

9.146—The setting will produce the waved effect in the comb-out.

Tapered Rollers

You can achieve practically the same styling results by using either cylinder or tapered rollers. However, since cylinder rollers must be placed slightly farther back from the point of distribution in a pie-shaped pattern, the movement of the hair might be weaker. The tapered roller, however, makes it possible to develop a stronger curvature movement.

Choose roller size according to the texture of your client's hair and the size of curl you desire. Fine hair requires smaller rollers; coarse hair needs larger rollers. (Figs. 9.147–9.149)

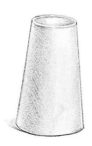

9.147—Tapered roller.

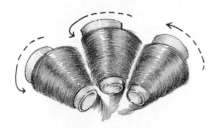

9.148—One-quarter circle setting using thinner rollers produces tighter comb-outs.

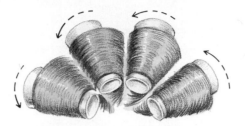

9.149—One-half circle setting using larger (thicker) rollers produces looser comb-outs.

Effect of Tapered Rollers

Tapered rollers set along the hairline produce a shell-shaped front with bangs or curled up ends. (Figs. 9.150, 9.151)

Tapered rollers set along the side of the head comb out in a forward movement. (Figs. 9.152, 9.153)

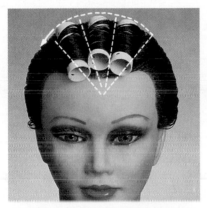

9.150—Tapered roller setting.

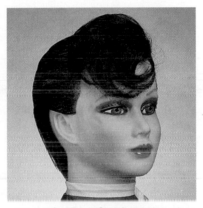

9.151—Comb-out.

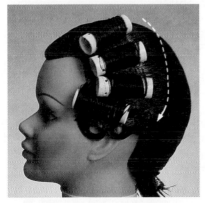

9.152—Side tapered roller setting.

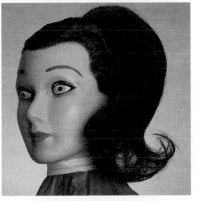

9.153—Comb-out.

People Skills

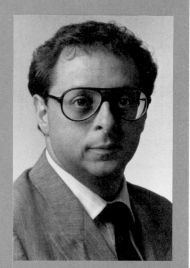

According to Larry Oskin, vice-president of marketing for Creative Hairdressers Inc. and its 300 Hair Cuttery salons, "difficult" clients are opportunities for success.

Says Oskin, "There are really no difficult clients, only difficult situations. Hairstyling can be a highly emotional experience for clients. They need to feel good about both you and their hair experience, or they won't like their new styles.

"If your client is unhappy with her service, remember that the customer is always right. Try to make her feel relaxed. Don't fight her emotional energy, or you'll lose the battle, and the client. Nod as you listen and don't interrupt. Show concern, sympathy, and empathy. Acknowledge her feelings, ask clarifying questions, and repeat back to her what she said, to be certain you understand her."

Oskin recommends a dialogue that shows both concern with how she feels and how you would like to make a professional recommendation to correct the situation. "Tell her what you can do, not what you can't," he adds. "Statistics show that 97% of clients leave an establishment because of the attitude of indifference toward them. People are leaving your competition every day because no one gave them special care or kindness. Building a clientele takes 20% technical skills and 80% people skills, which add up to 100% positive attitude. Go the extra mile, and you can turn many an unhappy client into a very, very loyal client. If you handle difficult situations as easily as you do regular ones, you'll have nothing but new opportunities for success."

COMB-OUT TECHNIQUES

Smooth and well-executed comb-outs result from perfect sets. To achieve success as a hairstylist, you must first master the skills of shaping and molding hair, then you must practice fast, simple, and effective methods for comb-outs.

Recommended Procedure

If you follow a definite system of combing out hairstyles, you will save time, be effective, and build an appreciative and loyal clientele. One procedure for combing out is outlined here.

1. After removing the rollers and clips, brush the hair through to integrate roller and pin curl settings, and relax the set. A cushioned paddle brush works well. Smooth and brush the hair into a semi-flat condition that permits you to position the lines for the planned hairstyle. It is essential that this procedure is correctly executed to achieve a smooth, flowing, finished coiffure.

2. After you have thoroughly brushed the hair, direct it into the general pattern desired. This can be accomplished by placing your hand on the client's head and gently pushing the hair forward in order that waves fall into the planned design. Lines of direction should be slightly over-emphasized to allow for some expected relaxation during the comb-out process.

3. Back comb areas that require volume and back brush sections that need to be integrated. Accentuate and develop lines and style. Take one section at a time, placing the proper lines, ridges, volume, and indentations into the hairstyle. You can create softness and evenness of flow by blending, smoothing, and combing. Exaggerations and overemphasis should be eliminated. Finished patterns should reveal rhythm, balance, and smoothness of line.

4. Final touches make hairstyles look professional; *take your time*. After completing the comb-out, you can use the tail of a comb to lift areas where the shape and form are not precise. Every touch during the final stage must be very lightly performed. When the finishing touches have been completed, check the entire set for structural balance and then *lightly* spray the hair.

Back-Combing and Back-Brushing Techniques

You might have to create areas of full volume in some hairstyles. Back-combing and back-brushing are the best means to achieve lift. These techniques incorporate the matting of the hair by combing or brushing it toward the scalp so that the shorter hair mats to form a cushion or base for the top or covering hair.

Back-combing is also called teasing, ratting, matting, or French lacing. It is a technique used to build a *firm* cushion on which to build full-volume curls or bouffant hairstyles.

After the basic comb-out has been directed into the desired pattern, analyze the areas that need volume.

1. Pick up a section of hair about ¾" (1.875 cm) wide and hold up firmly, away from the scalp.

2. Insert a fine-toothed comb into the strand about 1½" (3.75 cm) from its base, press to the scalp, and remove.

3. Repeat step 2 by inserting the comb into the strand a little farther away from the scalp and pressing firmly toward the scalp. Repeat this step as many times as necessary, using very small strokes until the desired volume of cushioned hair has been achieved.

4. Smooth the hair ends to conceal back-combing. (Figs. 9.154–9.156)

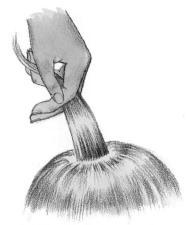
9.154—The hair properly held between the index and middle fingers.

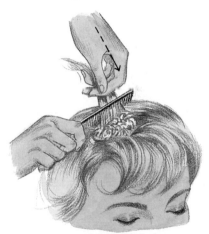
9.155—Back-combing on top of strand.

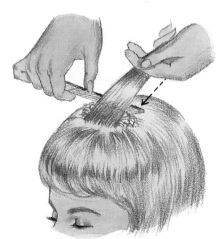
9.156—Back-combing in back of strand.

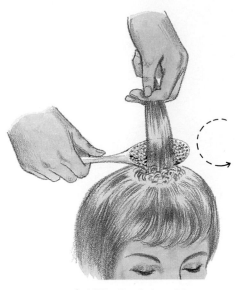

9.157—Back-brushing.

Back-brushing is also called ruffing. It is a technique used to build a *soft* cushion, or to mesh two or more curl patterns together for a uniform and smooth comb-out.

1. Pick up and hold a strand straight out from the scalp.
2. With a slight amount of slack in the strand, place a narrow brush near the base of the strand. Push and roll the inner edge of the brush with the wrist until it touches the scalp. For interlocking to occur, the brush must be rolled. Then remove the brush from the hair with a turn of the wrist, peeling back a layer of hair. The shorter ends of tapered hair are interlocked to form a cushion at the scalp.
3. Repeat this procedure by moving the brush about ½" (1.25 cm) farther away from the scalp with each stroke until the desired volume has been achieved. (Fig. 9.157)

BRAIDING

You will be asked to braid, plait, or corn-row the hair of children and adults alike. These styles must be done with a *firm* hand using even tension to all strands. It is advisable to braid on damp hair because some degree of stretch will assist in producing a long-lasting and neat style.

French Braiding

There are two different types of French braids: the *invisible braid* or regular braid and the *visible braid* or inverted braid.

Invisible braiding is performed by overlapping the strands on top.

1. Section the hair into two parts with a center part. (See Fig. 9.158)
2. Clamp one side and divide the other side into three strands. (See Fig. 9.159)

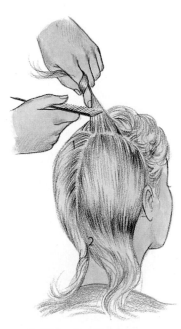

9.158—Section hair.

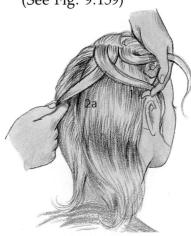

9.159—Divide into three strands.

3. Start the braid by taking strand 1 (from the left) and crossing it *over* strand 2 (center strand) (strand 1 becomes the center strand). (See Fig. 9.160)

4. Take strand 3 (from the right) and cross it *over* the center strand (it becomes the center strand). Hold the strands tightly. You have now completed the anchor point.

5. Pick up the strand on the left (original strand 2) and incorporate a small section (strand 2b), about ½″ (1.25 cm) wide, from the scalp. Join the new section with the left strand and together draw them over the center strand. (See Fig. 9.161)

6. Bring original strand 1 over the center hair. Bring a strand of scalp hair from the right, about ½″ (1.25 cm) wide, and place it with strand 1.

7. Continue to pick up strands and braid until all the hair in the section has been taken into the braid. (See Fig. 9.162)

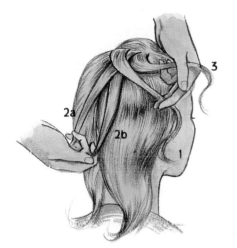

9.160—Starting the braiding.

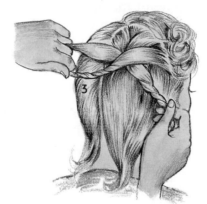

9.161—Drawing over center strand.

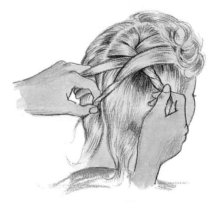

9.162—Pick up strand.

▶ NOTE: To keep the braid neat with all short hair ends in place, twist each strand toward the center as you put it in place.

8. Braid the other side in the same manner. (See Fig. 9.163)

9. If the hair is long you can:

- Continue to braid through to the ends. It can then be crossed and extended up the back of the head or left to hang loose.

- Stop the braid at the hairline and tie ribbons, allowing the ends to fall into curls.

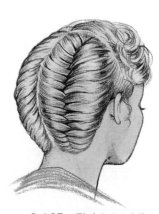

9.163—Finish braiding.

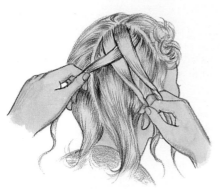

9.164—Divide into three sections and begin braiding.

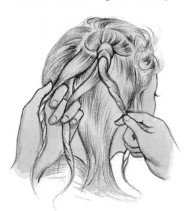

9.165—Drawing under center strand.

If the hair is not very long you can:

- Fasten the ends with a rubber band and tuck them under and pin in place with bobby pins.
- Create design lines that travel around the head from temple to temple, or form various patterns with the braids and parting lines.
- You might want to start the French braid at the nape and work toward the face. You can tuck the ends under or finish the style with curls.

Visible French braiding (inverted braid) is done by plaiting the strands under, thus making the braid visible. It is done in the same manner as the invisible braid except that strands are placed *under* the center strand.

Part and section the hair in the same manner as for regular French braid.

1. Divide the top right section evenly into three strands. Start to braid the hair strands by placing the right side strand under the center strand and the left side strand under this one. Draw strands tightly. (See Fig. 9.164)
2. Pick up ½" (1.25 cm) strand on the right side and combine with the right side strand. Place this combined strand under the center strand. Pick up ½" (1.25 cm) strand on the left side and combine with the left side strand. Place this combined strand under the center strand. (See Fig. 9.165)
3. Continue to pick up hair and braid as above. Finish braiding at nape, and hold in position with rubber bands. (See Fig. 9.166)
4. Braid left side of the head in the same manner as right side. (See Fig. 9.167)
5. The finished braids may be tucked under and held in place with hairpins or bobby pins. (See Fig. 9.168)

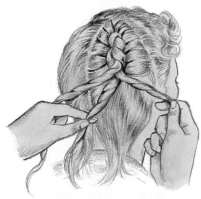

9.166—Continue braiding.

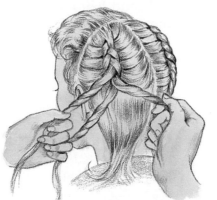

9.167—Finish braiding.

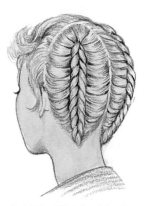

9.168—Finished look.

Corn-rowing is done in the same fashion as *visible French braiding* except that the sections are very narrow and form a predetermined style. It works well with overly curly hair and is popular with both children and adults. Corn-rowing should last for several weeks.

Preparation for Overly Curly Hair

If your client has overly curly hair, you can prepare to corn-row as follows:

1. Shampoo in the usual way.
2. Apply conditioner and distribute it well.
3. Tie a hair net over the hair to hold it flat.
4. Place your client under a hood dryer, or blow-dry the hair.
5. Follow the visible French braid procedure using narrower sections and more tension to form the corn-row braids. (Fig. 9.169)

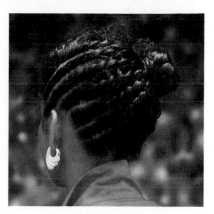

9.169—A finished corn-row style.

Artistry in Hairstyling

The principles of modern hairstyling and makeup are your guides to selecting what is most appropriate in order to achieve a beautiful appearance. The best results are obtained when each client's facial features are properly analyzed for strengths and shortcomings. Your job is to accentuate a client's best features and play down features that do not add to the person's attractiveness.

You must develop the ability to analyze hairstyles for your clients. Each client deserves a hairstyle that is properly proportioned to her body type, is correctly balanced to the head and facial features, and attractively frames the face. The essentials of an artistic and suitable hairstyle are based on the following general characteristics:

1. Shape of the head: front view (face shape), profile, and back view.
2. Characteristics of features: perfect as well as imperfect features, defects, or blemishes.
3. Body structure, posture, and poise.

FACIAL TYPES

Each client's facial shape is determined by the position and prominence of the facial bones. There are seven facial shapes: oval, round, square, oblong, pear-shaped, heart-shaped, and diamond-shaped. To recognize each facial shape and to be able to give correct advice, you should be acquainted with the outstanding characteristics of each.

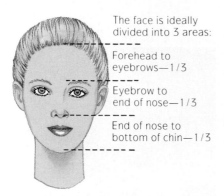

The face is ideally divided into 3 areas:

Forehead to eyebrows—1/3

Eyebrow to end of nose—1/3

End of nose to bottom of chin—1/3

9.170—Ideal facial proportions.

The face is divided into three zones: forehead to eyebrow, eyebrows to end of nose, and end of nose to bottom of chin. When creating a style for a client, you will be trying to create the illusion that each client has the ideal face shape. (Fig. 9.170)

Oval Facial Type

The oval-shaped face is generally recognized as the ideal shape. The contour and proportions of the oval face form the basis for modifying all other facial types.

Facial contour: The oval face is about 1½ times longer than its width across the brow. The forehead is slightly wider than the chin.

A person with an oval-shaped face can wear any hairstyle unless there are other considerations, such as eyeglasses, length and shape of nose, or profile. (See sections on special considerations.) (Fig. 9.171)

Round Facial Type

Facial contour: Round hairline and round chin line; wide face.

Aim: To create the illusion of length to the face.

Create a hairstyle with height by arranging the hair on top of the head. You can place some hair over the ears and cheeks, but it is also appropriate to keep the hair up on one side, leaving the ears exposed. Style the bangs to one side. (Fig. 9.172)

Square Facial Type

Facial contour: Straight hairline and square jawline; wide face.

Aims: To create the illusion of length; offset the square features.

The problems of the square facial type are similar to the round facial type. The style should lift off the forehead and come forward at the temples and jaw, creating the illusion of narrowness and softness in the face. Asymmetrical hairstyles work well. (Fig. 9.173)

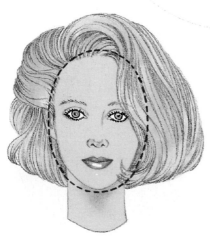

9.171—Oval face.

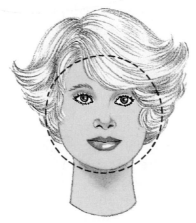

9.172—Round face.

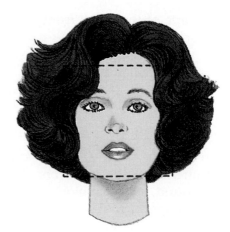

9.173—Square face.

Pear-Shaped Facial Type

Facial contour: Narrow forehead, wide jaw and chin line.

   Aim: To create the illusion of width in the forehead.

   Build a hairstyle that is fairly full and high. Cover the forehead partially with a fringe of soft hair. The hair should be worn with a semi-curl or soft wave effect cropped over the ears. This arrangement adds apparent width to the forehead. (Fig. 9.174)

Oblong Facial Type

Facial contour: Long, narrow face with hollow cheeks.

   Aim: To make the face appear shorter and wider.

   The hair should be styled fairly close to the top of the head with a fringe of curls and bangs, combined with fullness to the sides. Drawing the hair out from the cheeks creates the illusion of width. (Fig. 9.175)

Diamond Facial Type

Facial contour: Narrow forehead, extreme width through the cheekbones, and narrow chin.

   Aim: To reduce the width across the cheekbone line.

   Increasing the fullness across the jawline and forehead while keeping the hair close to the head at the cheekbone line helps create an oval appearance. Avoid hairstyles that lift away from the cheeks or move back from the hairline. (Fig. 9.176)

Heart-Shaped Facial Type

Facial contour: Wide forehead and narrow chin line.

   Aims: To decrease the width of the forehead and increase the width in the lower part of the face.

   To reduce the width of the forehead, a center part with bangs flipped up or a style slanted to one side is recommended. Add width and softness at the jawline. (Fig. 9.177)

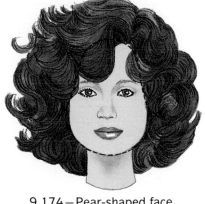

9.174—Pear-shaped face.

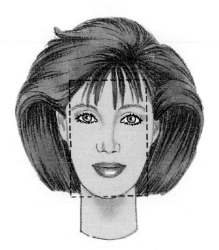

9.175—Oblong face.

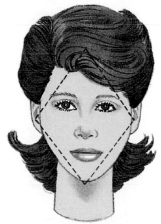

9.176—Diamond face.

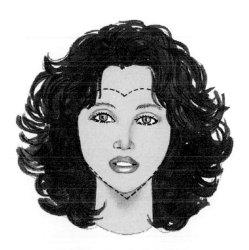

9.177—Heart-shaped face.

Profiles

Always look at your client's profile. When creating a hairstyle, the profile can be a good indicator as to the correct shape of hairstyle to choose.

Straight profile. This is considered the ideal. It is neither concave nor convex, with no unusual facial features. Usually, all hairstyles are becoming to the straight or normal profile. (Fig. 9.178)

Concave (prominent chin). The hair at the nape should be styled softly with a movement upward. Do not build hair out onto the forehead. (Fig. 9.179)

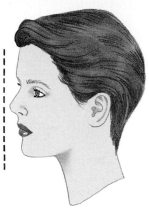
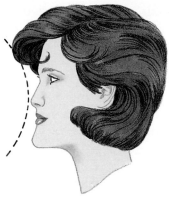

9.178—Straight profile.

9.179—Concave (prominent chin).

Convex (receding forehead, prominent nose, and receding chin). Place curls or bangs over the forehead. Keep the style close to the head at the nape. (Fig. 9.180)

Low forehead, protruding chin. Create an illusion of fullness to the forehead by building a fluffy bang with height. An upswept temple movement will add length to the face. Soft curls in the nape area soften the chin line. Do not end the style line at the nape—this draws attention to the chin line. Rather, create a line that is either higher or lower than the chin line. (Fig. 9.181)

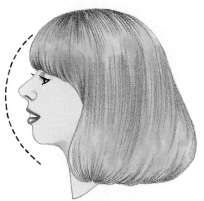
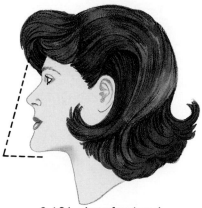

9.180—Convex (receding forehead, prominent nose, and receding chin).

9.181—Low forehead, protruding chin.

Nose Shapes

Nose shapes are closely related to profile. When studying your client's face, the nose must be considered both in profile and in full face. (Appropriate makeup for nose shapes will be found in the chapter on facial makeup.)

Turned-up nose. This type of nose is usually small and accompanied by a straight profile. The small nose is considered to be a childlike quality; therefore it is best to design a hairstyle that is not associated with children. The hair should be swept off the face creating a line from the nose to the ear. This will add length to the short nose. The top hair should move off the forehead to give the illusion of length to the nose. (Figs. 9.182, 9.183)

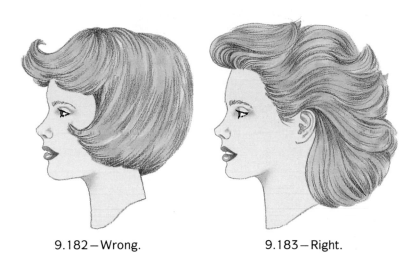

9.182—Wrong.   9.183—Right.

Prominent nose (hooked, large, or pointed). In order to draw attention away from the nose, bring the hair forward at the forehead with softness around the face. (Figs. 9.184, 9.185)

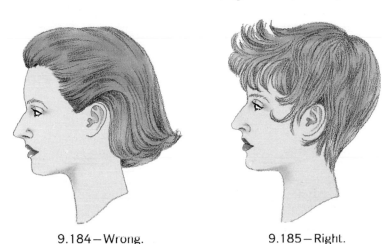

9.184—Wrong.   9.185—Right.

Crooked nose. To minimize the conspicuous crooked nose, style the hair in an off-center manner which will attract the eye away from the nose. Asymmetrical styles are best. Any well-balanced hairstyle will accentuate the fact that the face is not even. (Figs. 9.186, 9.187)

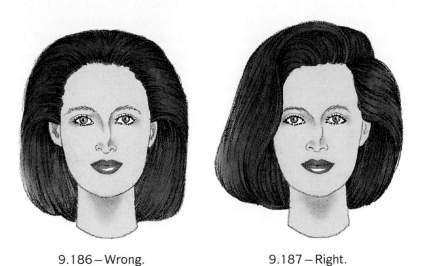

9.186 — Wrong.   9.187 — Right.

Wide, flat nose. A wide, flat nose tends to broaden the face. In order to minimize this effect, the hair should be drawn away from the face. In addition, a center part tends to narrow the nose, as well as draw attention away from the nose. (Figs. 9.188, 9.189)

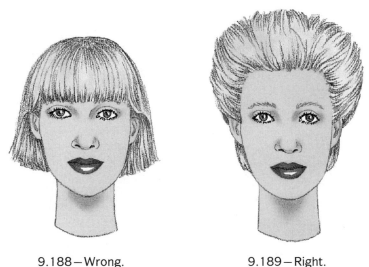

9.188 — Wrong.   9.189 — Right.

Eyes

The eyes are the focal point of a face. Be prepared to create hairstyles that bring out the best in a client's eyes.

Wide-set eyes are usually found on a round or square face. You can minimize the effect by lifting and fluffing the top of the hair and bang area. A side bang helps to draw attention away from the space between the eyes. (Figs. 9.190, 9.191)

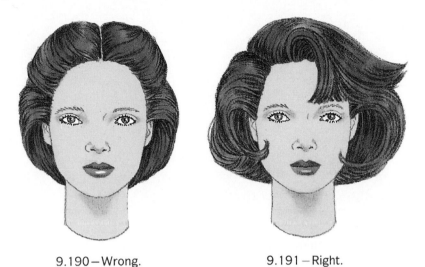

9.190—Wrong.   9.191—Right.

Close-set eyes are usually found on long, narrow faces. Try to open the face with the illusion of more space between the eyes. Style the hair fairly high with a side movement. The hair ends should turn outward and up. (Figs. 9.192, 9.193)

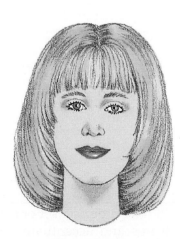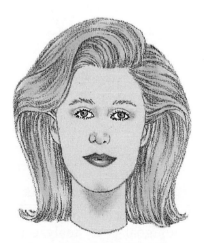

9.192—Wrong.   9.193—Right.

Head Shapes

The shape of your client's head is just as individual as other physical features. As with the face, the oval is considered the ideal shape. Your goal when designing hairstyles should be to give them the illusion of an oval. As you evaluate your client's head shape, mentally impose an oval picture over it. Where there is flatness, plan to build volume. (Figs. 9.194–9.199)

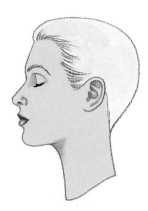

9.194—The perfect oval.

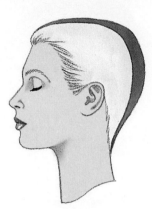

9.195—Narrow head— flat back.

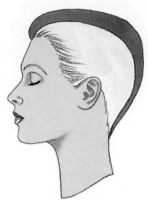

9.196—Flat crown.

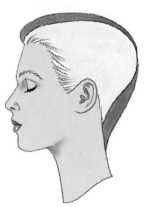

9.197—Pointed head, hollow nape.

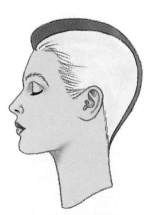

9.198—Flat top.

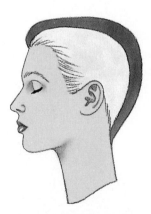

9.199—Small head.

Special Considerations

Very few, if any, of your clients will have a perfect set of features. Your goal is to analyze their features and accentuate the best ones. In addition you will need to consider the particular features of various ethnic groups.

Plump with short neck

   Aim: To create the illusion of length.

   Corrective hairstyle: Sweep the hair up to give length to the neck. Build height on top. Avoid hairstyles that give fullness to the back of the neck and hairstyles with horizontal lines. (Fig. 9.200)

Long, thin neck

   Aim: To minimize the appearance of the long neck.

   Corrective hairstyle: Cover the neck with soft waves. Avoid short or sculptured necklines. Keep the hair long and full at the nape. (Fig. 9.201)

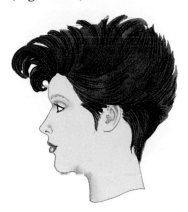

9.200—Plump with short neck.

9.201—Long, thin neck.

Thin features

   Aim: To give width to the face and neck.

   Corrective hairstyle: Lift sides up and away from the hairline, but keep the style soft and loose. The nape hair should be long and full to fill in at the neck. (Fig. 9.202)

Uneven features

   Aim: To minimize imperfect features.

   Corrective hairstyle: Any style that draws attention away from the imperfect features. If a face is smaller on one side than on the other, an asymmetrical style may balance it. (Fig. 9.203)

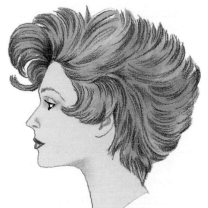

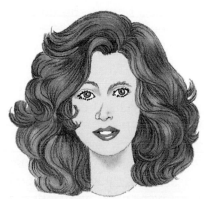

9.202—Thin features.

9.203—Uneven features.

Negroid features

Follow styling rules that relate to the particular face shape. If the hair has been straightened, set it on large rollers. If not, press it thermally with a large barrel iron (see chapter on thermal hairstyling). Either method will allow you to gain more control in order to style the hair according to hair art principles. (Fig. 9.204)

Oriental features

Follow styling rules that relate to the particular face shape. Keep in mind that oriental hair is usually strong and may require more precise handling. (Fig. 9.205)

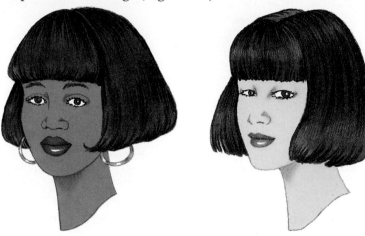

9.204—Negroid features.   9.205—Oriental features.

STYLING FOR PEOPLE WHO WEAR GLASSES

People who wear glasses have special issues regarding their hairstyling and makeup habits. A combination of a becoming hairstyle, the proper makeup, and the correct glasses will help to accentuate the wearer's best features.

The following are a number of basic good grooming rules that should be followed by all people who wear glasses:

1. Glass frames should be up-to-date, with large lenses for good vision.
2. Never wear gaudy, over-jewelled, or tricky frames.
3. Do not wear strip false eyelashes. They are too long and function like windshield wipers with every eye movement.
4. Do not use heavy eye makeup. It does not require heavy makeup to bring out the color and the best features of your eyes.
5. Hairstyles should fall naturally around the face, to make putting on and taking off glasses easy.
6. Over-styled hair with many tight curls is impractical for people with glasses.

The following are some of the "do's" for people who wear glasses:

The Round, Oval, or Square Face

Glasses. A person with big eyes should wear slender frames with large visual lenses to show off eyes and good eye makeup. The color of frames should be selected carefully to match hair color.

Hairstyle. A bouffant hairstyle in natural balance; a simple, uncluttered, casual style is best.

Bangs. A slashed bang freely touching the eyebrows is best.

Jewelry. If earrings are worn, they should be long and dangling. (Figs. 9.206, 9.207)

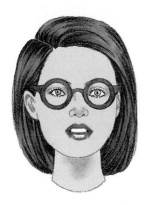
9.206—Wrong.

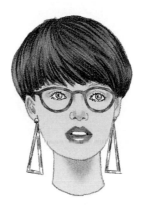
9.207—Right.

The Heart-Shaped or Diamond-Shaped Face

Glasses. The frames should be slender, of medium thickness, follow the eyebrows and rest gently against the face.

Makeup. Wear light makeup shades and delicate eye makeup.

Hairstyle. A full page boy style; or increase the width in the lower part of the face.

Bangs. Open bangs harmonize and balance with the lower part of the face. (Figs. 9.208, 9.209)

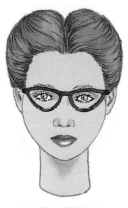
9.208—Wrong.

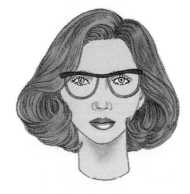
9.209—Right.

The Small, Narrow, or Oval Face

Glasses. Select large, up-to-date frames that are not too gaudy.

Makeup. Wear only natural tones of makeup. The eyes are seen and magnified through the glasses. Proper eye makeup emphasizes beautiful, sparkling eyes.

Hairstyle. Since the face is delicate in proportion, it is important that the hairstyle have width and height. The hairstyle should be short, with deep wave shapings on the sides, leaving freedom for control of glasses.

Bangs. A side wave bang caressing one eyebrow can compliment the eyes. (Figs. 9.210, 9.211)

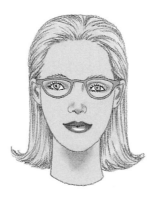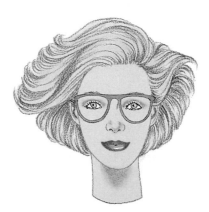

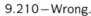

9.210—Wrong.   9.211—Right.

The Pear-Shaped Face

Glasses. Wear large, oval-shaped frames to let the glasses reveal eyes wearing appropriate makeup.

Hairstyle. This facial contour requires emphasis on length; therefore, wear the hair up and off the face, high in the front and crown. Soft bouffant styling around the face, with softness brushed forward on the cheeks, reduces width and adds beauty.

Bangs. A side wave bang over one eye will add expression and interest. (Figs. 9.212, 9.213)

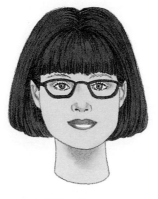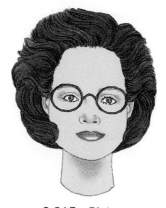

9.212—Wrong.   9.213—Right.

HAIR PARTINGS

Hair partings can be the focal point of a hairstyle. Because the eye is drawn to a part you must be careful how you use it. It must always be neat, without hairs straggling from one side or another, and it must be straight and directed positively. It is usually best to use a natural part if at all possible; however, you may want to create a parting according to your client's head shape, facial features, or desired hairstyle. It is often difficult to create a lasting hairstyle when working against the natural crown parting. You might be able to incorporate the natural parting into the finished style.

The following are suggestions for suitable hair partings for various facial types.

Partings for Bangs

1. *Rectangular* or *triangular partings* are most commonly used for children's bangs. The triangular parting distributes more hair to the temple area, which is often sparse in children.

2. *Diagonal part* used to give height to a round or square face. (Fig. 9.214)

3. *Curved rectangular part* used for receding hairline or high forehead. (Fig. 9.215)

4. *Center part* for popular children's hairstyle with bangs. (Fig. 9.216)

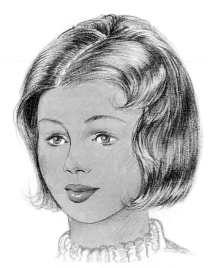 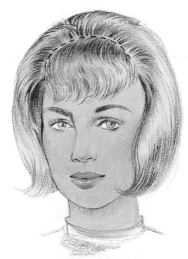 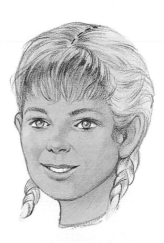

9.214—Diagonal part.   9.215—Curved rectangular part.   9.216—Center part for child.

Style Parts

1. *Concealed part,* used for height and a one-sided style effect. (Fig. 9.217)
2. *Side parts* are used for styles that are directed to one side. You might want to use a high side parting if your client has a wide forehead; and a low side parting or diagonal parting for a triangular, round, or square-shaped face. (Fig. 9.218)
3. *Center partings* are classical. They are usually used for an oval face, but give an oval illusion to wide, round, and heart-shaped faces. (Fig. 9.219)
4. Partings can be used on other parts of the head to create avant-garde looks. *Diagonal back parting* (Fig. 9.220), and *Natural crown partings* (Figs. 9.221, 9.222), used for clients with thin, long necks to create the illusion of width to the back of the head.

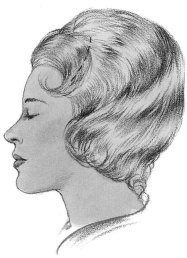

9.217—Concealed part.

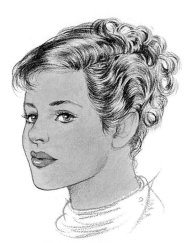

9.218—Side part.

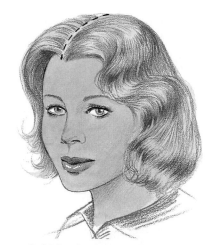

9.219—Center parting.

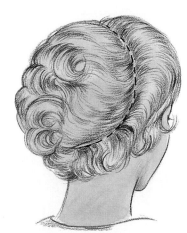

9.220—Diagonal back parting.

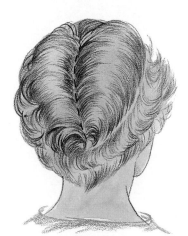

9.221—Natural crown parting—full length of head.

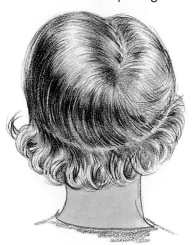

9.222—Natural crown parting—mid-way.

Learning to employ skills that produce predictable results will bring you success as a professional hairstylist. You can use the art and technique of shaping, molding, setting, and brushing and combing to create any hairstyle that comes into fashion. You will easily build an appreciative and loyal clientele if you are sensitive to and make suitable compensations for imperfections in your client's features.

Review Questions

WET HAIRSTYLING

1. What is hairstyling?
2. List the basic elements of art that you use to style hair.
3. What does a hairstyle consist of?
4. What four steps of analyzation are done prior to a shampoo?
5. List the implements employed in hair styling.
6. List the principal parts of a pin curl.
7. What is a shaping for pin curl placement and how is it classified?
8. List the most commonly used bases of a pin curl.
9. List the bases of a roller curl.
10. What ability must you develop to analyze your client?

10

THERMAL HAIRSTYLING

LEARNING OBJECTIVES

After completing this chapter, you should be able to:

1. Define the purpose of thermal waving and curling.
2. List safety measures used in thermal waving.
3. Demonstrate proper thermal wave techniques and implements.
4. Define blow-dry styling.
5. Demonstrate the use of implements, techniques, and cosmetics in blow-dry styling.
6. Define air waving.
7. Demonstrate the use of implements and techniques in air waving.

Introduction to Thermal Waving and Curling

The art and technique of using thermal irons for waving and curling was developed in 1875 by a Frenchman, Marcel Grateau. Thermal waving is still known as *marcel waving.*

Thermal waving and *curling* is the art of waving and curling straight or pressed hair (see chapter on thermal hair straightening) with thermal irons, either electrically heated or stove-heated, using special manipulative techniques. Modern implements have contributed to the continued success of these methods of waving and curling hair.

THERMAL IRONS

Thermal irons are an important implement in hairstyling. They provide an even heat that is completely controlled by the cosmetologist. Manipulative techniques are basically the same for electric irons or stove-heated irons.

The irons must be made of the best quality steel so that they hold an even temperature during the waving and curling process. The styling portion of the irons is composed of two parts: the rod (prong) and the shell (groove or bowl).

1. The *rod* is a perfectly round solid steel bar.
2. The *shell* is perfectly round with the inside grooved so that the rod can rest in it when the irons are closed.

The edge of the shell nearest the cosmetologist is called the *inner edge;* the one farthest from the cosmetologist is called the *outer edge.*

Thermal irons come in a variety of styles, sizes, and weights, from small to jumbo. They come in three different classifications:

1. Conventional (regular) stove-heated. (Fig. 10.1)
2. Electric self-heated. (Fig. 10.2)
3. Electric self-heated, vaporizing.

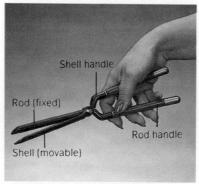

10.1—Conventional thermal (marcel) irons.

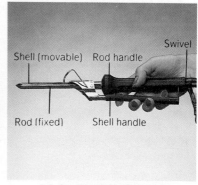

10.2—Electric thermal irons.

▶ **NOTE:** Do not use electric vaporizing irons on pressed hair; the moisture could cause the hair to revert to its natural overly curly state.

There is no one correct temperature used for the irons when thermal curling and waving the hair. Temperature setting for the irons depends on the texture of the hair, whether it is fine or coarse, or whether it has been lightened or tinted. Hair that has been lightened or tinted (also white hair) should be curled and waved with lukewarm irons. Coarse and gray hair, as a rule, can tolerate more heat than fine hair.

CAUTION

▶ *Do not use thermal irons on chemically treated hair; to do so could cause breakage.*

Testing Thermal Irons

After heating the irons to the desired temperature, test them on a piece of tissue paper. Clamp the heated irons over the tissue and hold for 5 seconds. If the paper scorches or turns brown, the irons are too hot. Let them cool somewhat before using. Remember that fine, lightened, or badly damaged hair withstands less heat than normal hair. (Fig. 10.3)

Care of Thermal Irons

Thermal irons should be kept clean and free from rust and carbon. To remove dirt or grease, wash the irons in a soap solution containing a few drops of ammonia. This cuts the oil and grease that usually adhere to the irons. Fine sandpaper, or steel wool with a little oil, helps to remove rust and carbon. It also polishes the irons. To permit greater facility in movement, oil the joint of the irons.

New thermal irons are *tempered* at the factory in order to hold heat uniformly. If you overheat the irons they usually lose their temper, and, in most cases, are ruined.

Holding the Thermal Irons

Hold the irons in a comfortable position that gives you complete control. Grasp the handles of the irons in the right hand, far enough away from the joint to avoid the heat. Place the three middle fingers on the back of the lower handle, the little finger in front of the lower handle, and the thumb in front of the upper handle.

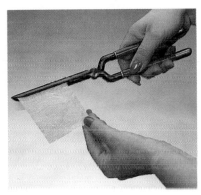

10.3—Testing the heat of thermal irons.

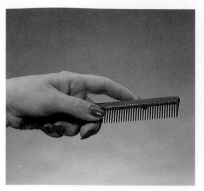

10.4—Holding the comb.

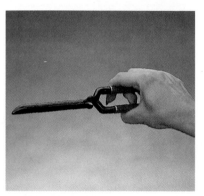

10.5—Rolling the irons.

Comb Used with Thermal Irons

The comb should be about 7″ (17.5 cm) long, made of hard rubber or another nonflammable substance, and should have fine teeth; fine teeth hold the hair more firmly than coarse teeth.

Holding the Comb

Hold the comb between the thumb and all four fingers of the left hand, with the index finger resting on the backbone of the comb for better control and one end of the comb resting against the outer edge of the palm. This position assures a strong hold and a firm movement. (Fig. 10.4)

Practicing with Cold Thermal Irons

Since thermal curling and waving is a somewhat difficult operation that uses heated irons, practice with cold irons on a mannequin or hairpiece pinned to a block until you have thoroughly mastered the technique.

Rolling the Thermal Irons

Practice rolling the cold thermal irons in the hand, first forward, then backward. The rolling movement should be done without any sway or motion in the arm; only the fingers are used to roll the handles in either direction. (Fig. 10.5)

Exercises with Cold Thermal Irons

Exercise 1

At the starting position the rod of the thermal iron will be on top of the hair strand. (Fig. 10.6a) To make the curl, rotate the iron one-half turn (Fig. 10.6b) and then one full turn to complete. (Fig. 10.6c)

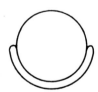

10.6a—Starting position.

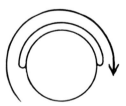

10.6b—One-half turn.

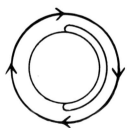

10.6c—Full turn.

Exercise 2

1. Insert hair in irons with rod on top (groove facing upward).
2. Turn irons forward for one-half turn (away from you).
3. Turn irons back to starting position.
4. Open irons slightly and slide down 1″ (2.5 cm), then clamp.
5. Turn irons backward for full turn (toward you).
6. Turn irons forward to starting position.
7. Release.

THERMAL WAVING WITH CONVENTIONAL THERMAL (MARCEL) IRONS

Thermal waving is the art of waving hair using conventional marcel irons. The process requires no setting creams or lotions.

Procedure for Left-Going Wave

Comb the hair thoroughly, following its directional growth. The natural growth will determine whether or not the first wave to be formed will be a left-going wave or a right-going wave. The procedure given here is for a left-going wave.

Before the wave is begun, comb the hair in the general shape desired by the client.

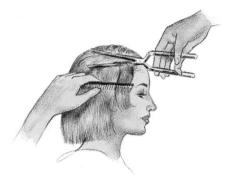

10.7 — Insert irons in the hair.

1. With the comb, pick up a strand of hair about 2″ (5 cm) in width. Insert the irons in the hair with the groove facing upward. (See Fig. 10.7)

2. Close irons and turn them about one-quarter turn forward (away from you). At the same time, draw the hair with the irons about ¼″ (.625 cm) to the left, (See Fig. 10.8) and direct the hair ¼″ (.625 cm) to the right with the comb. (See Fig. 10.9)

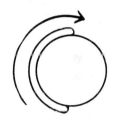

10.8 — One-quarter turn.

3. Roll the irons one full turn forward (away from you). (See Fig. 10.10) (In doing this, keep the hair uniform with the comb. You will find that the hair has rolled on a slight slant on the prong of the irons.) Keep position No. 3 for a few seconds in order to allow the hair to become sufficiently heated throughout.

4. Reverse movement No. 3 by simply unrolling the hair from the irons, bringing them back into their first resting position. (See Fig. 10.11) (When this movement is completed, you will find the comb resting somewhat away from the irons.)

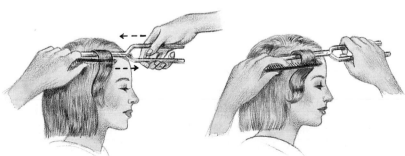

10.9 — Direct hair to the right with the comb.

10.10 — Roll irons one full turn forward.

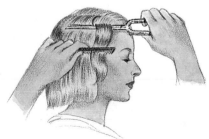

10.11 — Reverse movement.

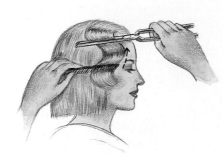

10.12—Start to form the curl.

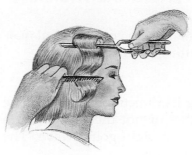

10.13—Form the hair into a half circle.

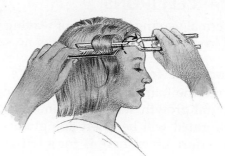

10.14—Roll irons one-half turn forward.

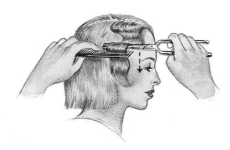

10.15—Slide irons down.

5. Open the irons with the little finger and place them just below the ridge, or crest, by swinging the rod of the irons toward you and then closing them. (See Fig. 10.12) (The outer edge of the groove should be directly underneath the ridge just produced by the inner ridge.)

6. Keep the irons perfectly still and direct the hair with the comb upward about 1" (2.5 cm), thus forming the hair into a half circle. (See Fig. 10.13) (You must remember that, in order to perform movement No. 6 properly, you do not move the comb from the position explained in movement No. 5.)

7. Without opening the irons, roll them one-half turn forward (from you). (See Fig. 10.14) (In this movement, keep the comb perfectly still and unchanged.)

8. Slide the irons down about 1" (2.5 cm). (See Fig. 10.15) (This movement is done by opening the irons slightly (loose grip) and then sliding them down the strand of hair.)

Right-Going Wave

After completing movement No. 8, you will find the irons and comb in a position to make the second ridge. This is the beginning of a right-going wave. As you might expect for a right-going wave, the hair is directed opposite to that of a left-going wave.

Joining or Matching the Waves

After completely waving one strand of hair, wave the next strand to match. When picking up the unwaved hair in the comb, include a small section of the waved strand as a guide to the formation of the new wave. (See Fig. 10.16)

When waving the second strand of hair, be sure that the comb and irons movements are the same as in the first strand of hair; otherwise the waves will not match.

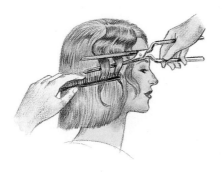

10.16—Matching the wave.

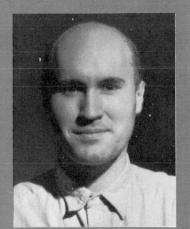
THERMAL CURLING WITH ELECTRIC THERMAL IRONS

Thermal curling is the art of creating curls in the hair using modern thermal irons and a comb. Since thermal curling requires no setting creams or lotions, it may be used to great advantage for the following:

1. *Straight hair*—permits quick styling. Thermal curling eliminates working with wet hair, use of rollers, and a long hair-drying process.
2. *Pressed hair*—permits styling the hair without the danger of its reverting to its former overly curly condition. Thermal curling prepares the hair for any desired style.
3. *Wigs* and *hairpieces*—presents a quick and effective method for their styling.

Curling Irons Manipulations

The following is a series of basic manipulative movements for using heated curling irons. Most other curling irons movements are variations of these basic movements.

The following illustrations show a grip with only the little finger used for opening the clamp. Some cosmetologists prefer to use the little finger plus the ring finger for this purpose. (See Figs. 10.17–10.24) Either method is correct.

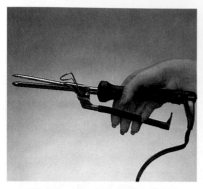

10.17—Use the little finger to open the clamp.

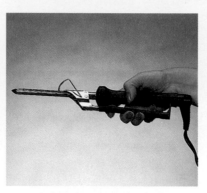

10.18—Use three middle fingers to close and manipulate irons.

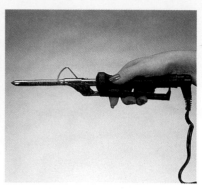

10.19—Shift the thumb when manipulating the irons.

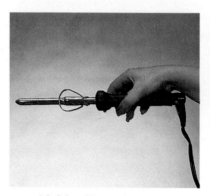

10.20—Close clamp and make a one-quarter turn downward.

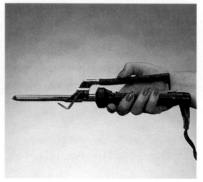

10.21—Irons have made a one-half turn. Use the thumb to open clamp and relax hair tension.

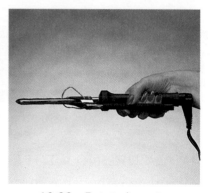

10.22—Rotate irons to three-quarters of a complete turn.

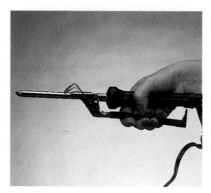

10.23—Full turn.

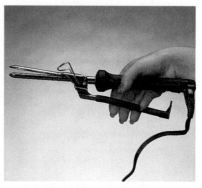

10.24—Alternate method— use little and ring fingers to open clamp.

The method of holding the irons is a matter of personal preference. The technique used should be the one that gives you the greatest ease, comfort, and facility of movement.

Practice in manipulating the curling irons is recommended to develop proficiency in their use. Remember to practice with cold irons. The following four exercises are designed to help achieve an effective use of the irons.

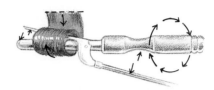

10.25—Rotating movement while opening and closing the irons.

1. Since it is important to develop a smooth rotating movement, practice turning the irons while opening and closing them at regular intervals. Practice rotating the irons in both directions. Examples: downward (toward you) and upward (away from you). (See Fig. 10.25)

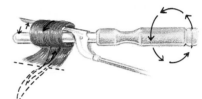

10.26—Guiding the hair strand into the center of the curl while rotating the irons.

2. Practice releasing the hair by opening and closing the irons in a quick, clicking movement.

3. Practice guiding the hair strand into the center of the curl as you rotate the irons. This exercise results in the end of the strand being firmly in the center of the curl. (See Fig. 10.26)

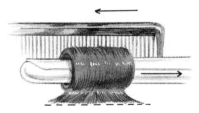

10.27—Removing the curl using comb as guide.

4. Practice removing the curl from the irons by drawing the comb to the left and the rod to the right. (See Fig. 10.27) Use the comb to protect the client's scalp from burns.

THERMAL IRONS CURLING METHODS

Today's thermal irons curling methods have improved over the older techniques. The following methods may be changed or modified to conform with your instructor's procedures.

Preparation

1. Comb the hair thoroughly, removing all tangles.
2. Divide the head into five sections.
    a) First section, about 2½" (6.25 cm) wide, extends from center of forehead to nape of neck.
    b) Divide two side panels in half, from top parting to neck, to provide four additional sections.
3. Heat thermal irons (large or jumbo size).
4. Subdivide sections into ¾" by 2½" (1.875 by 6.25 cm) subsections. (Fig. 10.28) The same procedure is followed for electric irons and stove-heated irons.

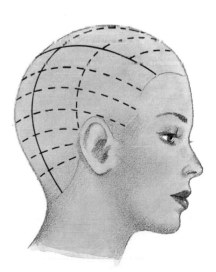

10.28—Hair sectioned and subdivided.

Curling Short Hair

The base of each curl is formed by sectioning and parting to conform with the size of the curl desired. It is important to consider hair length, density, and texture. The base is usually about 1½″ to 2″ (3.75 cm to 5 cm) in width and approximately ½″ (1.25 cm) in depth.

After sectioning off the base, comb the hair smooth and straight out from the scalp. The hair must be combed smooth in order that the heat and tension are the same for all hair in the section. Loose hairs may result in an uneven and ragged curl.

1. After the irons have been heated to the desired temperature, pick up a strand of hair and comb it up and smooth. With the groove on top, insert the irons about 1″ (2.5 cm) from the scalp and hold for a few seconds to form a base. (See Fig. 10.29)

2. Hold the ends of the hair strand with the thumb and two fingers of the left hand, using a medium degree of tension. Turn the irons downward (toward you) with the right hand. (See Fig. 10.30)

3. Open and close the irons rapidly as you turn, to prevent binding. Guide the ends of the strand into the center of the curl as you rotate the irons. (See Fig. 10.31)

4. The result of this procedure will be a smooth, finished curl, with the ends firmly fixed in the center. Remove the irons from the curl. (See Fig. 10.32)

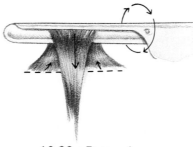

10.29—Form a base.

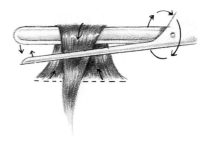

10.30—Turn irons downward.

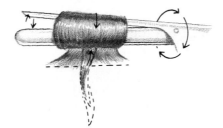

10.31—Rotate irons and guide ends of strand into center.

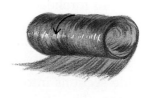

10.32—Finished curl.

Curling Medium Length Hair
(Using One Loop or "Figure 6")
Section and form the base of the curl as described for short hair.

1. Insert the hair into the open irons at the scalp. Pull the hair over the rod in the direction of the curl and close the shell. Hold irons in this position for about 5 seconds to heat the hair, and then slide irons up to 1" (2.5 cm) from the scalp. The shell must be on top. (See Fig. 10.33)

2. Turn irons downward one-half revolution; pull the end of the strand over the rod to the left and direct the strand toward the center of the curl. (See Fig. 10.34)

3. Complete the revolution of the irons, and continue directing the ends toward the center. (See Fig. 10.35)

4. Make another complete revolution of the irons. The entire strand has now been curled with the exception of the ends. Enlarge the curl by opening the shell. Insert the ends of the curl into the opening created between the shell and the rod. (See Fig. 10.36)

5. Close the shell and slide irons toward the handles. This technique will move the ends of the strand into the center of the curl. Rotate irons several times to even out the distribution of the hair in the curl. (See Fig. 10.37)

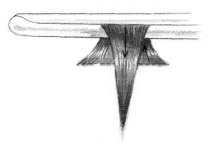

10.33—Insert the hair into open irons at the scalp.

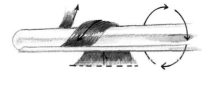

10.34—Turn irons downward one-half revolution.

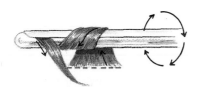

10.35—Complete the revolution of the irons.

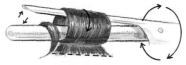

10.36—Make another complete revolution.

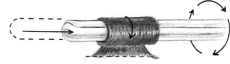

10.37—Close the shell and slide irons toward the handles.

CAUTION

▶ *To protect the client during the curling process, use the comb between the scalp and irons.*

When the curl is formed and the ends are freed from between the rod and the shell, make one complete revolution of the irons inside the curl. This final revolution smoothes the ends and loosens the hair away from the irons. The comb is then used to help remove the curl from the irons. The irons are drawn slowly in one direction, while the comb draws the hair in the opposite direction. In this way the curl is removed from the irons.

Curling Long Hair

(Using Two Loops or "Figure 8," Croquignole Technique)

Section and form the base of the curl as previously described.

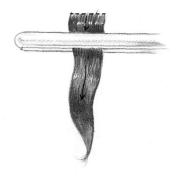

10.38—Insert hair about 1" (2.5 cm) from the scalp.

1. Insert the hair into the open irons about 1" (2.5 cm) from the scalp. Pull the hair over the rod in the direction in which the curl is to move and close the shell. Hold irons in this position for about 5 seconds, in order to heat the hair. Hold the strand of hair with a medium degree of tension (See Fig. 10.38)

2. Roll irons under. Click and roll the irons until the groove is facing you. (See Fig. 10.39)

3. With the left hand, pick up the ends of the hair. (See Fig. 10.40)

4. Continue to roll and click the irons, keeping them the same distance from the scalp. (See Fig. 10.41)

5. Draw the hair strand toward the tip of the irons. (See Fig. 10.42)

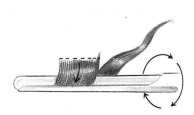

10.39—Roll irons under.

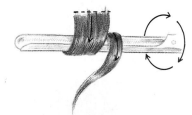

10.40—Pick up the ends of the hair.

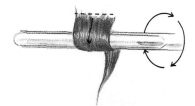

10.41—Continue to roll the irons.

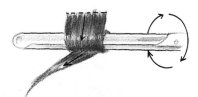

10.42—Draw hair strand toward the point of the irons.

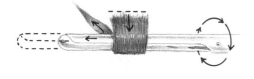

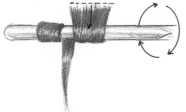

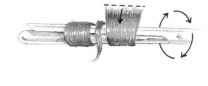

10.43—Draw strand right, push irons left.

10.44—Form two loops around the closed irons.

10.45—Roll irons until hair ends disappear.

6. Draw the strand a little to the right, and, at the same time, push the irons slightly to the left. (See Fig. 10.43)
7. By pushing irons forward and pushing the hair with the left hand, you form two loops around the closed irons, with the ends of the strand extending out between the loops. (See Fig. 10.44)
8. Roll under and click irons until the ends of the hair disappear. (See Fig. 10.45)
9. Rotate irons several times to even out the distribution of the hair in the curl and to facilitate the movement of the curl off the irons.

Other Types of Curls

Spiral curls are hanging curls that are suitable for long hairstyles.

Part the hair into as many sections as there will be curls and comb smooth. Insert the irons at an angle, with the bowl (groove) on top near the base of the strand, and rotate irons until all the hair is wound. Hold the curl in this position for 4 to 5 seconds, and remove the irons in the usual manner. (See Figs. 10.46–10.49)

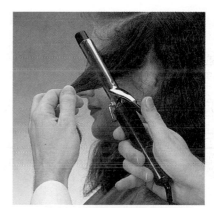

10.46—Insert irons at an angle.

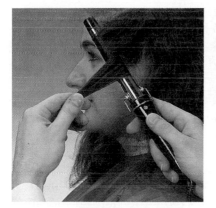

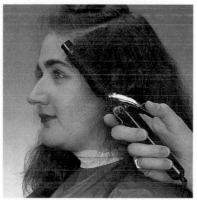

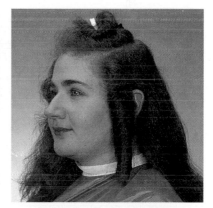

10.47—Rotate irons until hair is wound.

10.48—Hold curl in position.

10.49—Finished curl.

End curls can be used to give a finished appearance to hair ends. Long, medium length, or short hair may be styled with end curls. The hair ends can be turned under or over, as desired.

The position of the curling irons and the direction of their movements will determine whether the end curls will turn under or over. (Figs. 10.50, 10.51)

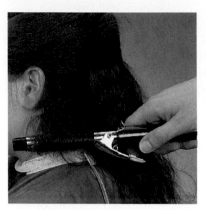 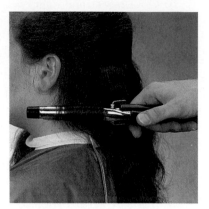

10.50—Turning irons under.

10.51—Turning irons over.

VOLUME THERMAL IRON CURLS

Volume thermal iron curls are used to create volume or lift in a finished hairstyle. The degree of lift desired determines the type of volume curls to be used.

Volume-Base Curls

Volume-base curls provide maximum lift or volume, since the curl is placed very high on its base. Section off the base as described on p. 172. Hold the curl strand at a 135° (2.36 rad.) angle. Slide irons over the strand about ½" (1.25 cm) from the scalp. Wrap the strand over the rod with medium tension. Maintain this position for approximately 5 seconds to heat the strand and set the base. Roll the curl in the usual manner and firmly place it forward and high on its base.

Full-Base Curls

The full-base curl provides a strong curl with full volume. Section off the base as described on p. 172. Hold the hair strand at a 125° (2.18 rad.) angle. Slide irons over the hair strand about ½" (1.25 cm) from the scalp. Wrap the strand over the rod with medium tension. Maintain this position for about 5 seconds to heat the strand and set the base. Roll the curl in the usual manner, and place it firmly in the center of its base. (Fig. 10.52)

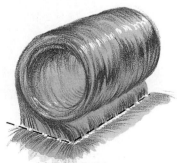

10.52—Full base.

Half-Base Curls

The half-base curl provides a strong curl with moderate lift or volume. Section off the base as described on p. 172. Hold the hair at a 90° (1.57 rad.) angle. Slide irons over the hair strand about ½″ (1.25 cm) from the scalp. Wrap the strand over the rod with medium tension. Maintain this position for about 5 seconds to heat the strand and set the base. Roll the curl in the usual manner, and place it half off its base. (Fig. 10.53)

Off-Base Curls

The off-base curl provides a strong curl with only slight lift or volume. Section off the base as described on p. 172. Hold the hair at a 70° (1.22 rad.) angle. Slide irons over the hair strand about ½″ (1.25 cm) from the scalp. Wrap the strand over the rod with medium tension. Maintain this position for about 5 seconds to heat the strand and set the base. Roll the curl in the usual manner, and place it completely off its base. (Fig. 10.54)

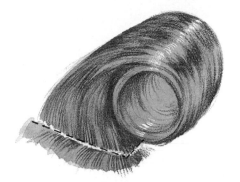
10.53—One-half off base.

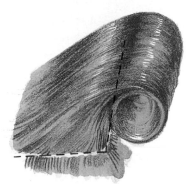
10.54—Off base.

FINISHED THERMAL CURL SETTINGS

For best results when giving a thermal setting, clip each curl in place until the whole head is complete and ready for styling. (Figs. 10.55–10.57)

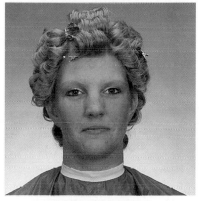
10.55—Front view completely curled.

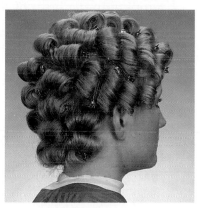
10.56—Side view.

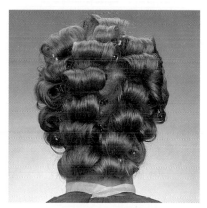
10.57—Back of head completely curled.

STYLING THE HAIR AFTER A THERMAL CURL OR WAVE

After thermal waving or curling, style the hair according to the client's wishes. Brush the hair, working up from the neckline; push the waves and curls into place as you progress over the entire head. If the hairstyle is to be finished with curls, do the bottom curls last. (Figs. 10.58–10.61)

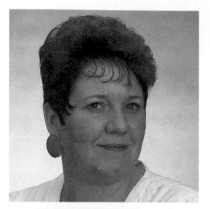

10.58—Finished thermal style for short hair.

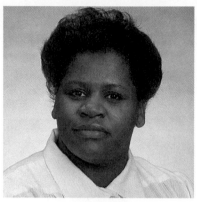

10.59—Finished thermal style for short hair.

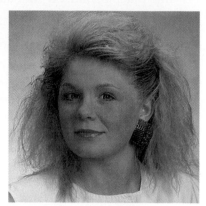

10.60—Finished thermal style for medium length hair.

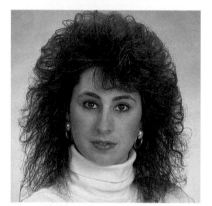

10.61—Finished thermal style for long hair.

SAFETY MEASURES

1. Keep thermal irons clean and the joint oiled.

2. Use thermal irons only after receiving instruction in their use.

3. Do not overheat the irons, because this can cause the metal to lose its temper.

4. Test the temperature of the irons on tissue paper before placing them on the hair. This will prevent the hair from being burned. Do not inhale the fumes of the irons because they are injurious to the lungs.

5. Do not place the hot irons near the face to test for temperature; a burn of the face can result.

6. Handle thermal irons carefully to avoid burning yourself or the client.

7. Place hot irons in a safe place to cool. Do not leave them where someone might accidentally come in contact with them and be burned.

8. When heating the irons, do not place handles too close to the heater. Your hand might be burned when removing the irons.

9. Make sure the irons are properly balanced in the heater, or they might fall and be damaged or injure someone.

10. Use only hard rubber or nonflammable combs. Celluloid combs must not be used in thermal curling; they are flammable.

11. Do not use metal combs; they can become hot and burn the scalp.

12. Do not use combs with broken teeth. They can break or split the hair or injure the scalp.

13. Place comb between scalp and thermal irons when curling or waving hair to prevent burning the scalp.

14. The client's hair must be clean to ensure a good thermal curl or wave.

15. If the hair is thick and bulky, thin and taper it first.

16. Never use hot pressing or thermal irons on lightened or tinted hair.

17. Do not allow the hair ends to protrude over the irons; to do so will cause fishhooks (hair that is bent or folded).

18. A first aid kit must be available in case of an accident.

19. Do not use vaporizing thermal irons on pressed hair because the hair will revert to its original overly curly state.

20. Do not use thermal irons on chemically straightened hair because they might cause damage to the hair.

Success Spotlight

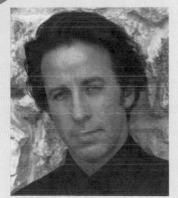

Diversification within your chosen field will magnify the quality of your work. Rocky Lyons, owner of the two busiest salons in Miami, Florida, found that taking an unusual path helped him become an in-demand platform artist and editorial source for many major magazines.

Lyons says, "Knowledge is king. Once you've become proficient at doing hair, you need to have your finger on the pulse of makeup and fashion."

He advises his colleagues and beginners alike to become well versed in all areas of the salon industry. "The professional who is articulate in all facets of beauty and fashion is the one who is destined for success," he says.

This drive led Lyons to pursue photography. Armed with the ability to create a permanent record of his salons' most outstanding total looks, he made his mark through the effective use of photo sessions.

"Everyone at my salons participates in shootings," Lyons explains. "When the photos are published in magazines around the world, our time and effort are rewarded by the recognition generated. If you're good enough, this could lead to a major contract for platform work with a manufacturer. It's also a way to share your vision with others."

In Lyons's case, diversifying his talent by being in touch with current tastes and trends and capturing the results on film have led to a thriving salon business and an international reputation for quality.

Blow-Dry Styling

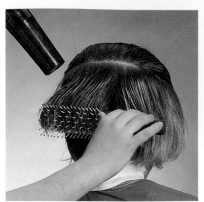

10.62—Blow-dry curling with a brush.

Blow-dry styling, often referred to as a "quick salon service," is the technique of drying and styling damp hair in one operation. This technique creates the basic structure of hairstyles without time-consuming setting, drying, and combing out. It helps to develop soft, natural hairstyles with free-flowing effects. These effects can also be achieved with the use of rollers and curls. (Fig. 10.62)

There are two basic techniques used in blow-dry styling:

1.   Blow-dry curling with a brush.
2.   Blow-dry waving with a comb.

This section covers these two basic techniques. Many other techniques can be developed with experience and advanced training.

▶ NOTE: Take special care when blow drying curled hair that is chemically treated or damaged. This type of hair has loss of elasticity; therefore, towel-dry the hair first to remove excess moisture.

EQUIPMENT, IMPLEMENTS, AND MATERIALS

The following equipment, implements, and materials are required for blow-dry styling:

Blow dryer (with or without attachments)
Combs (hard rubber or metal)
Shampoo

Styling lotions, gels, mousse
Conditioner
Hair spray

THE BLOW DRYER

The blow dryer (without attachments) is an electrical device especially designed for drying and styling the hair in a single operation. Its main parts are a handle, slotted nozzle, small fan, heating element, and controls. When in operation it produces a steady stream of temperature-controlled air. The various controls permit you to make necessary heat adjustments when operating the blow dryer. (Fig. 10.63)

COMBS AND BRUSHES

Both hard rubber combs and those made of metal are used for blow waving and air waving. Some stylists prefer to use metal combs, since they retain and transmit heat better. With metal combs the hair can be re-styled in the shortest possible time.

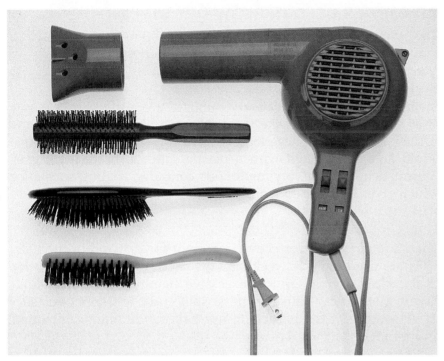

10.63—Implements for blow-dryer styling—from top to bottom: blow dryer; large round brush; wide rounded-shoulder brush; narrow rounded-shoulder brush.

Combs are available with coarse teeth, half coarse and half fine teeth, and all fine teeth.

Special narrow synthetic bristle brushes are used in blow-dry styling. It is often easier for the stylist to brush the hair into the desired style with a narrow brush. The smaller the diameter of the brush, the tighter the curl, with better staying qualities. (Fig. 10.64)

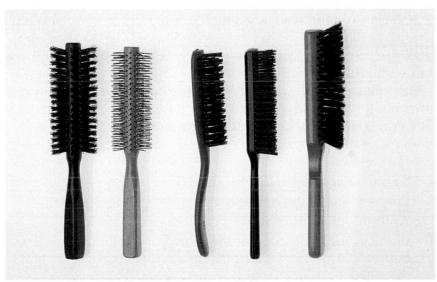

10.64—Brushes used in blow-dry styling.

COSMETICS USED IN BLOW-DRY STYLING

The principal cosmetics used in blow-dry styling include styling lotions, hair and scalp conditioners, and hair sprays.

Styling Lotions

Styling lotions such as gels and mousse are applied to the hair after shampooing to make the hair more manageable for blow curling or waving. These lotions have the consistency of dense liquid and are applied with a plastic squeeze bottle or trigger (pump) action bottle. Styling lotions contain a coating substance which gives blow-dried hair more body and staying qualities.

Hair Conditioners

These are used as a corrective treatment for dry and brittle hair. They are used daily or weekly by the client or immediately prior to the blow-drying service. Excessive hairstyling by the blow-drying method can cause dryness, split ends, and loss of elasticity. Therefore, it is advisable to use hair conditioners containing a lubricant.

Hair Sprays

These are applied to the hair to keep the finished hairstyle in place.

Be guided by the manufacturer's directions or by your instructor as to the proper usage of cosmetics on the client's hair and scalp.

BLOW CURLING WITH ROUND BRUSH

Blow curling is most successful on hair that is naturally curly or has received a permanent wave. The basis for all successful blow styling is the carefully planned hair shaping. In order to properly receive a blow-curling service, hair should be shaped with tapered ends. Successful blow curling is extremely difficult on hair with blunt-cut hair ends.

The following technique is offered as one method of creating a natural-looking, easy-to-wear, informal style with a brush and blower. (Your instructor's methods are equally correct.)

Procedure

1. Shampoo and towel-dry the hair.
2. Properly shape the hair leaving tapered ends.
3. Apply styling lotion and/or conditioner.
4. Pre-plan the style. Start at the crown or top of the head, as desired. Section the hair, pick up a wide strand, and comb through. (See Fig. 10.65)

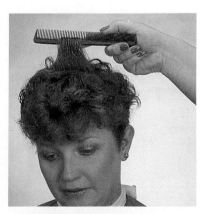

10.65—Section a wide strand and comb through.

5. Bring the comb out to the hair ends and insert the brush. Brush through the strand, bringing the brush out to the ends.

6. Roll the hair with the brush, making a complete downward turn, away from the face, until the brush rests on the scalp. Maintain this position and start the blower. Direct the blower very slowly through the curl in a back-and-forth movement. (See Fig. 10.66) When the hair section is completely dry, release the brush with a rounded movement. Use clippies to secure each curl as it is completed and to hold it in place until it is cooled off.

7. Continue making curls in the same manner across the crown and back of the head. Clip each curl as completed.

8. Shape the neckline curls with a comb, or make pin curls on the nape for a finished, close-to-the-head look.

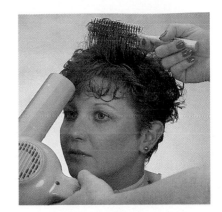

10.66—Roll the hair with brush and direct blower through the curl.

Reminders and Hints on Blow-Dry Styling

In order to achieve the best results from blow-dry styling, the hair should be in good condition. Permanently waved, chemically relaxed, tinted, or lightened hair should be partially towel dried before being blow curled or waved. (The hair stretches easily and could be damaged if very wet.) The hair should be shaped with tapered ends for successful blow curling or waving.

Styling lotion or mousse is important in blow waving and curling. Comb the hair thoroughly to spread the styling lotion evenly.

BLOW-DRYING THE HAIR

Hot air is directed straight onto the head only for rough drying. For successful blow-dry styling the air should be directed from the scalp area to the hair ends. (Fig. 10.67) The flow of air is directed to the top half of the brush in a back-and-forth movement. This method acts to deflect the hot air, reduce its heat, and dry the hair nearest the scalp.

Never hold the blower too long in one place. The blower should be directed so that the hot air flows in the same direction as the hair is wound. To avoid severe scalp burns, always direct the hot air away from the client's scalp. The hair must be thoroughly cooled before it is combed out. This can be accomplished by switching the dryer to cold and cooling the hair that has been dried.

In blow styling it is essential that when the hairstyle is completed the scalp should be thoroughly dry. The hairstyle will not hold if the scalp is damp.

Complete the blow-dry styling with a light application of hair spray to give shine and holding power to the hair.

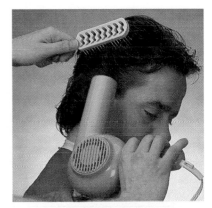

10.67—Direct air from the scalp to hair ends.

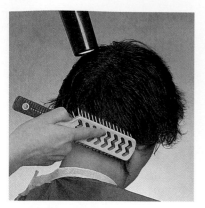

10.68—Blow-drying with a diameter brush.

BRUSHES AND COMBS

The actual styling is performed with the brush or comb. The blow dryer is an implement used for quickly drying the hair while the hair is being styled. The size of the styling brush used is determined by the style and length of the hair. As a general rule, short hair is styled with a small diameter brush. (Fig. 10.68) For medium or longer hair, best results are achieved with large diameter brushes. To avoid scalp burns, keep heated metal combs away from the scalp.

BLOW DRYER

Make sure that the blow dryer is perfectly clean and free of dirt, grease, hair, etc., before using. Dirt or hair can cause extreme heat and burn hair. The air intake at the back of the dryer must be kept clear at all times. If this intake is covered and air cannot pass through freely, the dryer element might burn out.

BLOW-DRYING TECHNIQUES

To give the crown hair a slight lift, a vent brush is used. This vent or open-back brush allows air from the dryer to pass through it easily. The dryer is kept on the move from side to side along the curl. Secure each curl with clippies as it is completed. (See Fig. 10.69)

To create a page boy effect, curl hair under with a brush and blow dry. (See Fig. 10.70)

To create a smooth top with flip, the hair ends are lifted by placing a brush close to the scalp. Rotate the brush. As the brush rotates, the hot air is directed to the base within the cupped area.

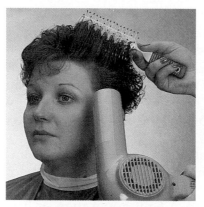

10.69—Crown hair lift.

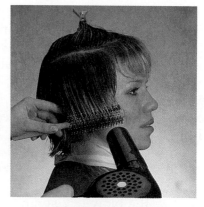

10.70—Page boy effect.

Air Waving

Another technique used to create attractive hairstyles without preliminary setting and drying of the hair is by the use of the electric air waver comb and styling comb. This technique is the same as finger waving, except that you use an electric air waver comb and styling comb. (Fig. 10.71)

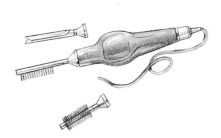

10.71—Air waver with comb attachment.

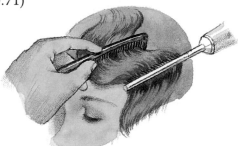

10.72—Comb hair in direction of wave desired.

The hair is styled after it has been shaped, shampooed, and towel dried. It is important to locate the natural wave formation in the hair. Comb the hair in the direction of the wave desired. This will help to establish the natural hair growth pattern. Comb the hair in the direction of the planned hairstyle. Comb the hair with the air waver until it is dry enough to hold a wave.

To achieve ridges and waves on various parts of the head, the hair must be slightly damp. Apply a light spray of styling lotion to assist in creating the desired hairstyle. Comb the hair in the desired direction. (See Fig. 10.72)

SHAPING HAIR WITH COMB

1. *Left side part.* Starting at the front section of the head, insert the styling comb into the hair about 1½" (3.75 cm) from the part. Draw the styling comb toward the back. Insert the air waver under the comb and draw the air waver comb toward the face to form a ridge. Hold both combs in this position until a firm ridge has been formed. (See Fig. 10.73) Continue toward the crown until the entire length of the ridge is completed.

   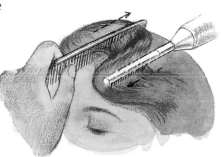

   10.73—Form ridge.

   Form the second ridge by starting at the crown and work toward the front. The ridge and shaping is made in reverse of the first ridge. (See Fig. 10.74) Support the completed ridgeline with the styling comb while the air waver comb lifts and designs the pattern.

2. *Right side part.* The procedure is exactly the same as for the left side part. The only exception is that the hand comb is held in the right hand and the air waver is controlled by the left hand. However, the waving should start at the crown and work forward toward the face.

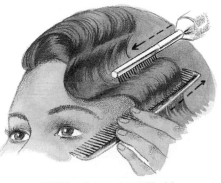

10.74—Form second ridge.

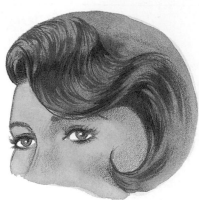

10.75—Finished style.

A finished wave is formed with the air waver comb and styling comb, taking advantage of the natural waving pattern of the hair. (See Fig. 10.75)

The air waver comb, when used in conjunction with the curling iron, presents many styling opportunities to the stylist. The number of styles and patterns that can be created with these implements working in harmony is limited only by the skill and imagination of the stylist.

SAFETY PRECAUTIONS

1. *Styling dryer.* Move moderately hot air back and forth on the hair and away from the scalp. Avoid holding the dryer too long in one place.
2. *Metal comb.* To avoid scalp burns, keep teeth of a heated metal comb away from the scalp.
3. *In all blow-dry styling* it is important that when the curling or waving is completed the scalp must be thoroughly dry. If the ends and the curls are dry but the scalp is damp, the hairstyle will not hold.

Review Questions

THERMAL HAIRSTYLING

1. Define thermal waving or curling.
2. List the three types of irons used in thermal waving.
3. To avoid burning the scalp, what procedure should you follow?
4. Define blow-dry styling.
5. List the implements used in blow-dry styling.
6. What cosmetics are used in blow-dry styling?

11

PERMANENT WAVING

LEARNING OBJECTIVES

After completing this chapter, you should be able to:

1. Define permanent waving.
2. Identify the chemistry of products used in permanent waving.
3. Describe the relationship between hair structure, perm chemistry, and perming techniques.
4. Demonstrate a client consultation.
5. Describe the purpose of waving lotions and neutralizers in the chemical process.
6. Demonstrate proper perming procedures.
7. List safety precautions required for permanent waving.

Introduction

Permanent waving (perming) is one of the most practical and lucrative techniques you will learn in cosmetology school. You'll use basic perming skills throughout your career as a salon stylist. The ability to create a beautiful perm style will bring you professional satisfaction and help build a loyal following of satisfied clients. A properly completed perm provides many valuable benefits to both the client and stylist:

1. Long-lasting style retention.
2. Easy manageability for the client when styling at home.
3. Additional volume and fullness for styling soft, fine hair textures.
4. Greater control in styling hair that is naturally coarse, wiry, and hard to manage.

History of Permanent Waving

Attempts to wave and curl straight hair date back to early civilization. Egyptian and Roman women were known to apply a mixture of soil and water to their hair, wrap it on crudely made wooden rollers, and then bake it in the sun. The results, of course, were not permanent.

THE MACHINE AGE OF PERMANENT WAVING

In 1905 Charles Nessler invented a heavily wired machine that supplied electrical current to metal rods around which hair strands were wrapped. These heavy units were heated during the perming process. They were kept from touching the scalp by a complex system of counterbalancing weights, suspended from an overhead chandelier mounted on a stand. (Fig. 11.1)

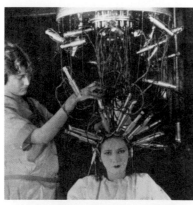

11.1—Machine permanent wave.

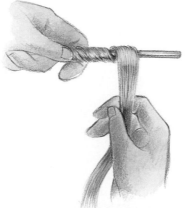

11.2—Spiral flat wrap.

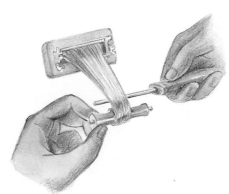

11.3—Croquignole wrap.

Two methods were used to wind hair strands around the metal units. Long hair was wound from the scalp to the ends, a technique called *spiral wrapping.* (Fig. 11.2) After World War I when many women cut their hair into the short bobbed style, the *cro-quignole* (**KROH**-ki-nohl) *wrapping* technique was introduced. Using this method, shorter hair was wound from the ends toward the scalp. The hair was then styled into deep waves with loose end curls. (Fig. 11.3)

The client's fear of being "tied" to an electrical contraption with the possibility of receiving a shock or burn led to the development of alternative methods of waving hair. In 1931, the *pre-heat* method of perming was introduced. Hair was wrapped using the croquignole method, and then clamps, pre-heated by a separate electrical unit, were placed over the wound curls.

THE FIRST MACHINELESS PERM

An alternative to the machine perm was introduced in 1932 when chemists Ralph L. Evans and Everett G. McDonough pioneered a method that used external heat generated by chemical reaction. Small, flexible pads containing a chemical mixture were wound around hair strands. When the pads were moistened with water, a chemical heat was released that created long-lasting curls. Thus, the first machineless permanent wave was born. Salon clients no longer were subjected to the dangers and discomforts of the Nessler machine.

COLD WAVES

In 1941 scientists discovered another method of permanent waving. They developed the waving **lotion**, a liquid that softens and expands the hair strand. After the waving lotion has done its work, another lotion called a **neutralizer** is applied. The neutralizer hardens and shrinks that hair strand, allowing it to conform to the shape of the rod around which the hair is wrapped. It also stops the action of the waving lotion.

Because this perm does not use heat, it is called a "cold wave." Cold waves replaced virtually all predecessors and competitors, and cold waving and permanent waving became almost synonymous terms. Modern versions of cold waves, usually referred to as alkaline perms, are still very popular today.

▶ NOTE: The word "perm" is now popularly used to indicate permanent waving with either an alkaline or acid-balanced solution.

ACID-BALANCED PERMS

For many years, manufacturers sought to develop a permanent wave solution that would minimize hair damage and permit hair that had been damaged by lightening or tinting services to receive a perm. To achieve these goals, they developed a waving lotion that was not as highly alkaline as earlier lotions.

Acid-balanced permanent waves with pH levels ranging from 4.5 to 7.9 were introduced in 1970. They did not contain strong alkalines and therefore were less damaging to the hair. Acid-balanced lotions were, however, slow to penetrate (to pass into or through; to enter by overcoming resistance) hair, and processing time was longer. To overcome this problem, the client is placed under a heated hood dryer to shorten the processing time.

Modern Perm Chemistry

Perm chemistry is constantly being refined and improved. Perms are available today in many different formulas for a wide variety of hair types. Waving lotions and neutralizers for both acid-balanced and alkaline perms are being formulated with new conditioners, proteins, and natural ingredients that help protect and condition the hair during and after perming.

Stop action processing is incorporated in many waving lotions to ensure optimum curl development. The curling takes place within a fixed time without the risk of overprocessing or damaging the hair. Special prewrapping lotions have also been developed to compensate for hair that is not equally porous all over.

Virtually all permanent waves are achieved with a two-step chemical process:

1. Waving lotion, which softens or breaks the internal structure of the hair.
2. Neutralizer, which rehardens or rebonds the internal structure of the hair.

ALKALINE PERMS

The main active ingredient or *reducing agent* in alkaline perms, *ammonium thioglycolate* (a-**MOHN**-nee-um theye-oh-**GLEYE**-coh-layt), is a chemical compound made up of ammonia and thioglycolic acid. The pH of alkaline waving lotions generally falls within the range of 8.2 to 9.6, depending on the amount of ammonia. Because the lotion is more alkaline, the cuticle layers swell slightly and open, allowing the solution to penetrate more quickly than acid-balanced lotions. Some alkaline perms are wrapped with waving lotion, others with water. Some require a plastic cap for processing, others do not. Therefore, it is extremely important to read the perm directions carefully before beginning.

The benefits of alkaline perms are:

*   Strong curl patterns (lotion wrapped alkaline perms are usually stronger than perms that are water wrapped).

- Fast processing time (varies from 5 minutes to 20 minutes).
- Room temperature processing.

Generally, alkaline perms should be used when:

- Perming resistant hair.
- A strong/tight curl is desired.
- The client has a history of early curl relaxation.

ACID-BALANCED PERMS

The main active ingredient in acid-balanced waving lotions is *glyceryl monothioglycolate*, which effectively reduces the pH. This lower pH is gentler on the hair and typically gives a softer curl than alkaline cold waves. Acid-balanced perms have a pH range of approximately 4.5 to 7.9 and usually penetrate the hair more slowly. Thus, they require a longer processing time and heat for curl development. Heat is used in one of two ways:

1. The perm is activated by heat created chemically within the product. This method is called *exothermic*.
2. The perm is activated by an outside heat source, usually a conventional hood-type hair dryer. This method is called *endothermic*.

Recent advances in acid-balanced perm chemistry, however, have made it possible to process some acid-balanced perms at room temperature without heat. These newer acid-balanced perms usually have a slightly higher pH but still contain glyceryl monothioglycolate as the active ingredient.

All acid-balanced perms are water wrapped, require a plastic cap, and may or may not require a pre-heated hood dryer for processing. Read the manufacturer's perm directions carefully before starting the perm.

The benefits of acid-balanced perms are:

- Softer curl patterns
- Slower, but more controllable processing time (usually 15 to 25 minutes)
- Gentler treatment for delicate hair types

Generally, acid-balanced perms should be used when:

- Perming delicate/fragile or color-treated hair
- Soft, natural curl or wave pattern is desired
- Style support, rather than strong curl, is required

THE CHEMISTRY OF NEUTRALIZERS

Neutralizers for both acid-balanced and alkaline perms have the same important function: to permanently establish the new curl shape. Neutralizing is a very important step in the perming process. If the hair is not properly neutralized, the curl will relax or straighten within one to two shampooings. Generally, today's neutralizers are composed of a relatively small percentage of hydrogen peroxide, an oxidizing agent, at an acidic pH. As with waving lotions, there are slightly different procedures recommended for individual products. To achieve the best possible results, read the directions carefully.

Hair Structure and Perming

Whether using an acid-balanced or alkaline formula, all perms subject the hair to two different actions:

1. Physical action—wrapping sections of hair around a perm rod.
2. Chemical action—created first by a reducing agent (waving lotion) and second by an oxidizing agent (neutralizer).

Since both of these actions work together to create a change in the internal structure of the hair, it is important to understand the composition of hair and how it is affected during perming.

PHYSICAL STRUCTURE OF HAIR

Each strand of hair is structurally subdivided into three major components:

1. The *cuticle* or outer covering consists of seven or more overlapping layers. Although it comprises a small percentage of the total weight of hair, the cuticle possesses unique structural properties that protect the hair. During perming, the waving lotion raises the cuticle layers and allows the active ingredients to enter the cortex.
2. The *cortex*, the major component of the hair structure, accounts for up to 90% of its total weight. The cortex gives hair its flexibility, elasticity, strength, resilience, and color. It is in the cortex that the physical and chemical actions take place during the perming process to restructure the hair into a new curl configuration.
3. The *medulla* is the innermost section of the hair structure. The function of the medulla, if any, is unknown. In fact, it is not at all unusual for an otherwise normal, healthy hair to be without a medulla. (Fig. 11.4)

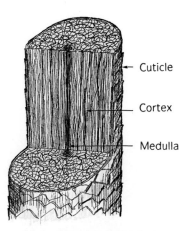

— Cuticle

— Cortex

— Medulla

11.4—Structure of a hair.

CHEMICAL COMPOSITION OF HAIR

The chemical composition of hair consists almost entirely of a protein material called *keratin* (**KER**-a-tin), which is made up of approximately nineteen amino acids. When many amino acids are bonded together, they form a *polypeptide* (pol-ee-**PEP**-teyed) *chain*. These chains intertwine around each other in a spiral fashion to assume a helical shape very similar to a spring. Hair contains a high concentration of the amino acid *cysteine* (**SIS**-teen), which is joined together crosswise with *disulfide* (deye-**SUL**-feyed) linkages or bonds. Disulfide bonds add strength to the keratin protein, and it is these bonds that must be broken down to allow the perming process to occur.

Processing. The chemical action of a waving lotion breaks the disulfide bonds and softens the hair. When the chemical action softens the inner structure of the hair enough, it can mold to the shape of the rod around which it is wound. (Fig. 11.5a–c)

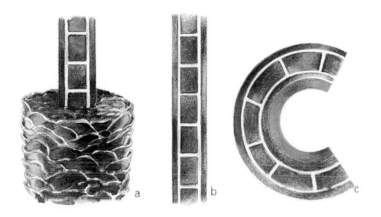

11.5a—Each hair strand is composed of many polypeptide chains. This series of illustrations shows the behavior of one such chain.

11.5b—Hair before processing. Chemical bonds (links) give hair its strength and firmness.

11.5c—Hair wound on rod. The hair bends to the curvature and size of the rod.

Neutralizing. When the hair has assumed the desired shape, the broken disulfide bonds must be chemically rebonded. Neutralizing rehardens the hair and fixes it into its new curl form. When the neutralizing action is completed, the hair is unwrapped from the rods, and you have a new curl formation. (Fig. 11.6a, b)

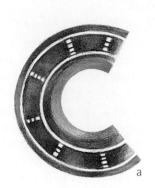
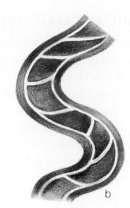

11.6a—During processing, waving lotion breaks the chemical cross-bonds (links), permitting the hair to adjust to the curvature of the rod while in this softened condition.

11.6b—The neutralizer re-forms the chemical bonds (links) to conform with the wound position of the hair, and rehardens the hair, thus creating the permanent wave.

CHOOSING THE RIGHT PERMING TECHNIQUE

How do you decide which perming technique is right for your client? You must be able to evaluate and analyze your client's hair. You must consult with your client to establish what the person expects to accomplish with a perm—a tight, curly look or a loose, wavy look. This information helps you to select the correct perm product and technique.

Basic Manual Perming Skills

Successful perming requires manual dexterity. With practice, your skills in handling and manipulating hair will improve. Before actually applying a perm, you will probably spend considerable time practicing pre-perming skills like blocking, sectioning, and wrapping. Your ability to give successful perms depends on mastering these important skills.

Client Consultation

Every perm client has a different expectation for how he or she wants the perm to look. The only way to meet your client's expectations is to determine what those expectations are. Talk to your client in a friendly, but professional way. Take a few minutes to discuss:

1. What hairstyle and how much curl your client wants. Photos or magazine pictures help to make this clearly understood by both of you.
2. Your client's life-style. Does he or she have leisure time, or a demanding schedule that requires a low-maintenance style?

3. How your client's hairstyle relates to overall personal image. Is your client concerned about current fashion trends?

4. Your client's previous experience with perming. What did he or she like or dislike about past perm services?

Once you learn what questions to ask and how to ask them, the consultation with your perm client takes only a few minutes. It is time well-spent, however, because the consultation helps establish your credibility as a professional. It inspires your client's confidence in your technical and creative abilities, and makes the perming experience more satisfactory for both of you.

Keep the vital information you learn during the client consultation as a written permanent record, along with other important data, including the client's address, home, and business phone numbers. Here is an example of an organized format for maintaining client records:

PERMANENT WAVE RECORD

Name .... Tel. ....

Address .... City .... State ....

DESCRIPTION OF HAIR   Zip ....

Length	**Texture**	**Type**	**Porosity**	
☐ short	☐ coarse	☐ normal	☐ very	☐ slightly
☐ medium	☐ medium	☐ resistant	porous	porous
☐ long	☐ fine	☐ tinted	☐ moderately	☐ resistant
		☐ highlighted	porous	
		☐ bleached	☐ normal	

Condition

☐ very good ☐ good ☐ fair ☐ poor ☐ dry ☐ oily

Tinted with ....

Previously permed with..

TYPE OF PERM

☐ alkaline ☐ acid ☐ body wave ☐ other..........................

No. of rods .... Lotion .... Strength ....

Results

☐ good ☐ poor ☐ too tight ☐ too loose

Date	Perm Used	Stylist	Date	Perm Used	Stylist
....	....	....	....	....	....
....	....	....	....	....	....
....	....	....	....	....	....

Other side of Record, continue with:

Date	Perm Used	Stylist	Date	Perm Used	Stylist

Business Tips

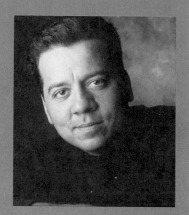

Chicago salon owner Lenny LaCour has made two distinctly different salons a success. One is located in Chicago's youthful Lincoln Park area, the second is on Michigan Avenue, along an upscale strip known as "the magnificent mile." What is LaCour's advice to cosmetology school graduates who hope to own their own business someday?

"The decision to be a stylist or an owner is up to the individual," says LaCour. "They are two very separate positions, and you shouldn't be fooled into thinking that you have to own your own business to be a success in life.

"The client pays the stylist, and it's your job to please him or her. As an owner, you pay your employees, and the control is in your hands. If working with hair and making clients look great is your first love, you should be aware that the successful owner cannot work behind the chair all the time and run a business, too. Breeding loyalty in nail technicians and managers alike is a lot different from building a loyal client following.

"A stylist who works behind the chair in a top salon can be much more successful than an owner who isn't wholly dedicated to business. The decision on which path to take is up to you, but whatever you choose, success comes to those who want it."

PRE-PERM ANALYSIS

After the client consultation, you must analyze the overall condition of your client's hair and scalp. This analysis is essential for you to determine:

1. If it is safe and advisable to proceed with the perm service. The hair must be in good condition and have the necessary strength to accept a chemical alteration to achieve a successful perm.
2. Which perm product should be chosen for the best results on the particular hair type.
3. Which perm technique should be used: rod and parting sizes and wrapping pattern.

First, examine the scalp for abrasions, irritations, or open sores. If any of these conditions exist, do not give the perm. Next, judge the physical characteristics of the hair with regard to these important criteria: porosity, elasticity, density, texture, length. Finally, determine the overall condition of the hair. Observe if the hair has been previously treated with chemicals: perm, tint, bleach, highlighting (frosting, dimensionally colored). This will guide you in choosing the appropriate perm.

CAUTION

▶ *If pre-perm analysis is not correct, poor curl development or hair damage can result.*

Determining Porosity

Porosity (po-**ROS**-i-tee) refers to the hair's capacity to absorb liquids. There is a direct relationship between the hair's porosity, the type of perm (acid-balanced or alkaline) you will use, and the strength of waving lotion you will choose.

The processing time for any perm depends more on hair porosity than on any other factor. The more porous the hair, the less processing time it takes, and a milder waving solution is required. The degree to which hair absorbs the waving lotion is related to its porosity, regardless of texture.

Hair porosity is affected by such factors as excessive exposure to sun and wind, use of harsh shampoos, tints, and lighteners, previous perms, and use of thermal styling appliances.

Porous hair might be dry—even very dry. If hair is tinted, bleached, has been exposed to sun, or was overprocessed by a previous perm, it will absorb liquids readily. Soft, fine, thin hair usually has a thin cuticle so it will absorb liquids quickly and easily. Rough, dull-looking hair and hair that tangles easily are also signs of porous hair.

While the hair is dry, check porosity in three different areas: front hairline, in front of the ear, and in the crown area. Select a single strand of hair, hold the end securely between the thumb and forefinger of one hand, and slide the thumb and forefinger of the other hand from the end to the scalp.

If the hair feels smooth and the cuticle is dense and hard, it is considered resistant and will not absorb liquids or perm lotion easily. If you can feel a slight roughness, this tells you that the cuticle is open and that the hair is porous and will absorb liquids more readily. (Fig. 11.7)

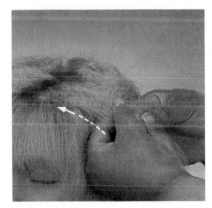

11.7—Testing for hair porosity.

Poor porosity (resistant hair). Hair with the cuticle layer lying close to the hair shaft. This type of hair absorbs waving lotion slowly and usually requires a longer processing time and/or a strong waving lotion.

Good porosity (normal hair). Hair with the cuticle layer slightly raised from the hair shaft. Hair of this type can absorb moisture or chemicals in an average amount of time.

Porous (tinted, lightened, or previously chemically treated hair). Hair that has been made porous by various treatments or styling. This type of hair absorbs lotion very quickly and requires the shortest processing time. Use either an acid-balanced perm or a very mild alkaline wave.

Over-porous hair (a result of overprocessing). This type of hair is very damaged, dry, fragile, and brittle. Until the hair has been reconditioned or the damaged part has been removed by cutting, it should not be permed.

If hair is unevenly porous (usually porous or over-porous at the ends with good to poor porosity near the scalp), a pre-wrap lotion, specifically designed to even out the porosity, is recommended to achieve even curl results and help prevent overprocessing porous ends. (Fig. 11.8a–d)

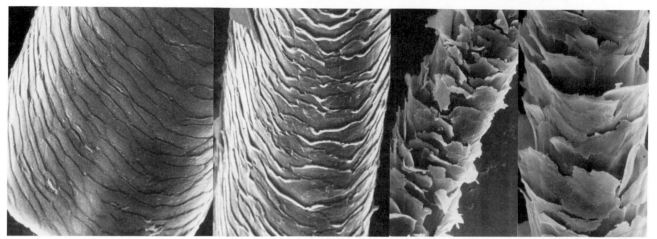

11.8a—Normal
(moderate porosity).   11.8b—Resistant
(poor porosity).   11.8c—Tinted
(extreme porosity).   11.8d—Damaged
(over-porous hair).

Determining Texture

Texture refers to how thick or thin (in diameter) each individual hair is. Fine hair has a small diameter; coarse hair has a large diameter. You can feel whether hair is fine, coarse, or medium when a single dry strand is held between the fingers.

The texture and porosity together are used to determine processing time of the waving lotion. Although porosity is the more important of the two, texture does play an important role in estimating processing time. Fine hair with a small diameter becomes saturated with waving lotion more quickly than coarse hair with a large diameter, even if both are of equal porosity. However, when coarse hair is porous, it processes faster than fine hair that is not porous.

A perm adds body to hair that appears limp, lifeless, and does not hold a style very long. For coarse, wiry hair, a perm provides greater manageability in styling. (Fig. 11.9a–c)

Testing Elasticity

Elasticity is the ability of hair to stretch and contract. To test for elasticity, stretch a single dry hair. If the hair breaks under very slight strain, it has little or no elasticity. Other signs of poor elas-

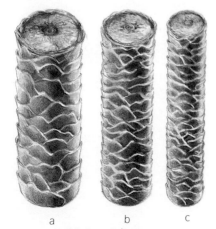

11.9a—Coarse.
11.9b—Medium.
11.9c—Fine.

ticity include a spongy feel when hair is wet and/or hair that tangles easily. When hair is completely lacking in elasticity (for example, extremely damaged hair), it will not take a satisfactory permanent wave because it has lost the ability to contract after stretching. The greater the degree of elasticity, the longer the wave will remain in the hair, because less relaxation of the hair occurs. Hair with good elastic qualities can be stretched 20% of its length without breaking. (Fig. 11.10)

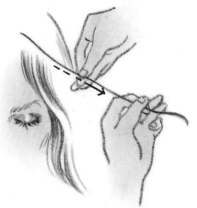

11.10—Testing for elasticity.

Assessing Density

Density, or thickness, refers to the number of hairs per square inch (6.452 sq. cm) on your client's head. Density is one characteristic that determines the size of the partings you will use. Thick hair (many hairs per square inch) will require small partings on each rod. Too much hair on the rod can result in a weak curl, especially at the scalp.

If hair is thin (fewer hairs per square inch), slightly larger partings can be used, but avoid stretching or pulling the hair toward the rod because this can cause hair breakage.

Hair Length and Perming

Hair that is 2″ to 6″ (5 to 15 cm) long is considered ideal for perming. Hair should be long enough to make at least 2½ turns around the rod. To perm hair longer than 6″ (15 cm), smaller partings must be used to allow the waving lotion and neutralizer to penetrate more easily and thoroughly.

PERM SELECTION

The type of perm you choose depends on the total evaluation of your client's hair and wishes during the consultation and pre-perm analysis. The following is a general guide to help you decide whether to use an alkaline or an acid-balanced perm.

Hair Type	Type of Perm
Coarse, resistant	Alkaline lotion wrap or alkaline water wrap
Fine, resistant	Alkaline lotion wrap or alkaline water wrap
Normal	Alkaline water wrap or acid-balanced
Normal, porous	Alkaline water wrap or acid-balanced
Normal, delicate	Acid-balanced
Tinted, non-porous	Alkaline water wrap or acid-balanced
Tinted, porous	Acid-balanced
Highlighted/frosted/ dimensionally colored	Acid-balanced
Highlighted, tinted	Acid-balanced
Bleached	Acid-balanced

Today's perm products offer a wide selection of special features and formulas for all hair types. There are alkaline formulas for bleached hair and acid-balanced formulas for resistant hair. Each formula gives excellent results if you choose the perm carefully and follow the product directions.

PRE-PERM SHAMPOOING

Today, there are shampoos specifically formulated for pre-perm cleansing that thoroughly yet gently cleanse the hair. Use of these shampoos is recommended for optimal perm results.

When analyzing a client's hair before perming, you might notice that the hair looks and feels coated. This coating might be the buildup of shampoo or conditioners, improper rinsing, resins from styling products or hair spray, or mineral deposits from hard water. This coating can prevent penetration of the waving lotion and interfere with perm results. It is very important for the hair to be free of all coatings before beginning any perm.

CAUTION

▶ *While shampooing or doing any pre-perm preparation of a client's hair, you should avoid vigorous brushing, combing, pulling, or rubbing that can cause the scalp to become sensitive to perm solutions.*

Begin the process by wetting the hair, applying the shampoo, and gently working it into a lather. If the hair is extremely coated, let the shampoo remain in the hair several minutes before rinsing. Rinse thoroughly to remove all shampoo and dissolved buildup. Towel blot excess water from hair.

PRE-PERM CUTTING OR SHAPING

If the client has chosen a hairstyle that is the same or very similar to the design he or she is currently wearing, reshape the style using either a scissors or razor. If the finished style requires texturizing or thinning of the ends, wait until after giving the perm to texturize. Tapered or thinned ends are more difficult to wrap smoothly and accurately.

If the client wants a completely new style, rough cut the hair into an approximation of the final shape. After the perm is completed, you can finish shaping the style more exactly.

PERM RODS

Proper selection of perm rod size is essential for successful perm results. The size of the rod controls the size of the curl created by the waving process. Perm rods are typically made of plastic and come in varying sizes. They range in diameter (distance through the center of the rod) from small to large (⅛″ to ¾″ [.3125 to 1.875 cm]). Rods are color coded to identify their size. Typically, the color/size designations are:

Small Rods	Medium Rods	Large Rods
Yellow	Gray	Beige
Blue	Black	Purple
Pink	White	Brown
		Orange

Perm rods are also available in various lengths: short, medium, and long (1¾″ to 3½″ [4.375 to 8.75 cm]). Rods of all diameters are available in long lengths. Medium and short lengths are not always available in all diameters. These shorter rods are used for wrapping small or awkward sections. (Fig. 11.11)

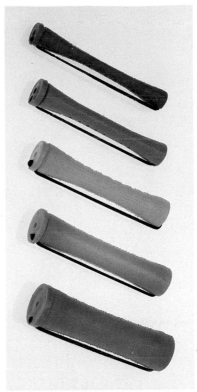

11.11—Types of rods—top to bottom: extra small, small, medium, large, extra large.

Types of Rods

There are two types of rods: concave and straight. Concave rods have a small diameter in the center area and gradually increase to their largest diameter at the ends, resulting in a tighter curl at the hair ends, with a looser, wider curl at the scalp. The diameter of the straight rods is the same throughout their length, creating the same size curl from end to scalp.

All rods have some means of securing the hair on the rod to prevent the curl from unwinding. Usually an elastic band, with a fastening button attached to the end, stretches across the wound hair and secures it when the button is inserted into the opposite end of the rod.

Selecting Rod Size

When selecting rod size, two things must be considered:

1. Amount of curl desired
2. Physical characteristics of the hair

Curl desired: The amount of wave, curl, or body needed is determined between you and the client during the consultation. Your success in creating a style depends primarily on the rod sizes you choose, the number of rods used, and where the rods are placed on the head.

Hair characteristics: Of the hair characteristics described earlier, three are important to rod size selection:

1. Hair length
2. Hair elasticity
3. Hair texture

Suggested Hair Parting and Rod Sizes

Although the hair length, elasticity, and texture must be considered in the choice of rods, the texture should be the determining factor.

Coarse texture, good elasticity. Requires smaller (narrower) partings and larger rods to permit better placement of rods for a definite wave pattern.

Medium texture, average elasticity. Medium or average textured hair requires average size partings and medium size rods.

Fine texture, poor elasticity. Requires smaller than average partings and small to medium size rods to prevent hair strain or breakage.

Hair in nape area. Use smaller partings and smaller rods.

Long hair. To permanently wave hair longer than 6″ (15 cm), use small partings and wrap smoothly and close to the scalp. The use of smaller partings permits the waving lotion and neutralizer to penetrate more easily and thoroughly.

SECTIONING AND PARTING

Sectioning is the dividing of hair into uniform working areas at the top, front, crown, sides, back, and nape. Sectioning makes your work easier because you can pin up all sections out of your way except the section you are working with.

Parting, also known as *blocking,* is the overall plan for rod placement. You block so that you know where to place the rods in order to give the design the support, direction, and curl pattern it needs. It is important that the blocking is done in uniform sections. You should use the following guidelines to help you:

1. Uniformly arrange sections.
2. Equally subdivide sections (blockings).
3. Create clean and uniform partings (length and width).
4. The average parting should match the diameter (size) of the rod being used.
5. The length of the blocking should be the same as or a little shorter, but never longer, than the length of the rod. (Figs. 11.12–11.14)

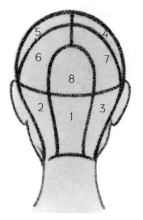

11.12—Sectioning.

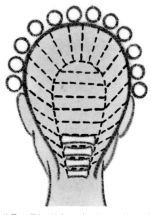

11.13—Blocking (subsections).

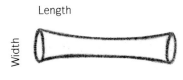

Length

Width

11.14—Length denotes span of blocking. Width refers to the depth of the blocking. Small or large blockings usually refer to their width.

WRAPPING PATTERNS

Just as the rod size and parting size determine the size of the curl, the wrapping pattern determines the direction or flow of the curl.

Six popular wrapping patterns are:

1. Single halo
2. Double halo (double horseshoe)
3. Straight back
4. Dropped crown
5. Spiral wrap
6. Stack perm

These are known by other names in different areas of the country.

The following sections and partings are suggested for these wrapping patterns. Your instructor might suggest different sections, which are equally correct.

Single Halo

The single halo wrap is commonly used for average size heads to create even curls. (Figs. 11.15–11.18)

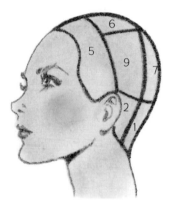

11.15—Sectioning side.

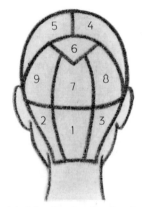

11.16—Sectioning back.

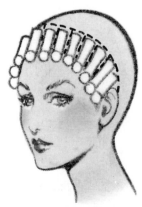

11.17—Blocking side.

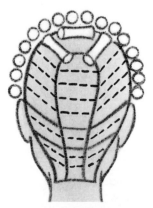

11.18—Blocking back.

Double Halo

The double halo wrap is usually used for larger size heads. (Figs. 11.19–11.22)

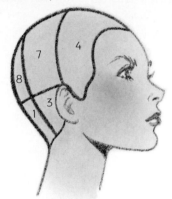

11.19—Sectioning side.

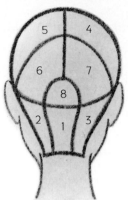

11.20—Sectioning back.

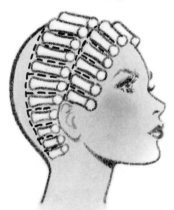

11.21—Blocking side.

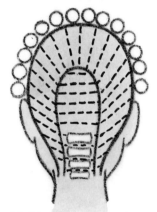

11.22—Blocking back.

Straight Back

The straight back wrap is used to create a rather soft, full, and high style effect, directed off the face. (Figs. 11.23, 11.24)

To create *bangs* on the forehead, the first two top front curls are wrapped in a forward direction (see directional wrapping, pages 218–220). (Fig. 11.25)

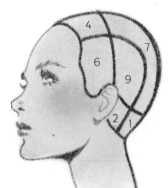

11.23—Sectioning side.

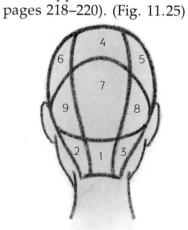

11.24—Sectioning back.

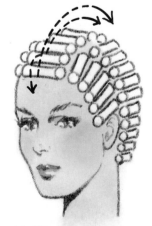

11.25—Setting for bangs.

Dropped Crown

The dropped crown wrap is usually used for longer hair and for a smooth crown effect.

The hair is sectioned in the same way as for the straight back pattern. However, in the back area that is not numbered on the illustration, larger hair sections are made, depending on the amount of hair in that section. Only the hair ends are wrapped and the rods rest on the smaller rods in the nape area (sections 2, 1, 3). Be guided by your instructor. (Figs. 11.26–11.29)

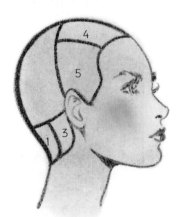

11.26 — Sectioning side.

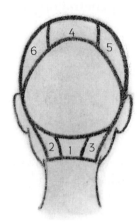

11.27 — Sectioning back.

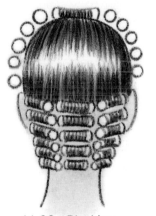

11.28 — Blocking (subsectioning) pattern.

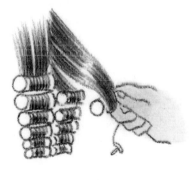

11.29 — Wrapping hair ends of crown area.

Spiral Wrap

The spiral wrap is used for long hair to create tight, springy curls. (Fig. 11.30)

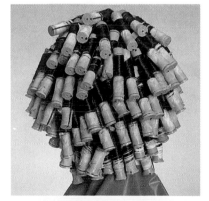

11.30 — Spiral wrap.

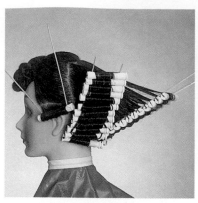

11.31—Stack perm.

Stack Perm

The stack technique is usually used for greater curl at the nape. (Fig. 11.31)

WRAPPING THE HAIR

To create a uniform wave or curl pattern, the hair must be wrapped smoothly and neatly on each perm rod *without stretching*. As noted earlier, the action of the waving lotion expands the hair. Hair that is tightly wrapped interferes with this action and prevents penetration of the waving lotion and neutralizer.

Hair Strand Parting in Relation to the Head

Base refers to the head or scalp and where the rod is placed in relation to the head. The rods can be wrapped on-base, off-base, or one-half off-base. Each of these rod positions creates a slightly different scalp wave direction, which will influence the overall curl pattern results.

Curl on-base. When the strand is held in an upward position and wound on the rod, the curl will rest on-base. (See Fig. 11.32) Hair wound in this manner will produce curls that start close to the scalp for hairstyles that require fullness, height, and upward movement.

Curl off-base. When the strand is held in a downward position and wound on a rod, the curl will rest off-base. (See Fig. 11.33) Hair wound in this manner will produce a curl that starts farther away from the scalp than hair wound on base. Off-base winding produces close-to-the-head hairstyles that do not require fullness or height.

Curl one-half off-base. When the strand is held straight out from the head and wound on a rod, the curl will rest one-half off-base. (See Fig. 11.34) Hair wound in this manner is adaptable to many hairstyles.

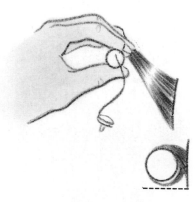

11.32—Curl on-base.

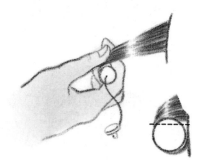

11.33—Curl off-base.

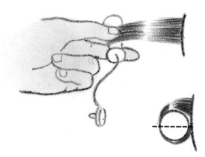

11.34—Curl one-half off-base.

End Wraps

End wraps or end papers are porous papers used to cover the ends of the hair to ensure smooth, even wrapping. End wraps minimize the danger of hair breakage and help to form smooth, even curls and waves. They are especially important in helping to wrap uneven hair lengths smoothly.

There are three methods of end wrap application in general use today. Each method is equally effective, if properly used.

1. Double end paper wrap
2. Single end paper wrap
3. Book end wrap

▶ **NOTE:** Hair should be shampooed and left moist (not saturated) for wrapping. Section hair, then begin by making your first parting. Remember, each parting should be no longer than the length of the rod. If the parting is too long, the hair will not wave evenly. If the hair should become dry while you are wrapping, mist the hair lightly with water.

Double End Paper Wrap

1. Part off and comb the parting up and out until all hair is smooth and evenly distributed. (See Fig. 11.35)

2. Place one end wrap under the hair strand so that it extends below the ends of the hair. Place the other end wrap on top. (See Fig. 11.36)

3. With your right hand, place the rod under the double end wraps, parallel with the parting at the scalp. (See Fig. 11.37)

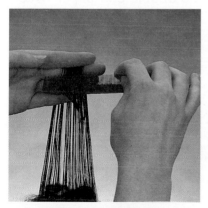

11.35—Comb and distribute strand evenly.

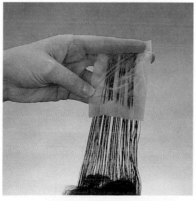

11.36—Position end papers.

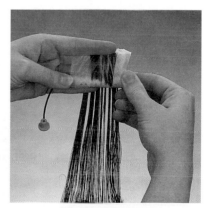

11.37—Position rod.

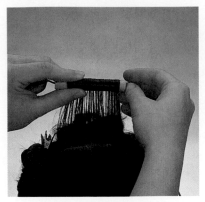

11.38—Wind the strand.

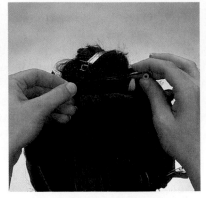

11.39—Fasten band.

4. Wind the strand smoothly on the rod to the scalp without tension. (See Fig. 11.38)
5. Fasten band at top of rod. (See Fig. 11.39)

CAUTION

▶ *To prevent breakage, the band should not press into the hair near the scalp or be twisted against the wound hair.*

The preparation and winding of curls for the single end paper wrap and book end wrap are the same as the double end paper wrap, with the following exceptions:

Single end paper wrap. Place only one end wrap on top of the hair strand and hold it flat between the index and middle fingers to prevent bunching. (See Fig. 11.40) The hair is wound in the same manner as the double end paper wrap.

Book end wrap. Hold the strand between the index and middle fingers; fold and place an end paper over the strand, forming an envelope. Wind the curl as in the double end paper wrap. (See Fig. 11.41)

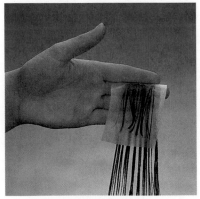

11.40—Single end paper wrap.

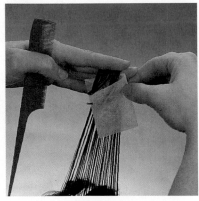

11.41—Book end wrap.

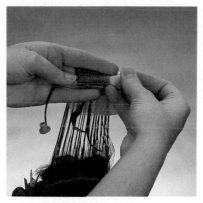

11.42—Position porous end papers.

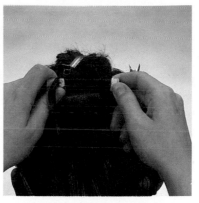

11.43—Start wrapping.

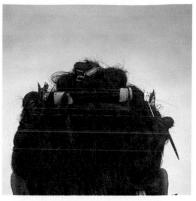

11.44—Secure the wrapped rod.

The Piggyback (Double Rod) Wrap

The piggyback (double rod) method of wrapping is especially suitable for extra long hair. This wrapping technique permits maximum control of the size and tightness of the curl from the scalp to the hair ends. Control of the amount of curl can be exercised by the size of the rods selected. Thus, the use of larger rods will result in a loose, wide wave; while small, or medium rods will give tighter curls. The following is the procedure for wrapping in the piggyback (double rod) method:

1. Section the head in the usual manner (9 sections).
2. Select the desired size rods. The rods used in the midpoint to the scalp area should be at least one size larger than those used for the hair ends.
3. About halfway up the strand, place porous end papers one on top and one underneath. (See Fig. 11.42)
4. Start at the midpoint part of the strand. Place the larger rod underneath the hair strand and start wrapping. (See Fig. 11.43)
5. Roll the rod toward the scalp and, at the same time, control the hair ends by holding them to the left away from the rod.
6. Secure the wrapped rod at the scalp, leaving the hair ends dangling free from the rod. (See Fig. 11.44)
7. Place an end paper on the hair strand covering the ends. Using the smaller size rod, wrap the hair ends up to the above larger rod. (See Fig. 11.45)
8. Secure the second rod to rest against the first one in piggyback fashion. (See Fig. 11.46)
9. To maintain better control over the wrapping and processing, it is advisable to complete the wrapping of each hair strand before proceeding to the next one.

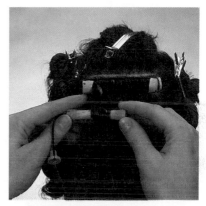

11.45—Wrap the remaining hair ends.

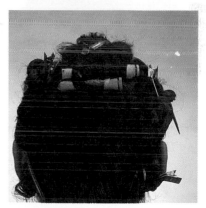

11.46—Secure the second rod beneath the first rod.

10. Test curls should be taken from the rods closer to the scalp because the hair in this area is more resistant and might require additional processing.

▶ **NOTE:** When wrapping hair, always avoid bulkiness on the rod. Bulkiness prevents the formation of a good curl because the hair cannot conform to the shape of the rod, and the waving lotion and neutralizer cannot penetrate evenly and thoroughly. To ensure a smooth wave formation and avoid fishhook ends, the first turn on the rod should be the end wraps without any of the hair ends between them.

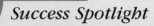

Success Spotlight

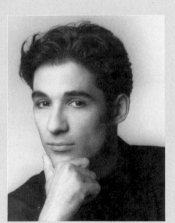

Sam Brocato has been described as a preacher, teacher, artist, and businessman, but whichever talent you zero in on, one thing is for certain—Brocato is one of the youngest American hairdressers ever to make his mark on the professional salon industry.

Armed with $900 and high hopes, Brocato started his own business in Baton Rouge, Louisiana, at the age of 22. Today, Lockworks USA is a high-fashion, high-return beauty corporation that includes four full-service salons, two training academies, a warehouse, corporate offices, and 150 highly motivated employees. Brocato attributes this success to the philosophy that, "You don't grow businesses, you grow people."

Brocato and his company have been the recipients of numerous awards including Business of the Year, Marketer of the Year, American Hairdresser of the Year, and World's Top Fashion Hairstylist.

Not content to take the money and run, Brocato wanted to share his successes and his knowledge with others. As president and founder of Brocato International hair care products, Brocato has extended his career to yet another facet of the beauty business. According to Brocato, professional growth is the result of education, promotion, and motivation.

PRELIMINARY TEST CURLS

Preliminary test curls help determine how your client's hair will react to a perm. It is advisable to do a test on hair that is tinted, bleached, over-porous, or shows any signs of damage.

Also, before applying waving lotion, be sure to check with your instructor or state board to find out if you are required to wear protective gloves during application.

Preliminary testing gives you the following additional information:

- Actual processing time needed to achieve optimum curl results
- Curl results based on the rod size and perm product you have selected

Procedure

1. Shampoo the hair and towel dry.
2. Following the perm directions, wrap two or three rods in the most delicate areas of the hair.
3. Wrap a coil of cotton around the rod.
4. Apply waving lotion to wrapped curls, being very careful not to allow the waving lotion to come in contact with unwrapped hair.
5. Set a timer and process the hair according to the perm directions.
6. Check the hair frequently.

To check a test curl, unfasten a rod and carefully (remember— hair is in a softened state) unwind the curl about 1½ turns of the rod. Do not permit the hair to become loose or unwound from the rod completely. Hold the hair firmly by placing a thumb at each end of the rod. Move the rod gently toward the scalp so that the hair falls loosely into the wave pattern. Continue checking the rods until a firm and definite "S" is formed. The "S" reflects the size of the rod used. (Fig. 11.47) Be guided by the manufacturer's direction.

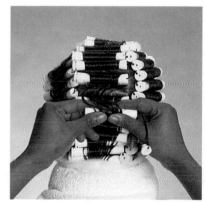

11.47—Unwinding hair carefully, without pulling or pushing.

▶ **NOTE:** When judging test curls, different hair textures with varying degrees of elasticity will have slightly different "S" formations. Fine, thin hair is generally softer and has less bulk. The wave ridge might be less defined and more difficult to read. Coarse, thick hair has better elasticity and seems to reinforce itself, falling into the wave pattern more readily. The wave ridge will be stronger and better defined. Long hair may produce a wider scalp wave than short hair, because larger rods are used and the diameter of the wave widens toward the scalp.

When the optimum curl has been formed, rinse the curls with warm water, blot the curls thoroughly, apply, process and rinse the neutralizer according to the perm directions and gently dry these test curls. Evaluate the curl results. If the hair is overprocessed, do not perm the rest of the hair until it is in better condition. If the test curl results are good, proceed with the perm, but *do not re-perm these preliminary test curls.*

Overprocessing

Any lotion that can properly process the hair also can overprocess it, causing dryness, frizziness, or hair damage. Overprocessed hair is easily detected. It is very curly when wet, but frizzy when dry. It cannot be combed into a suitable wave pattern, because the elasticity of the hair has been excessively damaged, and the hair feels harsh after being dried. Reconditioning treatments should begin immediately.

Causes of overprocessing are:

1. Lotion left on too long.
2. Improperly judged pre-perm hair analysis and/or waving lotion that was too strong.
3. Test curls were not made frequently enough or were judged improperly.

Underprocessing

Underprocessing is caused by insufficient processing time of the waving lotion. After perming, underprocessed hair has a limp or weak wave formation. The ridges are not well defined, and the hair retains little or no wave formation. Typically, after a few shampooings, the hair will have no curl pattern at all. (Fig. 11.48a–e)

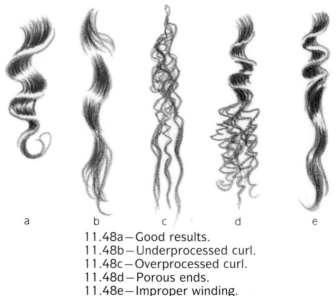

a   b   c   d   e

11.48a – Good results.
11.48b – Underprocessed curl.
11.48c – Overprocessed curl.
11.48d – Porous ends.
11.48e – Improper winding.

CAUTION

▶ *Underprocessed hair, even if there is no curl, has been chemically treated. If, in your professional judgment, you decide the hair can be re-permed, condition it first, choose a milder waving lotion, and test the curls frequently.*

Important Safety Precautions

Remember that the lotions used for perming contain chemically active ingredients and therefore must be used carefully to avoid injury to you and your client. The following precautions should always be taken:

1. Protect the client's clothing with a plastic shampoo cape, or ask the client to change into a smock.
2. Ask the client to remove glasses, earrings, and necklaces to prevent damage.
3. Do not give a perm to a client who has experienced an allergic reaction to a previous perm.
4. Do not save any opened, unused waving lotion or neutralizer. These lotions can change in strength and effectiveness if not used within a few hours after opening the container.
5. Do not dilute or add anything to the waving lotion or neutralizer unless the product directions tell you to do so.
6. Keep waving lotion out of eyes and away from the skin. If waving lotion should contact these areas, rinse *thoroughly* with cool water.
7. Do not perm and apply hair color to a client on the same day. Perm the hair first, wait one week, then apply hair color.

Perming Techniques

Before you begin perming, make sure you have all the necessary supplies at hand. Good organization and planning will help you develop precision and speed in completing a perm. At your station, the following equipment should be laid out in an organized, easily accessible fashion:

- The perm product
- Rods (organized by size)
- End wraps
- Cotton coil
- Towels
- Plastic hair clips and pins
- Tail comb
- Protective gloves

Always Read and Follow the Product Directions Carefully. Some alkaline perm product directions call for water wrapping, some are lotion wrapped, and others require pre-wrap lotions. Some wave lotions come in two parts that must be mixed just prior to use. Some need dryer heat. (*Note:* Dryer should be pre-heated.) Some perms require that a plastic cap be placed over the rods during the processing, others do not. Considering all the variables, it is not a good idea to trust your memory. Make it a practice to check the printed directions that accompany every perm *each time you give a perm*.

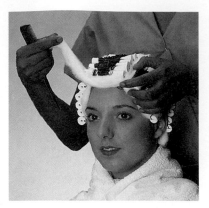

11.49—Hairline protected by cotton strips or neutralizing band.

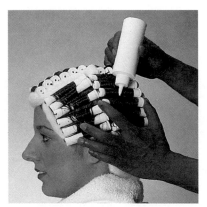

11.50—Applying waving lotion.

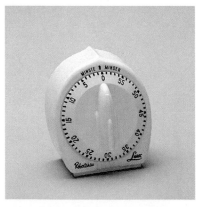

11.51—Processing timer.

APPLYING WAVING LOTION

After shampooing, shaping, and wrapping the hair, place a coil or band of cotton around the entire hairline. This safety precaution prevents waving lotion from coming into contact with the skin and possibly causing irritation. If lotion is applied accurately there should be a minimum of dripping, but the cotton is assurance of your client's comfort and safety. After the waving lotion has been applied, remove the cotton, gently pat the skin with water-soaked cotton, and replace with dry cotton. (Fig. 11.49)

Unless otherwise specified in the product instructions, apply waving lotion liberally to the top and underside of each wound rod. Start at the crown area and progress systematically down each section. Be sure that the surface area of the wound curls is wet with lotion so penetration is even. (Fig. 11.50)

Processing Time

Processing time is the length of time required for the hair strands to absorb the waving lotion (softening) and for the hair to re-curl (rearrangement of chemical bonds). It depends on the hair type (porosity, elasticity, length, density, texture, and overall condition) and the specific perm you are using. Again, follow the manufacturer's directions explicitly. It is usually safe to anticipate the processing time to be less than suggested by the manufacturer or a client's previous record card. Some perms have stop-action processing so that all you have to do is set a timer. (Fig. 11.51) Some perms give you a general timetable to follow and require that you do a test curl during processing. It is very important to accurately time the perm process to help prevent over- or under-processing.

The ability of the hair to absorb moisture may vary from time to time in the same individual, even when the same lotions and procedures are used. A record of the previous processing time is desirable, but should be used only as a guide.

Often, it is necessary to resaturate all the rods a second time during the processing time. This might be due to:

1. Evaporation of the lotion or dryness of the hair.
2. Hair poorly saturated by the cosmetologist.
3. No wave development after the maximum time indicated by the manufacturer.
4. Improper selection of solution strength for the client's hair.
5. Failure to follow the manufacturer's directions for a specific formula.

A reapplication of the lotion will hasten processing. Watch the wave development closely. ***Negligence can result in hair damage.***

Most manufacturers provide instructions with their product. Here are some you will encounter:

1. ***Place a plastic cap over the wrapped rods.*** Be sure that the plastic cap covers all the rods and that the cap is airtight. Secure the cap with a plastic clip. The cap holds in heat. If it is too loose or if all the rods are not covered, processing might take longer. (Fig. 11.52)

2. ***Pre-heated dryer.*** Turn the hood dryer to the high setting and medium airflow. Allow the dryer to warm up for approximately 5 minutes before placing your client under the dryer. (***Note:*** Dryer filters should be cleaned frequently so that optimum heat and airflow will remain constant.) (Fig. 11.53)

3. ***Process at room temperature.*** Make sure the client is not sitting in a draft or too close to an air-conditioner. A room that is too cool slows the processing time.

Testing Curls during Processing

Optimum curl development occurs only once during the processing time. The ability to read a test curl "S" formation and recognize proper wave development will help you avoid two of the most common problems in perming: overprocessing and underprocessing. Three test curls should be taken: in the crown, on top of the head, and on the side of the head. These three locations will allow you to judge the progress of curl development on the most resistant and the least resistant areas of the head. Follow the procedure for unwinding the rod and checking the "S" pattern formation described in the preliminary test curl section (pages 210–211). (Fig. 11.54)

Water Rinsing

Rinsing the waving lotion from the hair is extremely important. Any lotion left in the hair can cause poor perm results. When your test curl indicates that optimum curl has been achieved, remove the cotton from around the hairline. Rinse the hair thoroughly with a moderate force of warm water. The manufacturer's perm directions will indicate how long you should rinse—usually 3 to 5 minutes. Always set your timer for the exact time. Remember, you are rinsing the lotion *out* of the internal hair structure, not merely off the surface. Make sure that all rods are thoroughly rinsed. Pay special attention to the rods at the nape of the neck. They are a little difficult to reach, but they must be rinsed as well as all the other rods. Long hair and thick hair usually require the

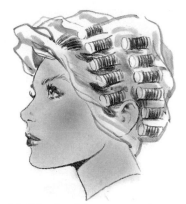

11.52—Applying processing cap.

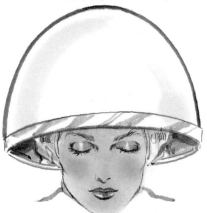

11.53—Putting client under pre-heated dryer.

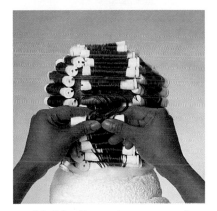

11.54—Properly processed strand opens up into "S" formation.

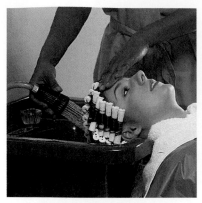

11.55—Rinsing waving lotion from the hair.

maximum rinsing time (5 minutes) to make sure that the lotion has been removed from all the hair wrapped around the rods. (Fig. 11.55)

Undesirable effects of improper or incomplete rinsing include:

1. *Early curl relaxation.* Even if the perm has been processed correctly, any waving lotion left in the hair can interfere with the action of the neutralizer. If the neutralizer is not able to properly rebond the hair, the curl will be weak or will not last very long.

2. *Lightening of hair color (natural or tint).* Rinsing helps reduce the pH of the hair and helps to close the cuticle layer. If the hair is not rinsed properly, the hydrogen peroxide in the neutralizer can react with waving lotion left in the hair and cause the hair color to lighten. This lightening effect is usually seen on the hair ends.

3. *Residual perm odor.* If any waving lotion is left in the hair, it will become trapped inside the hair when the neutralizer is applied. This is especially true of acid-balanced perms. Unpleasant odors may be evident each time the hair gets wet or damp.

Blotting after Water Rinsing

Careful blotting assures that the neutralizer will penetrate the hair immediately and completely: Do not omit this important step. To obtain the best results from towel blotting, carefully press a towel between each curl, using your fingers. Do not rock or roll the rods while blotting. When the hair is in a softened state, any such movement can cause hair breakage. Change to dry towels frequently in order to remove as much excess water as possible. Excess water left in the hair can dilute or weaken the action of the neutralizer. If this happens the curl can be either weak or relaxed. (Fig. 11.56)

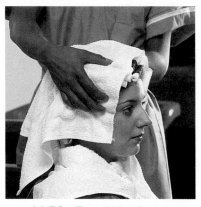

11.56—Towel blotting.

After rinsing and blotting has been completed, place a fresh, clean band of cotton around the hairline before applying neutralizer.

NEUTRALIZING

Neutralizing procedures can vary according to the perm product you are using. Again, follow the manufacturer's directions explicitly. In general, the following procedure is the accepted method for neutralizing:

1. Apply neutralizer to the top and underside of all rods. Apply to the top of the rod, then gently turn the rod up and apply to the underside of the rod in the same manner you applied the waving lotion.

2. Repeat the entire application a second time.

3. Wait 5 minutes to allow for optimum rebonding. Set a timer for accuracy. (Figs. 11.57, 11.58)

4. Remove the rods carefully and gently.

5. Work any remaining neutralizer through the hair gently with the palms of your hands.

6. Remove cotton from hairline and rinse the hair thoroughly with warm water.

7. Towel blot the hair.

Post-Perm Precautions

After blotting, your new perm is ready for final shaping and styling. It is important to avoid shampooing, conditioning, stretching, or excessive manipulations of freshly permed hair. When styling, do not pull on the hair or use intense heat that could result in curl relaxation. Generally, hair should not be shampooed, conditioned, or treated harshly for 48 hours after perming. This special care will help ensure that the perm does not relax.

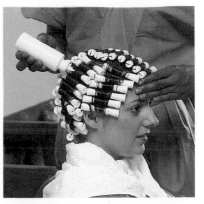

11.57 — Neutralizing — direct or on-the-rod method.

TEN POINTERS FOR A PERFECT PERM

1. Consult with the client.

2. Analyze the hair and scalp carefully.

3. Select the correct rod size for the desired style.

4. Choose the appropriate perm product for the hair type and final design. Follow the manufacturer's directions carefully.

5. Section and make accurate partings for each rod. Wrap specifically for the style chosen.

6. Apply waving lotion to the top and underside of all wound rods. Saturate thoroughly.

7. If the perm product requires a test curl, be sure the result is a firmly formed "S" shape.

8. Water rinse for at least 3 to 5 minutes and carefully towel blot each rod.

9. Apply neutralizer to the top and underside of all rods. Saturate thoroughly.

10. Wait 5 minutes, remove the rods carefully, apply any remaining neutralizer, and gently work through the hair. Rinse with warm water.

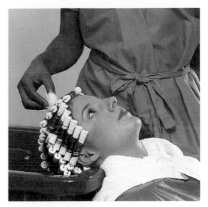

11.58 — Neutralizing — splash-on method.

CLEANUP

1. Discard all used supplies.

2. Clean up the work area.

3. Thoroughly clean and sanitize the rods and implements.

4. Wash and sanitize your hands.

5. Complete the client record card.

Special Perming Techniques

DIRECTIONAL WRAPPING

Directional wrapping refers to the angle of the partings, placement of the rods, and the wrapping pattern you choose to create specific direction or movement in the final design. There are six basic directions in which hair can be wrapped. (Figs. 11.59–11.70)

By using a combination of these basic wrapping directions you will be able to create very specific designs. Directional wrapping allows for lamp or natural drying and easier styling, particularly for the client. Use the following method for directional wrapping:

1. While the hair is wet, comb it in the direction that you want in your final design, including a part if one is required.
2. Use your fingers and a comb to mold a wave pattern as if you were finger waving.
3. Wrap the hair based on the direction of the design pattern.

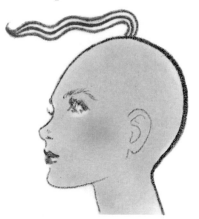

11.59—Vertical direction (forward).

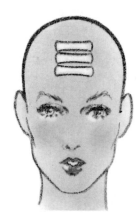

11.60—Forward blocking.

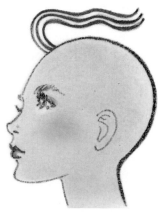

11.61—Vertical direction (back).

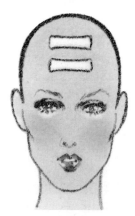

11.62—Back blocking.

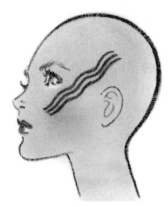

11.63—Horizontal direction (forward).

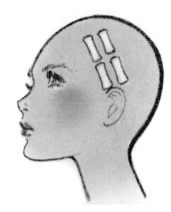

11.64—Forward blocking.

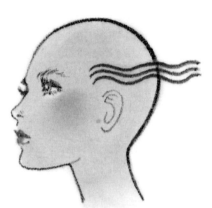

11.65—Horizontal direction (back).

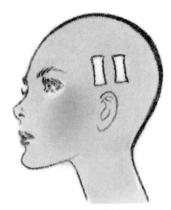

11.66—Back blocking.

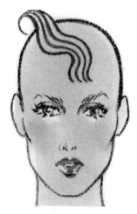

11.67—Diagonal direction (down).

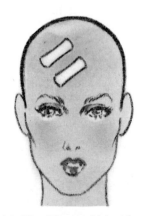

11.68—Diagonal blocking (down).

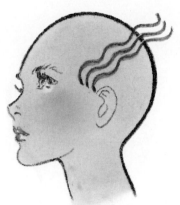

11.69—Diagonal direction (up).

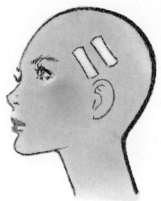

11.70—Diagonal blocking (up).

BODY WAVES

A body wave is a perm that gives support to a style, without definite curl. Large or extra large rods are used to give the hair softer, wider waves. Body waves are given when a softer curl or wave is desired. The wrapping patterns and techniques used for body waves are the same as those used for perming. Generally, the difference between perming and body waving is the size of rods. This affects the size of the final curl results.

The following are important considerations when giving a body wave:

1. Use large to extra large rods and make slightly larger partings. Do not take extra large partings or the waving lotion and neutralizer will not be able to penetrate all of the hair on the rod to properly form the curl/wave.
2. Follow perm directions regarding procedure, especially the processing time. Never reduce processing time to produce a softer curl/wave. Although the wave will be softer, it will be underprocessed and will not last very long.
3. Use straight rather than concave rods for body waving. The straight rods will give a more uniform wave from scalp to ends.

▶ NOTE: Body waves are softer and wider than regular perm curls because the physical force (hair wrapped around a very large rod) is not as great as in the standard perming method. The wave results from body waving will relax faster than a curl.

PARTIAL PERMING

Perming only a section of a whole head of hair is called *partial perming*. Partial perming can be used on:

1. Clients (male and female) who have long hair on the top and crown and very short, tapered sides and nape.
2. Clients who need volume and lift only in certain areas.
3. Designs that require curl support in the nape area but a smooth, sleek surface.

Partial perming uses the same techniques and wrapping patterns that you have already learned. There are a few extra considerations:

1. When you are wrapping the hair and reach the area that will be left unpermed, go to the next larger rod size so that the curl pattern of the permed hair will blend into the unpermed hair.
2. After wrapping the area to be permed, place a coil of cotton around the wrapped rods as well as around the entire hairline.
3. Before applying the waving lotion, apply a heavy, creamy conditioner to the sections that *will not* be permed to protect this hair from the effects of the waving lotion (waving lotion softens and straightens unwrapped hair).

PERMS FOR MEN

Many of your male clients need the added texture and fullness that only a perm can give. A perm can also help overcome common hair problems. A perm can redirect a cowlick, help limp or unmanageable hair more easily maintain a style, and make sparse hair look fuller.

Perming techniques are basically the same for both men and women. Most often, the partial perm technique gives you and your male clients the best results.

Keep in mind that men want waves for control. (Figs. 11.71–11.73)

HEATED CLAMP METHOD

This technique of perming involves the use of heated clamps applied directly over each wound rod. After the hair is wound on rods and thoroughly saturated with the waving lotion, a preheated clamp is placed on each curl. Processing begins as soon as the heat is applied. After the hair has been processed for a

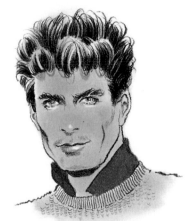

11.71—Man's short, curly style.

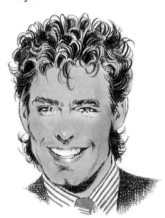

11.72—Man's medium length style.

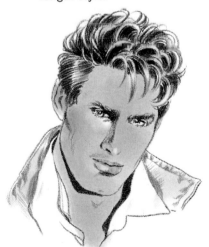

11.73—Man's short, wavy style.

pre-determined period of time, the clamps are removed and the hair is rinsed and neutralized in the usual manner.

There are three special control features of the heated clamp method:

1. The temperature of the rods is strictly controlled.
2. The processing does not start until the heat is applied.
3. All curls are processed for exactly the same length of time.

SPECIAL SITUATIONS

There are certain hair types and conditions that require special attention. There also are hair types that should not be permed. If you have any doubt about perming the hair successfully, make a preliminary test curl.

1. Hair that shows signs of damage or breakage should not be permed. If the hair is excessively dry, brittle, or over-porous, it should be given reconditioning treatments until the condition improves and the damaged areas can be cut off. When you determine that the condition of the hair has improved, choose a mild perm formula and make a complete preliminary test curl before giving the perm.
2. Hair that has been previously treated with a sodium hydroxide or "no lye" relaxer (or any hair straightener that does not require a neutralizing step) should not be permed. Relaxers and perms break different bonds in the hair structure. Since the bonds are not all completely re-formed, the use of both products on the same hair can result in severe hair damage or breakage.
3. Tinted, bleached, highlighted/frosted, or previously permed hair in good condition can usually be permed successfully if the correct perm formula is chosen. Generally, these hair types vary in porosity so a product with a pre-wrap lotion to fill in porous areas is usually the best choice.

▶ **NOTE:** Tinted hair usually refers to hair that has been treated with a permanent hair color that is mixed with 20 volume peroxide. If the hair has been tinted with an ultralight shade or higher than 20 volume peroxide, it should be treated as bleached hair, which is usually more delicate and porous.

4. Hair treated with a semi-permanent hair color (color that is not mixed with peroxide/developer and therefore does not lighten the natural color) is frequently resistant to perming because semi-permanent color coats the surface of the hair and slows down penetration of the waving lotion. Hair

treated with a semi-permanent color should be considered more resistant than tinted or color-treated (tint mixed with peroxide) hair. Perming can also cause discoloration of semi-permanent color. If you perm hair that has been treated with a semi-permanent color, it might be necessary to apply a temporary rinse after perming in order to even out the color. One week after perming you may reapply the semi-permanent color to achieve more acceptable and long-lasting color results.

5. Hair color restorers or progressive hair color darkeners contain metallic salts. These metallic salts form a residue on the hair, which interferes with the action of the waving lotion and can result in very uneven curls, severe discoloration, or hair damage.

   To determine if hair has been treated with a hair color restorer or darkener, a 1-20 test is recommended. In a glass bowl, mix 1 oz (30 ml) of 20 volume peroxide and 20 drops of 28% ammonia. Into this mixture immerse at least 20 strands of hair for 30 minutes.

   • If there are no metallic salts present, the hair will lighten slightly. You can perm the hair.
   • If hair strands lighten very rapidly, the hair contains lead. Do not perm.
   • If there is no reaction after 30 minutes, the hair contains silver. Do not perm.
   • If the solution begins to boil within a few minutes and a very unpleasant odor is evident, plus the hair pulls apart easily, then the hair contains copper. Do not perm.

   Hair coated with metallic salts must not be permed. Do not perm until the product has been cut out of the hair. Rerun the 1-20 test to be sure that the hair is no longer coated with metallic salts before perming.

6. Unmanageable, naturally curly hair with an uneven curl pattern can be permed to form larger, more defined curls that are easier to manage. Generally, the procedure for a body wave (page 220) is the best approach. Keep in mind that naturally curly hair, even if it is coarse and dense, can be very porous, so choose the perm formula carefully.

7. Once the hair is permed, your client should return for another perm every 3 to 4 months depending on how quickly the hair grows, the type of curl given, and how frequently the hair is cut. Before re-perming, carefully analyze the hair again, and if necessary, use a pre-wrap lotion and/or a milder waving lotion formula. Note the product and procedure used and the results achieved on the client's record card.

Review Questions

PERMANENT WAVING

1. Why is permanent waving beneficial to the client?
2. What is spiral wrapping?
3. What is croquignole wrapping?
4. What is a cold wave?
5. What is the purpose of a) waving lotion, b) neutralizer?
6. Define an acid-balanced perm.
7. What is "stop-action" processing?
8. What is an alkaline perm?
9. What is the main active ingredient or "reducing agent" in an a) alkaline perm, b) acid-balanced perm?
10. Name the acid-balanced perm that is heat activated by a chemical within the product.
11. What is the main ingredient in neutralizers?
12. What are the two main actions in permanent waving?
13. Define the three major components of hair.
14. Hair is composed almost entirely of a protein material called _____ .
15. What bonds must be broken in order for the perming process to occur?
16. How do you decide which perming technique is right for your client?
17. Why is pre-perm analysis important?
18. What is hair porosity?
19. What is a pre-wrap lotion?
20. What is hair texture?
21. What two factors determine processing time?
22. What is hair elasticity?
23. Define hair density.
24. What factor determines the size of a curl?
25. Name two types of permanent wave rods.
26. Name two factors that must be considered in choosing rod size.
27. Why is sectioning and blocking important in permanent waving?
28. Name two rules to follow when wrapping a perm rod.
29. How must the hair be wrapped on a perm rod?
30. What is the purpose of end wraps?
31. What are the three methods of end wrap application?
32. What is a test curl and how is it taken?

12

HAIR COLORING

LEARNING OBJECTIVES

After completing this chapter, you should be able to:

1. Explain the principles of color theory, and relate their importance to hair coloring.

2. List the classifications of hair color, explain their activity on the hair, and give examples of their use.

3. Demonstrate the correct preparation for hair coloring, including consultation and strand test procedures.

4. List the safety precautions to follow during hair coloring procedures.

5. Explain the activity of hydrogen peroxide in hair coloring.

6. Explain the uses of hair lighteners, and give examples when each type of lightener would be preferred.

7. List preventative and corrective steps to avoid or solve hair coloring problems.

225

Introduction

Hair coloring is both the science and art of changing the color of hair. Hair coloring includes the processes of:

1. Adding artificial pigment to the natural hair color.
2. Adding artificial pigment to previously colored hair.
3. Adding artificial pigment to pre-lightened hair.
4. Diffusing natural pigment and adding artificial pigment in one step.

(The terms "tinting" and "coloring" are used interchangeably in this text.)

Hair lightening involves the diffusing of the natural pigment or artificial color from the hair.

Skill in hair coloring and lightening is accomplished through continuous practice and study. These are profitable sources of salon income because coloring represents repeat business. The client who has tinted or lightened hair usually returns for retouching at regular intervals. Satisfactory service encourages the client to return to the same salon.

The principal reasons for coloring or lightening hair are:

1. To restore gray hair to its original color.
2. To change the natural color of hair to a more attractive shade.
3. To restore hair to its natural color.
4. To create decorative effects.
5. To enhance or create highlights.

Typical clients are:

1. Women and men who enjoy fashion changes.
2. Men and women with prematurely gray hair.
3. Women and men who wish to maintain a youthful appearance for business or personal reasons.

As a successful cosmetologist you should understand:

1. The composition of the hair and scalp.
2. The proper selection and application of coloring and lightening products.
3. The chemical reactions of tints and lighteners on hair.

▶ **NOTE:** This chapter contains many technical terms. You should refer to the Hair Coloring Glossary on page 272. This glossary was prepared by the International Haircolor Exchange for the purpose of providing a standard vocabulary of hair coloring for our industry.

Color Theory

It is important that you understand the theory of color pigment before you begin applying hair coloring products to clients' hair. It is only through knowledge of color theory that you can think your way through color problems to the correct color formulation for each situation.

Color is created by the movement of rays of light, as they are either absorbed or reflected by artificial pigment added to the hair in the tinting process or by natural pigment found in the hair.

Natural hair color is created by the reflection or absorption of light rays by melanin. Melanin is the type of pigment found in the cortex of the hair shaft. The size, amount, and distribution of melanin determine the color of the hair. Greater amounts of large melanin molecules distributed throughout the cortex create dark colors. Lesser amounts of smaller melanin molecules distributed throughout the cortex create light colors. The great variety of combinations in the size, amount, and distribution of melanin create all natural hair colors.

This phenomenon of nature is simulated in the hair coloring process to create colors that almost duplicate nature. It is the selective absorption or reflection of light rays by certain pigment molecules that creates every color in the world. For example, when we see the color red, it means that the yellow, red, and orange light rays are reflected to the eye while the blue, green, and violet rays are absorbed by the pigment.

Color scientists have used this phenomenon as a basis to establish certain laws of light reflection and absorption. These laws, known as the *laws of color*, provide the basic concepts by which cosmetologists, artists, fashion designers, paint manufacturers, and anyone else using color can understand the way that different colors are formed.

THE LAWS OF COLOR

The laws of color regulate the mixing of dyes and pigment to make other colors. They are based in science and adapted to art. The laws of color serve as guidelines for harmonious color mixing. (Fig. 12.1)

Primary Colors

Primary colors are basic or true colors that are not created by combining other colors. The three primary colors are yellow, red, and blue. All other colors are created by some combination of red, yellow, or blue. (Fig. 12.1)

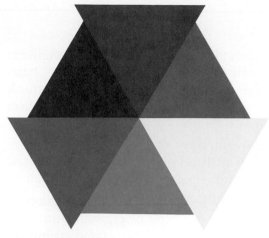

Primary

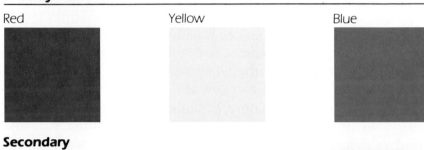

Secondary

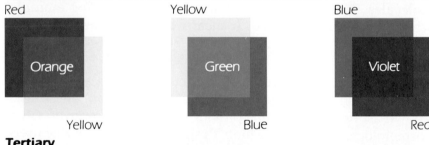

Tertiary

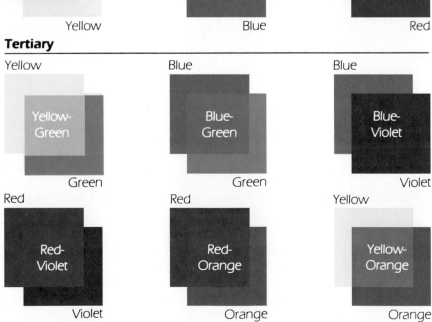

12.1 — The laws of color.

Secondary Colors

Secondary colors are created by mixing equal amounts of two primary colors. Mixed in equal parts, yellow and blue create green, blue and red create violet, and red and yellow create orange. (Fig. 12.1)

Tertiary Colors

Tertiary colors are created by mixing equal amounts of one primary color with one of its adjacent secondary colors. The tertiary colors are red-violet, blue-violet, blue-green, yellow-green, yellow-orange, and red-orange. (Fig. 12.1)

Quaternary Colors

Quaternary colors are all other combinations that create any color that has not been previously described.

Complementary Colors

Complementary colors are any two colors situated directly across from each other on the color wheel. When mixed together their action is to neutralize each other. For example, when mixed in equal amounts, red and green neutralize each other, creating brown. Orange and blue neutralize each other, and yellow and violet neutralize each other. Complementary colors are always composed of a primary and a secondary color. Complementary pairs always consist of all three primary colors. For example, if you look at the color wheel, you see that the complement of red (a primary color) is green (a secondary color). Green is made up of blue and yellow (both primary colors)—so all three primaries are represented in this complementary pair.

Tone

Tone refers to whether a color is warm or cool. The warm colors—also known as highlighting colors—are red, orange, and yellow. The cool colors—also known as ash or drab—are blue, green, and violet.

Level

Level indicates the degree of lightness or darkness of a color. Every color can be made either lighter or darker, thus changing the level, by the addition of white or black. Hair colors, both natural and color treated, are classified by level on a scale of 1 to 10, 1 indicating black and 10 indicating the lightest blonde.

Saturation

Saturation refers to the degree of concentration or amount of pigment in the color. For example, a saturated red is very vivid. Any color can be more saturated or less saturated. A more saturated product creates a dramatic change in hair color.

Classifications of Hair Coloring

Hair coloring falls into three main categories: temporary, semi-permanent, and permanent. These classifications refer primarily to color fastness. As a professional colorist you should understand the differences between each classification.

TEMPORARY HAIR COLORING

Temporary hair colorings are designed to remain on the hair from shampoo to shampoo. Temporary color can only deposit pigment; it cannot lighten. (Fig. 12.2) On excessively porous hair this type of hair coloring lasts longer, gradually fading with each shampoo. A patch test is usually not necessary for this type of hair color. Consult the manufacturer's directions.

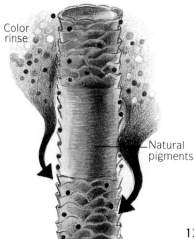

Color rinse

Natural pigments

12.2—Action of temporary hair color.

Types of Temporary Hair Coloring

1. Color rinses are prepared rinses used either to highlight or add color to the hair. These rinses contain *certified colors*, and remain on the hair until the next shampoo.

    Color rinses are now available as creams and gels, and have been added to lightweight setting agents in the form of mousses.
2. Highlighting color shampoos combine the action of a color rinse with that of a shampoo. These shampoos add highlights and color tones to the hair.
3. Crayons and mascara are temporary colors used to add color to eyebrows and lashes.
4. Hair color sprays are applied to dry hair from aerosol containers. These are generally used for special or party effects.

SEMI-PERMANENT HAIR COLORING

Semi-permanent hair colorings are formulated to last three to four weeks. They have a mild penetrating action that results in a gentle addition of color in the cortex as well as some coating of the cuticle. Semi-permanent colors do not change the basic structure of the hair and therefore cannot lighten the natural color of the hair.

Semi-permanent colors are used:

1. To cover or blend partially gray hair without affecting its natural color. Most semi-permanent colors are designed to cover hair that is 25% or less gray.
2. To enhance or blend partially gray hair without affecting its natural color. This can be done successfully on almost any percentage of gray, depending upon the desired color.
3. To highlight and enhance the color tones of the hair. Semi-permanent colors can be used to add golden or red highlights, and to deepen the color of the hair. This type of color is especially effective on ethnic clients and clients whose natural hair color is too light or too drab to set off their complexions.
4. To serve as a non-peroxide toner for pre-lightened hair. Pre-lightened hair is porous and the toner will penetrate.

The following illustration (Fig. 12.3) indicates how this type of hair coloring works on the hair shaft.

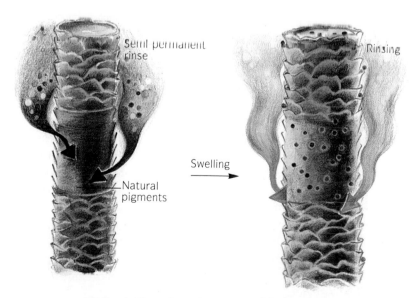

12.3—Action of semi-permanent hair color.

PERMANENT HAIR COLORING

Permanent hair colorings are designed to penetrate the cuticle and deposit molecules into the cortex. Due to the penetration and the addition of peroxide, these colors can both *lift* and *deposit*. (Fig. 12.4)

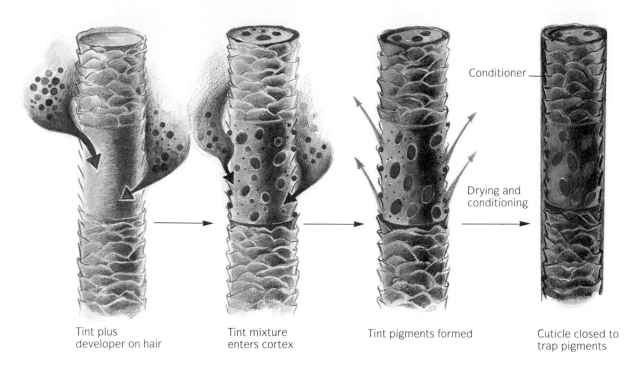

Tint plus developer on hair

Tint mixture enters cortex

Tint pigments formed

Conditioner

Drying and conditioning

Cuticle closed to trap pigments

12.4—Action of permanent hair color.

Permanent hair colors fall into four classifications: oxidation tints, vegetable tints, metallic dyes, and compound dyes.

1. *Oxidation tints* are also known as *aniline derivative tints, penetrating tints, synthetic-organic tints,* and *amino tints.* Tints can lighten and deposit color in a single process and are available in a wide variety of colors. Toners also fall into the category of permanent color. Toners are aniline derivative products of pale, delicate shades designed for use on pre-lightened hair.

    Most oxidation tints contain aniline derivatives and require a *predisposition test* before the service. As long as the hair is of normal strength and kept in good condition, oxidation tints are compatible with other professional chemical services.

Oxidation tints are sold in bottles, canisters, and tubes in either a semi-liquid or cream form. These products must be mixed with hydrogen peroxide, which activates the chemical reaction known as oxidation. This reaction begins as soon as the two compounds are combined, so the mixed tint must be used immediately. Any leftover tint must be discarded since it deteriorates quickly.

Timing the application of the tint depends upon the product and the volume of peroxide selected. Consult the manufacturer's directions and your instructor for assistance. A test strand should always be taken to ensure satisfactory results.

2. *Vegetable tints* are hair coloring products made from various plants, such as herbs and flowers. In the past, indigo, camomile, sage, Egyptian henna, and other plants were used to color the hair. Henna is still used as a professional hair coloring product, but it should be used with some caution. Henna has a coating action that, if overused, can build up on the hair and prevent penetration of other chemicals. Henna also penetrates the cortex and attaches to the salt bonds. Both of these actions may leave the hair unfit for other professional treatments.

3. *Metallic* or *mineral dyes* are advertised as "color restorers" or "progressive colors." The metallic ingredients, such as lead acetate or silver nitrate, react with the keratin in the hair, turning it brown. This reaction creates a colored film coating which creates a dull metallic appearance. Repeated treatments damage the hair and can react adversely with many professional chemical services. Metallic dyes are *not* professional coloring products.

4. *Compound dyes* are a combination of metallic or mineral dyes with a vegetable tint. The metallic salts are added to give the product more staying power and to create different colors. Like metallic dyes, compound dyes are *not* used professionally.

Many clients buy and use hair coloring products at home. Therefore, you must be able to recognize and understand their effects. Such coloring agents must be removed and the hair reconditioned prior to any other chemical service.

Hair treated with a metallic or any other coating dye looks dry and dull. It is generally harsh and brittle to the touch. These colorings usually fade to unnatural tones. Silver dyes have a greenish cast, lead dyes leave a purple color, and those containing copper turn red.

TEST FOR METALLIC SALTS AND COATING DYES

1. In a glass container, mix one ounce (30 ml) of 20 volume (6%) peroxide and 20 drops of 28% ammonia water.
2. Cut a strand of the client's hair, bind it with tape, and immerse in the solution for 30 minutes.
3. Remove, towel dry, and observe the strand.

Hair dyed with lead will lighten immediately. Hair treated with silver will show no reaction at all. This indicates that other chemicals will not be successful because they will not be able to penetrate the coating.

Hair treated with copper will start to boil, and will pull apart easily. This hair would be severely damaged or destroyed if other chemicals such as those found in permanent colors or perm solutions were applied to it.

Hair treated with a coating dye either will not change color or will lighten in spots. This hair will not receive chemical services easily, and the length of time necessary for penetration may very well damage the hair.

REMOVING COATINGS FROM THE HAIR

Preparations designed to remove metallics, and non-peroxide dye solvents may assist in the removal of metallic and coating dyes from the hair. The most effective guarantee of future successful chemical services is to cut the tinted hair off.

TEST FOR ALLERGY

Allergy to aniline derivative tints is unpredictable. Some clients may be sensitive, and others may suddenly develop a sensitivity after years of use. To identify an allergic client, the U.S. Federal Food, Drug, and Cosmetic Act prescribes that a patch or predisposition test be given 24 to 48 hours prior to each application of an aniline derivative tint or toner.

CAUTION

▶ *Aniline derivative tints must never be used on the eyelashes or eyebrows. To do so may cause blindness.*

Preparation for Hair Coloring

CONSULTATION

Consultation is one of the most important steps in the hair coloring service. The finest formulation combined with the most talented application will still result in color failure if the client is dissatisfied.

Always record the consultation on the client's record card. Perform the consultation in a well-lighted room, preferably with natural lighting. If this is not possible, arrange lighting so that there is incandescent in front of the client (around the mirror) and fluorescent behind the colorist (ceiling fixtures).

When talking with the client, consider what colors will suit the skin tones, and how those tones may change with maturity. Also consider the client's personality and life-style. For example, a coloring procedure that requires a great deal of care may be impractical for a very active person. Pale blonde may be the wrong choice for someone who swims regularly (pool chemicals can turn blonde hair green). An iridescent eggplant color could be inadvisable for someone who works in a conservative law firm. Advise your clients to use a high-quality shampoo at home that will not strip the color, as well as conditioners to maintain the condition of the hair.

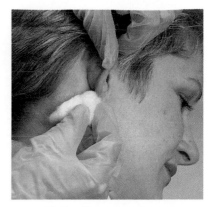

12.5—Clean patch test area.

PREDISPOSITION TEST

The patch test, or predisposition test, must be given 24 to 48 hours before each tinting or toner treatment. The tint used for the skin test must be the same formula as that used for the hair coloring service.

Procedure

1. Select test area, behind one ear, extending into the hairline.
2. Cleanse an area about the size of a quarter. (Fig. 12.5) Be guided by your state board of cosmetology and your instructor as to the correct solution to use for cleansing.
3. Dry the area.
4. Prepare the test solution according to the manufacturer's directions. (Fig. 12.6)
5. Apply to test area with a sterile cotton swab. (Fig. 12.7)
6. Leave the area undisturbed for 24 to 48 hours.
7. Examine the test area.
8. Note results on client's record card.

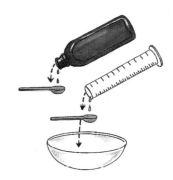

12.6—Mix tint and peroxide.

Alternate Method

A patch test can also be given on the arm.

A negative skin test will show no sign of inflammation, and an aniline tint may be safely applied.

If the skin test is positive you will see redness, swelling, burning, itching, and blisters. A client with these symptoms is allergic, and under no circumstances should receive an aniline derivative tint. Application of an aniline tint in this instance could result in a serious reaction for the client, and a malpractice suit for the hair colorist.

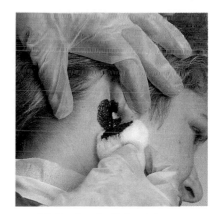

12.7—Apply tint mixture.

EXAMINING SCALP AND HAIR

Carefully examine the scalp and hair to determine if it is safe to use a hair coloring product, and whether any special hair problems exist.

The results of such an examination may indicate the need for any of the following:

1. Reconditioning treatments.
2. Color removal.
3. Removal of metallic coloring.
4. Postponement of service due to breakage, or some other problem.

An aniline derivative tint should not be used if the following conditions are noted:

Positive skin test
Scalp irritations or eruptions
Contagious scalp or hair disorders
Presence of metallic or compound dyes

All information about the condition of a client's hair should be recorded on the client's record card.

FORMULATING COLORS

The laws of color should be considered as you begin to formulate colors for application to a client's hair. Most hair colors represent a balance of colors, which means that they generally contain a balance of each of the primary colors. However, colors will have a predominant base and a level of lightness or darkness that must be identified before formulating a tint for the hair.

Oxidation tints are classified by the predominant base and the level of color formulated by the manufacturer. Most manufacturers provide literature that identifies the level and base color for you. As a professional cosmetologist you may identify the level and base color of the client's hair by comparing it to the manufacturer's color identification chart. Cool colors are formulated with blue, green, or violet as their predominant base color. Warm colors are formulated with yellow, orange, or red as their predominant base color. All colors—warm, cool, or neutral—can be formulated in tones that range from the lightest blonde to the darkest black.

The following chart will help you in your selection. Remember that each person is unique, however, and consult with your instructor. (See also Fig. 12.8, The Color Key System)

HAIR COLOR SELECTION CHART

Skin Tone Range	Eye Color	Hair Color Options
Warm, Yellow-red Undertones such as:		
Ivory, Peaches and cream, Creamy beige, Light golden brown, Café au lait, Tawny, Coppery, Deep golden brown, Golden-red brown	Blue, Blue-green, Hazel, Green, Topaz, Amber, Cinnamon, Coffee bean	Golden highlights, Golden with red highlights, Golden brown, Honey brown, Chestnut, Copper, Auburn, Mahogany, Warm tones of gray, Warm tones of white
Cool, Blue-red Undertones such as:		
Alabaster, Rosy pink, Rose beige, Light pearl, Light olive (green), Dark olive (green), Gray-brown (light to dark), Dark brown, Ebony	Light blue, Gray-blue, Gray-green, Blue-green, Deep blue, Deep green, Brown (medium to dark), Black	Plum, Burgundy highlights, Ash, Platinum blonde, Ash brown (medium to dark), Dark brown, Black, Slate, Salt and pepper, Pure white

BASIC RULES FOR COLOR SELECTION

1. Make sure the client's hair is clean and dry.
2. Look through the hair. To see depth as well as highlights, raise the hair by pushing it up with the hands against the scalp.
3. Analyze the depth present in the hair. Does the client want to go lighter or darker?
4. Analyze the depth of the desired color. Add or subtract from the natural color to determine the level of color necessary.
5. What are the natural highlights? What highlights does the client want? Select the color within the level that will supply those highlights, or determine what primary additive should be used.

Color Key 1

YOUR NATURAL EYE COLORS

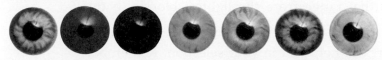

YOUR NATURAL HAIR COLORS AND MOST FLATTERING TINTS

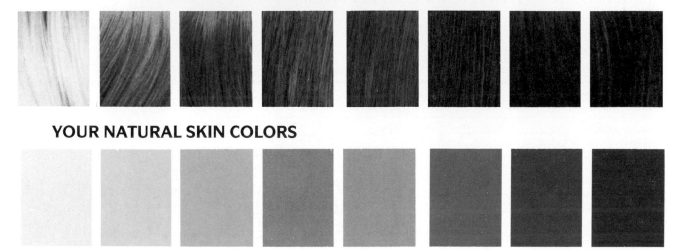

YOUR NATURAL SKIN COLORS

MAKEUP AND WARDROBE COLORS FOR PERSONS IN COLOR KEY 1

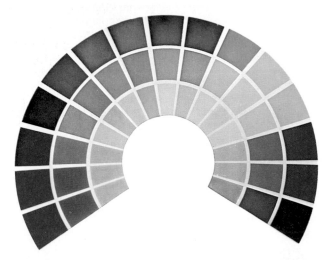

The purpose of this chart is to help you select your client's best colors for makeup, hair color and wardrobe; colors that will harmonize with their complexion tones. In Color Key 1, blue pigmentation predominates the undertones of the skin. When selecting a person's Color Key, the natural eye colors in the chart will be helpful in determining their correct Color Key. Light-skinned people who have a blue-pink undertone to their complexions, therefore, fall into Color Key 1. Some people in Color Key 1 have an olive undertone. Dark-skinned people in Color Key 1 may have a charcoal, or occasionally an ashen gray hue to their dark complexions. If you determine that a client's personal coloring is in Color Key 1, always choose colors from the Color Key 1 selection.

12.8—The Color Key System.

Color Key 2

YOUR NATURAL EYE COLORS

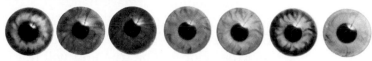

YOUR NATURAL HAIR COLORS AND MOST FLATTERING TINTS

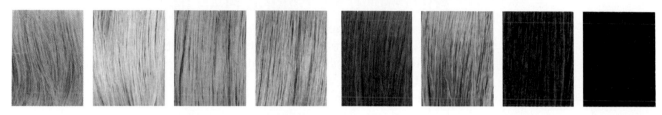

YOUR NATURAL SKIN COLORS

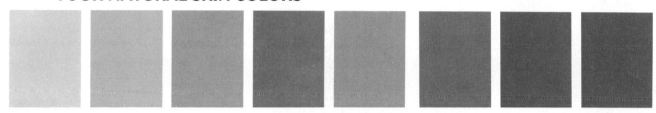

MAKEUP AND WARDROBE COLORS FOR PERSONS IN COLOR KEY 2

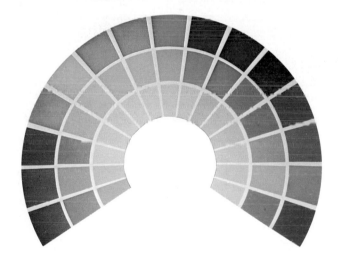

The purpose of this chart is to help you select your client's best colors for makeup, hair color and wardrobe; colors that will harmonize with their complexion tones. In Color Key 2, yellow pigmentation predominates. Light-skinned people with a peach-pink undertone to their complexion will, therefore, fall into Color Key 2. Dark-skinned people in Color Key 2 have a golden undertone. If you determine that a client's personal coloring is in Color Key 2, always choose colors from the Color Key 2 selection.

6. Know the properties of the product you are using. Consult the manufacturer's information on each color when applied to light, medium, or dark hair.

7. Analyze the condition of the hair, especially its porosity. Does the hair need to be conditioned prior to the service so that the color will be true and will not fade?

FOLLOWING A WORKING PLAN IN TINTING

For successful hair coloring services, the technician must follow a definite procedure. A system makes for the greatest efficiency, and the most satisfactory results. Without such a plan, the work will take longer, results will be uneven, and mistakes will be made.

A working plan includes the materials and supplies needed for the tinting service, and a thorough knowledge of the product to be used.

Keep a permanent record of each client's color service.

Business Tips

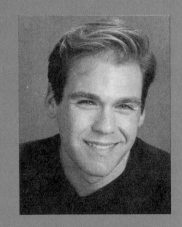

Once you know how to do color, you have to learn to sell color. According to Michael Stinchcomb, color director at Yves Claude Salon, New York City, the key to selling is conducting a successful consultation.

Says Stinchcomb, who sees over 100 color clients a week, "Most women want to sit down and simply ask you what's best. Don't answer this question too quickly, because if you tell her she'd make a great redhead and she hates red, she'll think that you can't ever see her as she sees herself. Instead, ask her what she likes and dislikes about her color and listen for clues about her lifestyle and self-image.

"Once you know that the client wants a new color, or to go brighter or darker, offer some options. Cients have a built-in prejudice about peroxide and are afraid of becoming slaves to color. A little education about semi-permanent, permanent, and no-peroxide colors will gain their confidence and show that there are ways to achieve hair color without a commitment to constant touch-ups. Tell your clients what they can't have, too. For instance, if a woman wants to cover gray but avoid outgrowth, let her know this isn't possible, but that if you add highlights, the outgrowth will be camouflaged and the hair won't need a retouch as often.

"As you select an actual color, look through magazines with her. Swatches are too exact and she'll expect a perfect match. Also, looking at magazines will tell you what she's drawn to and will give you a common language. You'll know something about her preferences and if what you call 'ash,' she calls 'golden.'

"When you select the actual color, always use skin tone and eye color to determine your tonal value and you'll never go wrong."

KEEPING HAIR COLOR RECORDS

It is of the utmost importance to keep an accurate record so that successful services can be repeated and any difficulties encountered in one service may be avoided in the next. A complete record should be kept, containing all analysis notes, strand test and whole head results, timing, and suggestions for the next service. A sample hair color record is shown.

```
┌──────────────── HAIR COLOR RECORD ─────────────────┐
│ Name ..........................  Tel. .............. │
│ Address .......................  City .............. │
│ Patch Test: Negative ☐  Positive ☐    Date ........ │
│ DESCRIPTION OF HAIR                                  │
│                                                      │
│ Form        Length     Texture      Porosity         │
│ ☐ straight  ☐ short    ☐ coarse    ☐ very porous  ☐ resistant │
│ ☐ wavy      ☐ medium   ☐ medium    ☐ porous       ☐ very resistant │
│ ☐ curly     ☐ long     ☐ fine      ☐ normal       ☐ perm. waved │
│                                                      │
│ Natural hair color ................................. │
│                                                      │
│ Condition                                            │
│ ☐ normal  ☐ dry  ☐ oily  ☐ faded  ☐ streaked  ...... % gray │
│ Previously lightened with ............... for...... (time) │
│ Previously tinted with ............. for ........ (time) │
│ ☐ original sample enclosed   ☐ not enclosed         │
│ Desired hair color ................................. │
│ CORRECTIVE TREATMENTS                                │
│ Color filler used .......... Corrective treatments with ...... │
│ HAIR TINTING PROCESS                                 │
│ whole head ....... retouch ....... inches (cm) shade desired ...... │
│ Formula: color .......... lightener ................ │
│ Results:                                             │
│ ☐ good   ☐ poor   ☐ too light   ☐ too dark   ☐ streaked │
│   Date   Operator   Price    Date   Operator   Price │
│   ...................    .................... │
│   ...................    .................... │
│   ...................    .................... │
└──────────────────────────────────────────────────────┘
```

STRAND TEST TO CONFIRM COLOR SELECTION

Before applying a tint, conduct a preliminary strand test to confirm your selection. You will learn the following information:

1. Whether the proper color selection was made.
2. Timing needed to achieve desired results.

3. If further pre-conditioning treatments are needed.
4. If it is necessary to apply a *filler*.

Strand Test Procedure

1. Mix a small amount of color with peroxide according to the manufacturer's directions.
2. Apply mixture to a ½" (1.25 cm) section, usually in the crown area of the head.

▶ NOTE: It is important that the hair has received all pre-treatments necessary according to your analysis before the strand test is given, so that the results will be accurate.

3. Process with or without heat according to the manufacturer's directions, keeping careful records of timing on the client's record card.
4. Rinse strand, shampoo, towel dry, and examine results. Adjust formula, timing, or pre-conditioning necessary and proceed with tinting on entire head.
5. If results are unsatisfactory, adjust the formula and repeat the process on a new test strand.

RELEASE STATEMENT

A release statement is used for chemical services. It releases the school or salon owner from responsibility for accidents or damages, and is required for some malpractice insurance. A sample release is provided.

RELEASE FORM

I, the undersigned, ...
(name)

residing at . . . .
(street, address)

. . . .
(city, state and zip)

about to receive services in the Clinical Department of

. . . .

and having been advised that the services shall be performed by either students, graduate students and/or instructors of the school, in consideration of the nominal charge for such services, hereby release the school, its students, graduate students, instructors, agents, representatives and/or employees, from any and all claims arising out of and in any way connected with the performance of these services.

The Proprietor Is Not Responsible For Personal Property

Signed . . . .

Date . . . .

Witnessed . . . .

THIS RELEASE FORM MUST BE SIGNED BY THE PARENT OR GUARDIAN IF THE CLIENT BEING SERVED IS UNDER 21 YEARS OF AGE.

Temporary Coloring

Temporary color coats the cuticle of the hair with a film of color pigment. Since the color remains on the cuticle and does not penetrate into the cortex, it lasts only from shampoo to shampoo. However, excessive porosity can allow temporary color to penetrate, making it last much longer. Temporary colors usually contain certified colors, colors which have been approved by the FDA for use in cosmetics.

Temporary colors can be used for the following advantages:

1. To bring out highlights in the hair.
2. To temporarily restore faded hair to its natural color.
3. To neutralize the yellowish tinge in white or gray hair.
4. To tone down overlightened hair.
5. To temporarily add color to the hair without changing the condition of the hair.
6. To perform hair coloring without a required skin test.

Temporary hair colorings also have several disadvantages:

1. Color is of short duration; it must be applied after every shampoo.
2. Coating is thin and may not cover hair evenly.
3. Color may rub off on pillow, collar, etc., and may run with perspiration or other moisture.
4. They can only add color; they cannot lift.
5. Staining may result if the hair is porous, or if a dark color is used on very light hair.

For the clients who want to highlight the color of their hair or glamorize gray hair, a temporary color is very helpful. Temporary colors come in a wide array of colors from light to dark, warm to cool. They are applied easily and are valuable as an introduction to hair coloring.

METHODS OF APPLICATION

There are many methods of application, depending upon the product used. Your instructor will help you interpret the manufacturer's directions.

Implements and Materials

Neck strip	Towels	Protective gloves
Shampoo cape	Comb	Applicator bottle (optional)
Temporary color	Shampoo	Record card

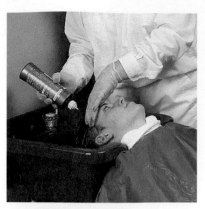

12.9—Apply temporary rinse.

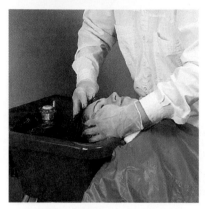

12.10—Blend rinse through hair.

Procedure

The hair is first shampooed and towel dried. Make sure that the client is protected with the neck strip and cape as temporary coloring can easily stain skin and clothing.

1. Client should be comfortably reclined at the shampoo bowl.
2. Apply color. Use an applicator bottle as directed by your instructor. (Fig. 12.9)
3. Apply rinse through entire hair shaft and comb through. (Fig. 12.10)
4. Blend the color with a comb, applying more color as necessary.
5. *Do not* rinse hair.
6. Proceed with styling as desired.

Cleanup

1. Discard all disposable supplies and materials.
2. Close containers, wipe them off, and store in proper place.
3. Clean and sanitize implements.
4. Organize and sanitize work area.
5. Wash and sanitize hands.
6. Record results and file record card.

Alternate Methods

Temporary color is also available in the form of gels, mousses, foams, and sprays. To apply, return the client to your work area and apply color as directed by the manufacturer.

Semi-Permanent Coloring

Semi-permanent color offers a form of hair coloring suitable for the client who is reluctant to have a permanent color change. The semi-permanent color is formulated to be more lasting than temporary but milder than permanent color techniques.

Semi-permanent color may be excellent for the client who feels that his or her hair is dull, drab, or showing gray, but is not ready to begin permanent hair coloring. Semi-permanent color can add highlights, blend gray, and deepen color tones without altering the natural color, since there is no lightening action on the hair.

Semi-permanent color is often chosen by younger clients as fashion trends change. Semi-permanent color can deposit a dramatic color, or even be used for special effect streaks in bright colors. The color will naturally fade without a regrowth, so the client can change the color at any time, or discontinue the effect.

Semi-permanent color is available in a wide range of shades. It can be purchased as a gel, cream, liquid, or mousse. Results depend on the original color of the hair, the porosity, processing time, and technique.

Semi-permanent hair color is formulated to last 4 to 6 shampoos. No hydrogen peroxide is required. The color molecules penetrate the cuticle somewhat so that the color gradually fades with each shampoo. No retouching is required. If the hair is extremely porous, or if heat is used with some types of semi-permanent color, the results can be more permanent.

Semi-permanent coloring can have the following advantages:

1. The color is self-penetrating.
2. The color is applied the same way each time.
3. Retouching is not necessary.
4. Color does not rub off on pillow or clothing.
5. Hair returns to its natural color after 4 to 6 shampoos.

Semi-permanent tints containing aniline derivatives require a patch test. Follow the manufacturer's directions carefully.

TYPES

1. Semi-permanent tints that cover gray completely, but do not affect the remaining pigmented hair.
2. Semi-permanent tints that enhance gray hair without changing the natural pigment.
3. Semi-permanent tints that add color and highlights to hair that is not gray.
4. Translucent tints that add gloss, highlights, and sometimes special effects to the hair. These colors vary in their effect according to porosity, heat application, and timing. Consult your instructor and product information for assistance with these products.

Implements and Materials

Neck strip	Applicator bottle or brush	Finishing rinse
Towels		Plastic clips
Tint cape	Cotton	Plastic cap (optional)
Protective gloves	Mild shampoo	Protective cream
Comb	Selected color	Record card
Timer	Color chart	

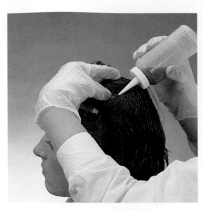

12.11—Apply semi-permanent color.

Preliminary Steps

1. Give preliminary patch test if required. Proceed only if test is negative.
2. Thoroughly analyze hair and scalp. Record results on client's record card.
3. Assemble all necessary supplies.
4. Prepare client. Protect clothing with towel and tint cape. Ask client to remove jewelry and put safely away.
5. Apply protective cream around hairline and over ears.
6. Put on protective gloves.
7. Perform a strand test.
8. Record results on client's card.

Procedure

1. Give a mild shampoo, if required.
2. Towel dry hair.
3. Put on protective gloves.
4. Apply semi-permanent tint to entire hair shaft, (Fig. 12.11) starting near the scalp and gently working color through ends. (Fig. 12.12) Apply with bottle or brush according to the consistency of the color selected and your instructor's directions. (Fig. 12.13)
5. Pile hair loosely on top of head.
6. Follow the manufacturer's directions about using a plastic cap or heat. (Fig. 12.14)

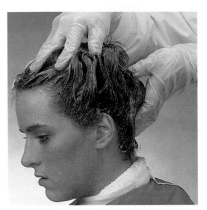

12.12—Gently work color through hair.

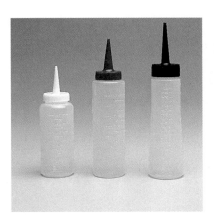

12.13—Tint bottles.

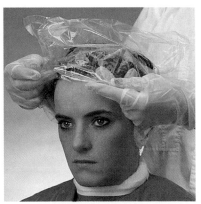

12.14—Use plastic cover if required.

7. Process according to strand test results.
8. According to the timing instructions provided by the manufacturer, when color has developed, wet hair with warm water and lather.

9. Rinse, then shampoo, if the manufacturer recommends it, then rinse again with warm water until water is clear. (Fig. 12.15)
10. Use a finishing rinse to close the cuticle and set color. (Fig. 12.16)
11. Rinse and towel blot hair. Style as desired.
12. Complete record card and file.

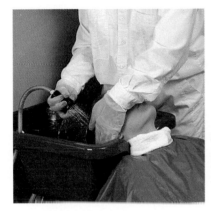
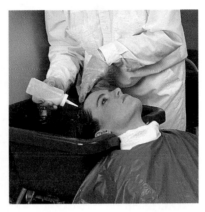

12.15—Rinse hair with warm water until it is clear.

12.16—Give a finishing rinse.

Cleanup

1. Discard all disposable supplies and materials.
2. Close containers, wipe them off, and store safely.
3. Clean and sanitize implements.
4. Clean and sanitize tint cape.
5. Sanitize work area.
6. Wash and sanitize hands.

Permanent Hair Coloring

Practically all permanent hair coloring is done with the use of oxidizing penetrating tints which contain aniline derivatives.

These tints penetrate the cuticle of the hair and enter the cortical layer. Here, they are oxidized by the peroxide added into color pigments. These pigments are distributed throughout the hair shaft much like natural pigment.

APPLICATION CLASSIFICATIONS

Permanent hair color applications are classified as either single-process coloring or double-process coloring.

Single-process coloring achieves the desired color with one application. While the application itself may have several different steps, the desired color is achieved with a single application. Single-process coloring is also known as single-application tinting and one-step coloring. Some examples are virgin tint applications, tint retouch applications.

Double-process coloring achieves the desired color upon completion of two separate applications of products. It is also known as double-application tinting and two-step coloring. Two examples are bleaching followed by a toner application and pre-softening followed by a tint application.

CAUTION

A predisposition test must be given before coloring the hair with an aniline derivative product. The client should be draped to protect clothing. You should protect yourself from allergic reactions by wearing gloves until the product is completely removed from the client's hair.

SINGLE-PROCESS TINTS

Single-process tints have the ability to both lighten and deposit pigment at one time to achieve the desired color. Pre-lightening or pre-softening is not required.

Single-process tints usually contain a lightening agent, a shampoo, an aniline derivative tint, and an alkalizing agent to activate the peroxide which is added. Most color is formulated to be used with 20 volume peroxide. Color results are altered when other volumes are used.

The advantages of single-process tints are that they:

1. Can produce shades from the deepest black to the lightest blonde.
2. Can color the hair lighter or darker than the client's original shade.
3. Can blend white or gray hair to a natural hair shade.
4. Can correct streaks, off-shades, discolorations, and faded ends.
5. Are available as creams, liquids, and gels.

SINGLE-PROCESS TINT FOR LIGHTENING VIRGIN HAIR

Virgin hair is hair that has had no chemical services and has not been damaged by natural factors such as wind and sun.

The procedure that follows is a basic color procedure. Your instructor may have another technique just as correct for the particular color used.

Implements and Materials

Towels	Plastic or glass bowl	Finishing rinse
Tint cape	Timer	Protective cream
Protective gloves	Mild shampoo	Cotton
Comb	Selected tint	Record card
Applicator bottle or brush	Hydrogen peroxide	
	Color chart	

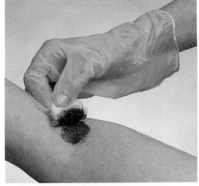

12.17—Give a patch test.

Preliminary Steps

1. Give patch test 24 to 48 hours before the service. (Fig. 12.17) Proceed only if test is negative. (Fig. 12.18)
2. Thoroughly analyze scalp and hair. Perform any necessary pre-conditioning treatments, and record results on client's record card.
3. Assemble all necessary supplies.
4. Prepare client. Protect clothing with a towel and tint cape. Ask client to remove all jewelry and place safely away.
5. Apply protective cream around hairline and over ears.
6. Put on protective gloves.
7. Perform a strand test.
8. Record results on record card.

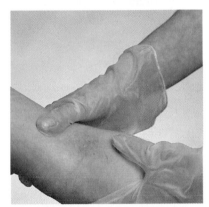

12.18—Proceed if test is negative.

Procedure

1. Section the hair into four quarters. (Fig. 12.19)
2. Prepare tint formula for either bottle or brush application. (Fig. 12.20)
3. Begin in section where color change will be greatest or hair is most resistant. (Fig. 12.21)

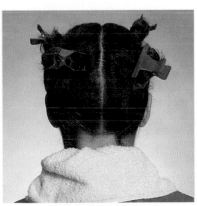

12.19—Hair sectioned into four quarters.

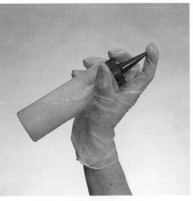

12.20—Prepare and mix tint formula.

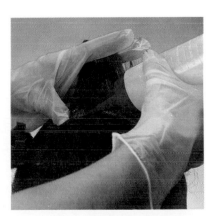

12.21—Begin applying color.

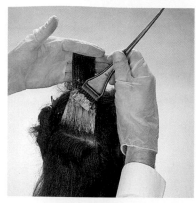

12.22—Apply tint to the hair ends.

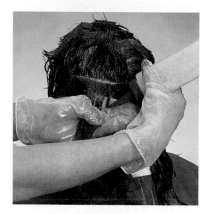

12.23—Blend tint to hair ends.

4.   Part off ¼″ (.625 cm) subsection with applicator.
5.   Lift subsection and apply tint to hair ½″ (1.25 cm) from scalp up through ends. (Fig. 12.22)

▶ NOTE: The hair at the scalp will process faster due to body heat and incomplete keratinization. For this reason the tint is applied in the scalp area after being applied to the shaft. Your strand test will determine the application procedure and timing for even color development.

6.   Process according to strand test results. Check for color development by removing color as described in the strand test procedure on page 242.
7.   Apply tint mixture to hair at scalp.
8.   Blend tint to hair ends. (Fig. 12.23)
9.   Lightly rinse with lukewarm water. Massage color to lather and rinse thoroughly.
10. Remove any stains around hairline with remaining tint mixture, shampoo, or stain remover. Use cotton or terry towel to gently remove stains.
11. Shampoo hair thoroughly with a mild (acid-balanced) shampoo.
12. Apply an acid or a finishing rinse to close the cuticle, restore pH, and prevent fading.
13. Style hair.
14. Complete record card and file.

Cleanup
1.   Discard all disposable supplies and materials.
2.   Close containers tightly, wipe them off, and put them in their proper places.
3.   Clean and sanitize implements.
4.   Sanitize tint cape.
5.   Sanitize work area.
6.   Wash and sanitize hands.

SINGLE-PROCESS TINT FOR DARKENING VIRGIN HAIR

When tinting close to, or darker than natural hair color, follow the same preparation and procedure as for a lighter shade. Then proceed as follows:

1.   Select appropriate color.
2.   Application begins where the hair is the most resistant. (If gray is present, application most likely will begin in the front. If no gray is evident, then begin in the back.)

3. Apply tint from scalp to the porous ends using ¼″ (.625 cm) subpartings.

4. Process according to strand test results.

5. When color has developed to desired degree, distribute the tint through the ends with a large-toothed comb to ensure complete coverage.

6. Continue processing according to strand test results.

7. Shampoo color off and complete styling and cleanup in usual manner.

SINGLE-PROCESS TINT FOR LONG HAIR

The same preparation and procedure are used for long hair as for short hair. Condition the ends according to your analysis. You will probably need more color material than you used for short hair.

SINGLE-PROCESS TINT RETOUCH

As the hair grows, you will need to do a "retouch" so the hair looks attractive and not two-toned. After you assemble the materials and implements as for a virgin tint, follow the procedure below.

Preliminary Steps

1. Give a patch test 24 to 48 hours before the service. Proceed only if test is negative.

2. Assemble all necessary supplies.

3. Prepare client. Protect clothing with a towel and tint cape. Ask client to remove all jewelry and put safely away.

4. Take out client's record card. Consult with client to see if she or he liked the original color. Carefully analyze hair and condition previously tinted hair as needed.

5. Apply protective cream around hairline and over ears.

6. Perform a strand test.

7. Record all results on record card.

Procedure

1. Section the hair into four quarters.

2. Prepare tint formula.

3. Begin in section where color was begun in the virgin application.

4. Part off ¼″ (.625 cm) subsection with applicator.

5. Apply tint to new growth only. (Fig. 12.24) *Do not overlap.* Overlapping of color can cause breakage and create lines of *demarcation* (visible lines separating colored hair from regrowth).

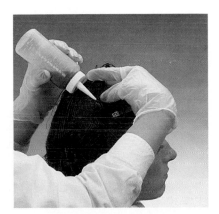

12.24—Apply tint to new growth only.

6.   Confirm color development by strand testing.
7.   Apply diluted color formula to ends according to your analysis and strand test results. Dilute the remaining tint mixture with distilled water, shampoo, or conditioner. (This step is done only if color is faded.)
8.   Lightly rinse with lukewarm water. Massage color to lather and rinse thoroughly.
9.   Remove any stains around hairline with remaining tint mixture, shampoo, or stain remover. Use cotton to gently remove stains.
10.   Shampoo hair thoroughly with a mild (acid-balanced) shampoo.
11.   Apply an acid or a finishing rinse to close the cuticle, restore pH, and prevent fading.
12.   Style hair.
13.   Complete record card and file.
14.   Clean up in the usual manner.

HIGHLIGHTING SHAMPOO COLOR

Highlighting shampoo tints are prepared by combining aniline derivative tints, hydrogen peroxide, and shampoo. They are used when a very slight change in hair shade is desired, or when the client's hair processes very rapidly. These tints highlight the hair's natural color in a single application. A patch test is required.

Highlighting shampoos are a mixture of shampoo and hydrogen peroxide. The natural color is slightly lightened. No patch test is required.

Procedure

Perform consultation and analysis as for a regular color procedure. If highlighting shampoo tint is to be used, a patch test must have been performed 24 to 48 hours before.

1.   Drape client and take to shampoo bowl.
2.   Distribute the color over clean, damp hair. Gently lather and process for 8 to 15 minutes.
3.   Complete as for a regular tint procedure.

DOUBLE-PROCESS TINT
Pre-Lightening
If the client desires a drastically lighter color, the hair should first be pre-lightened. The pre-lightener is applied in the same manner as for a regular hair lightening treatment. After the pre-lightening has reached the desired shade, the hair is lightly shampooed, acidified, and towel dried. The color is then applied in the usual manner after a strand test has been taken.

Pre-Softening
If the client's hair is gray and resistant, the hair should be pre-softened with *hydrogen peroxide* in order for it to readily absorb the tint. Pre-softening is also effective on nongray resistant hair.

Apply the softener from the scalp to the hair ends as in regular lightening and process a few minutes. Little color change will take place, but the cuticle is opened so that the hair is more receptive to color. Do not rinse softener from hair. Towel blot and apply color as the manufacturer directs.

SAFETY PRECAUTIONS
1. Give a patch test 24 to 48 hours prior to any application of aniline derivative.
2. Apply tint only if patch test is negative.
3. Do not apply tint if abrasions are present.
4. Do not apply tint if metallic or compound dye is present.
5. Do not brush hair prior to applying color.
6. Always read and follow manufacturer's directions.
7. Use sanitized applicator bottles, brushes, combs, and towels.
8. Protect client's clothing by proper draping.
9. Perform a strand test for color, breakage, and/or discoloration.
10. Use an applicator bottle or bowl (glass or plastic) for mixing the tint.
11. Do not mix tint before you are ready to use it; discard leftover tint.
12. Wear gloves to protect your hands.
13. Do not permit the color to come in contact with the client's eyes.
14. Do not overlap during a tint retouch.
15. Do not use water that is too hot; use lukewarm water for removing color.
16. Use a mild shampoo. If an alkaline or harsh shampoo is used, it will strip the color.
17. Always wash hands before and after serving a client.

Hydrogen Peroxide

Hydrogen peroxide serves as the oxidizing agent most commonly used in hair coloring. An oxidizer is a substance that causes oxygen to combine with another substance, such as melanin. As the oxygen and melanin combine, the peroxide solution begins to diffuse (break apart and spread out) and lighten the melanin within the hair shaft. This new smaller structure and spread-out distribution of the diffused melanin gives the hair its light appearance.

Peroxide alone creates a relatively mild lightening of the hair color. To lighten the hair significantly, heat must be applied, or the solution must be left on a longer amount of time or mixed with other ingredients to create a stronger formula.

Hydrogen peroxide is distributed for cosmetology use under a variety of names such as *oxidizer, generator*, and *catalyst*. Regardless of which name is used, hydrogen peroxide comes in three forms: dry, cream, and liquid.

Dry peroxide, in either tablet or powder form, is dissolved in liquid hydrogen peroxide to boost the volume. The availability of liquid peroxides in a variety of volumes has made this product somewhat obsolete.

Cream peroxides contain additives such as thickeners, *drabbers*, conditioners, and an acid for stabilization. The thickeners help to create a product that is easy to control. However, the additives may dilute the strength of the formula and make it undesirable when full strength is needed such as in tinting to cover gray.

Liquid hydrogen peroxide contains only a stabilizing acid which brings the pH to 3.5–4.0.

STRENGTHS OF HYDROGEN PEROXIDE

A variety of strengths of peroxide are available for your use as a professional cosmetologist. Consult your manufacturer's directions for the recommended strength.

The majority of permanent coloring products use 20 volume hydrogen peroxide for proper color development. Those that recommend the use of 40 volume are designed to achieve a greater breakdown of melanin, resulting in a lighter color than may be achieved with a standard lightening tint formula. Formulas recommending the use of less than 20 volume are designed to allow more deposit than lift. Such formulas may be used when there is no need for breakdown of melanin to achieve the desired color.

CAUTION

▶ *Increasing the strength or volume used in a formula beyond the manufacturer's recommended directions may cause excessive damage to the hair and chemical burns to the skin and scalp.*

A hydrometer can be used to measure the volume of liquid peroxide for the purpose of adjusting its strength or simply confirming that the product is still potent. It is important to use clean implements in measuring, using, and storing hydrogen peroxide. Even a small amount of dirt or impurity can cause peroxide to deteriorate.

Never measure the needed amount of hydrogen peroxide by pouring it into the lid of another product. The residue will cause the container to oxidize as it sits on the shelf, thus making it unusable. Also, do not allow hydrogen peroxide formulations to come in contact with metal. Metal causes the oxidation process to occur too quickly to allow proper color development.

Hair lightening, removing pigment from the hair, is always a popular salon service. Changing styles determine if the entire head is lightened, or just one area, or if a special effect is created. Hair lightening is especially popular for people involved with TV, photography, or competition modeling. Lighter strands draw light and attract attention to the individual. (Fig. 12.25)

Hair Lightening

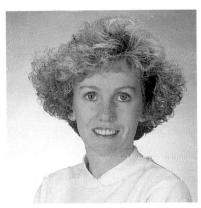

12.25—Special effects hair lightening.

ACTION OF LIGHTENERS

Lighteners may be used for two purposes:
1. As a color treatment, to lighten the hair to the final shade.
2. As a preliminary treatment, to prepare the hair for the application of a toner or tint (double-process application).
   a) *Toner*—A lightener is always necessary before applying delicate toner shades.
   b) *Tint*—If the client desires a shade much lighter than the natural shade, a lightener can be used to remove some color before the tint is applied.

Lightening creates a desired color foundation. This new color foundation may be the finished result or it may be the first step of a double-process application. Before beginning the lightening process, it is important to understand that achieving the desired shade requires that you consider not only the virgin hair color, how long the product should be left on to achieve the desired stage of lightening, and the resulting porosity of the hair shaft, but also selection of the appropriate product to achieve the desired color foundation.

CAUTION

▶ *Clients with dark hair may not be able to be lightened to a very pale blonde color without extreme damage to their hair.*

Hair lighteners, used according to the manufacturer's directions, can:

1. Lighten the entire head of hair for toner application.
2. Lighten hair to a particular shade.
3. Brighten and lighten existing shade.
4. Lighten only certain parts of the hair.
5. Lighten hair that has already been tinted.
6. Remove undesirable casts and off-shades.
7. Correct dark streaks or spots in lightened or tinted hair.

EFFECTS OF LIGHTENERS

A lightening product is used to diffuse pigment. (Fig. 12.26) The hair pigment goes through different changing stages of color as it lightens. The amount of change depends on how much pigment the hair has and the length of time the lightening agent is processed. Hair goes through seven stages of lightening from the darkest to the lightest: A natural head of black hair will go from black to brown, to red, to red-gold, to gold, to yellow, and finally to pale yellow (almost white). (Fig. 12.27)

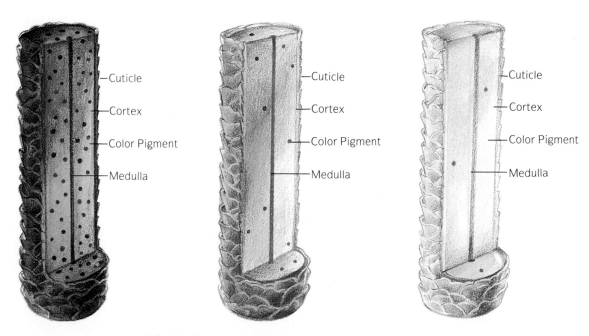

12.26—Hair lighteners are used to diffuse pigment.

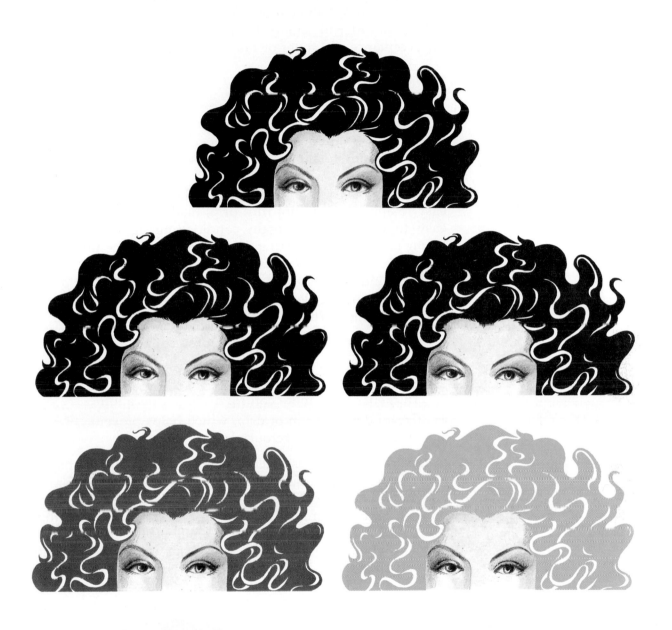
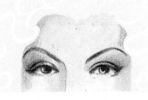
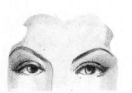

12.27—Seven stages of hair lightening.

The hair also becomes more porous during the lightening treatment, a condition necessary to permit penetration of a toner.

Even naturally light hair or gray hair may need a pre-lightening process in order to achieve the necessary degree of porosity for the acceptance of a toner or tint.

TYPES OF LIGHTENERS

Lighteners are available in liquid, cream, and powder forms.

Liquid lighteners are made of ammonia mixed with hydrogen peroxide. They are designed to be used for lightening the entire head. Caution should be exercised as these lighteners can run and drip.

Cream lighteners are the most popular type because they are easy to apply and do not run, drip, or dry out easily. They are easy to control and contain conditioning agents, sometimes *bluing* (a temporary coloring used to neutralize the unbecoming yellowish tinge in gray or white hair), and thickener.

Liquid and cream lighteners are generally mixed with accelerators, sometimes called boosters or activators, to increase the lightening action. The benefits of cream lighteners are that:

1. Conditioning agents give some protection to the hair and scalp.
2. Bluing agent helps to drab red and gold tones.
3. Thickener gives more control during application.
4. Cream does not run or drip, which helps prevent overlapping during retouch.

Powder lighteners, also called quick lighteners, contain oxygen-releasing boosters for quicker and stronger action. They may dry out more quickly, but they do not run or drip. Because most powder lighteners are too harsh to use on the hair closest to the scalp, they are used generally for special effects lightening. Most powder lighteners expand and spread out as processing continues and should not be used for retouch services. Powder lighteners are recommended for off-the-scalp applications on resistant hair.

LIGHTENING VIRGIN HAIR

A preliminary strand test is necessary before lightening in order to determine the processing time needed, the condition of the hair after lightening, and the end results. Carefully record all data on client record card.

Preliminary Test Results

1. If test shows the hair is not light enough:
    a) Increase strength of mixture and/or:
    b) Increase processing time.

2. If hair strand is too light:
   a) Decrease strength of mixture and/or:
   b) Decrease processing time.
3. Watch strand carefully for reaction to lightening mixture and for discoloration or breakage. Reconditioning may be required prior to toning.
4. If color and condition are good, proceed with lightening.

▶ **NOTE:** A patch test must be taken 24 to 48 hours prior to the application of a toner containing aniline derivatives. To save the client's time, the strand test for lightening should be made the same day as the patch test.

Implements and Materials

Towels	Comb	Protective gloves
Plastic clips	Tint cape	Plastic or glass bowl
Shampoo	Peroxide	Acid or finishing
Cotton	Protective cream	rinse
Lightener	Applicator bottle	Record card
Timer	or brush	

Procedure

The following general instructions may be changed by your instructor for particular lightening effects or products.

1. Prepare client. Protect client's clothing with towel and tint cape.
2. Analyze scalp and hair, and record on client's card. Do not perform the service if the client has abrasions or inflammation of the scalp.
3. Do not brush hair.
4. Check patch test area if toner is to be used. Proceed only if test results are negative.
5. Section hair into four quarters.
6. Apply protective cream around hairline and over ears.
7. Put on gloves to protect your hands.
8. Prepare lightening formula. Use immediately to prevent deterioration.
9. Apply lightener. Begin application where hair seems resistant or especially dark, usually the back of the head.
   Use ⅛" (.3125 cm) partings to apply lightener. Start ½" (1.25 cm) from the scalp and extend lightener through the ends. Apply lightener to top and underside of subsection in quick, rhythmic movements. (Fig. 12.28)

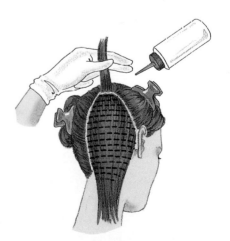

12.28—Apply lightener to underside of strand.

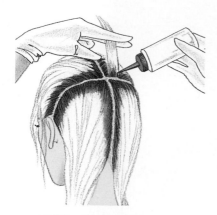

12.29—Apply lightener at scalp.

10. Continue to apply lightener. Double check application, adding more lightener if necessary. Do not comb lightener through hair.

    Keep lightener moist during development by misting the hair lightly with a spray bottle or reapplying lightener as the mixture dries.

11. Test for lightening action. Make first check about 15 minutes before time indicated by preliminary strand test. Remove mixture from the strand with damp towel. Towel dry and examine. If strand is not light enough, reapply mixture and continue testing frequently until desired level is reached.

12. Apply lightener to hair near scalp with ⅛" (.3125 cm) parting. (Fig. 12.29) If necessary, prepare fresh lightener. Process and strand test until entire shaft has reached desired stage.

13. Remove lightener. Rinse thoroughly with cool water. Shampoo gently with acid-balanced shampoo. Shampoo with hands under hair to avoid tangling.

14. Neutralize the alkalinity of the hair with an acid or a normalizing rinse. Recondition if necessary.

15. Towel dry hair, or dry completely under cool dryer if manufacturer requires it.

16. Examine scalp for abrasions. Analyze condition of hair.

17. Proceed with toner application.

18. Complete record card and file.

19. Clean up in usual manner.

LIGHTENER RETOUCH

As the hair grows, dark regrowth will be very obvious. A lightener retouch corrects this problem and matches the regrowth to the rest of the lightened hair.

During the retouch, the lightener is applied to the new growth only, with the following exceptions:

1. If another color is desired.
2. If a lighter shade is desired.
3. If color has become dull from repeated applications.

In each case, lighten the regrowth first. Then bring remaining lightener mixture gently through the hair shaft. Process for 1 to 5 minutes until problem is corrected.

Procedure
Always consult the client's record card to tell you about lightener formula, timing, and other pertinent information. The procedure

for a lightener retouch is the same as that for lightening a virgin head of hair, except that the mixture is applied only to the new growth of hair. (Figs. 12.30–12.32)

A cream lightener is generally used for a lightener retouch because its consistency helps prevent overlapping of previously lightened hair, and it is gentler on the scalp. Overlapping can cause severe breakage and lines of demarcation.

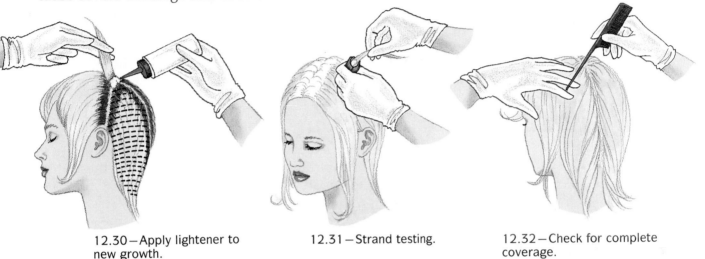

12.30—Apply lightener to new growth.

12.31—Strand testing.

12.32—Check for complete coverage.

SAFETY PRECAUTIONS

1. Give a patch test 24 to 48 hours before toner application.
2. Read manufacturer's directions before preparing lightener.
3. Always wash your hands before and after servicing a client.
4. Drape client properly to protect clothing.
5. Examine scalp carefully. Do not apply lightener if irritation or abrasions are present.
6. Do not brush hair. If shampoo is required, avoid irritating scalp.
7. Analyze condition of hair and give any necessary reconditioning treatments.
8. Wear protective gloves.
9. Use only sanitized applicators and towels.
10. Conduct strand test prior to lightener retouch.
11. Cream lightener should be the thickness of whipped cream to avoid dripping, running, or overlapping.
12. Always use lightener immediately after mixing. Discard leftover lightener.
13. Apply lightener to resistant areas first. Use ⅛" partings to ensure accurate coverage.
14. Apply rapidly and neatly for even lightening.

15. Give frequent strand tests until desired stage is reached.
16. Check skin and scalp after application and gently remove any lightener with cool, damp towel.
17. Lightener can be safely left on the scalp area a maximum of 1 hour.
18. If towel around client's neck becomes saturated, remove and replace to avoid skin irritation.
19. Cool water and mild shampoo should be used to remove lightener. Avoid tangling fragile hair.
20. Cap all bottles to avoid contamination. Store carefully.
21. Complete record card and file.

SPOT LIGHTENING

Uneven lightening, streaking, or dark spots are usually due to careless lightener application. It is necessary to correct these areas prior to toning to ensure even color.

To correct streaked hair:

1. Prepare lightening formula.
2. Apply mixture only to the darker areas.
3. Allow mixture to remain on hair until all streaks are removed.
4. Shampoo lightener from hair.

TONERS

Toners are aniline derivative tints and require a 24 to 48 hour patch test. They consist of pale and delicate colors.

Toners require a double-process application:

1. The first process is the lightener.
2. The second process is the toner.

Pre-Lightening to Create a Foundation for Toners

After the hair goes through the seven stages of lightening, the color left in the hair is known as its "foundation." Achieving the correct foundation is necessary for proper toner development.

Manufacturers of toners provide literature that recommend the proper foundation to achieve your desired color. As a general rule, the paler the desired color, the lighter the foundation must be. It is important to follow the guide closely because:

1. Over-lightened hair will "grab" the base color of the toner.
2. Under-lightened hair will appear to have more red, yellow, or orange than the intended color.

Focus On: Beth Minardi, Hair Colorist

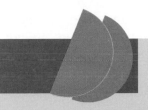

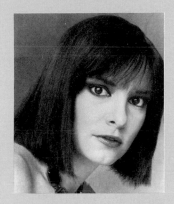

"It's a wonderful challenge to come to work," says Beth Minardi, a highly successful hair colorist whose sense of "adventure" has taken her to new heights in the world of beauty. "Hair coloring is always different on every head," she explains. "I love the creativity."

Minardi, who has recently won the Hair Colorist of the Year Award sponsored by *American Salon,* is also co-owner with husband Carmine of Minardi Minardi Imagemakers in New York City. Her beauty tips have appeared in *Vogue, Self, Glamour,* and *Mademoiselle.* In addition, she teaches private color seminars, is a national television spokesperson for Clairol, tours the United States teaching color, and services a host of celebrity clients.

Minardi made the unusual decision to go to cosmetology school after getting a college degree in theater and education because she "thought it would be fun to be involved in beauty." But it was her initial frustration with executing color that sparked her success in the field. "Nobody knew enough about hair color," she recalls. "A good hair color could look really lovely, but it was always guesswork as to whether it would come out right." She determined to fine-tune that process.

"I practiced coloring over and over. It's the first ten thousand that are the toughest. You just have to keep going."

She began as an entry-level trainee at Clairol and rose to the position of director of education, and then on to her own exclusive salon which, naturally, boasts an outstanding color department. Says Minardi, "Lots of people know a little about color, few know it thoroughly. If you do, there's no reason why you can't earn as much as a doctor or lawyer and have job security for life."

Her advice for those who want to put color in their lives is to learn all that they can about color, attend all the generic and company-sponsored educational shows they're able to, and to buy all the hair color videos and books they can. "Then, go to a salon known for color and tell the owner that you want a career in hair color," says Minardi. "Other colorists love to hear this. There's a real need for well-educated colorists and it's a great career. Color has come of age," Minardi says proudly.

Refer to the laws of color to select a toner that will neutralize or tone the pre-lightened hair to the desired shade.

In addition to achieving the correct foundation stage for toning, you must also achieve sufficient porosity for toner development. Occasionally, virgin blonde, gray, or white hair reaches the correct color foundation without achieving sufficient porosity. You must make adjustments in your color mixture to achieve the desired color.

Preliminary Toner Application

1. Give 24 to 48 hour patch test prior to toner application.
2. Strand test to predetermine results may be given on same day as patch test to save time.
3. Proceed with application only if test results are negative and hair is in good condition.

Implements and Materials

Towels	Comb	Protective gloves
Plastic clips	Tint cape	Plastic or glass bowl
Shampoo	Peroxide	Acid or finishing rinse
Cotton	Protective cream	Record card
Toner	Applicator bottle	
Timer	or brush	

Preparation

1. Arrange all supplies.
2. Prepare client.
3. Wear gloves to protect your hands.
4. Pre-lighten hair to desired stage.
5. Shampoo hair lightly, rinse, and towel dry.
6. Acidify and recondition as necessary.
7. Select desired toner shade.
8. Apply protective cream around hairline and over ears.
9. Strand test and record results on client's card.
10. Prepare formula. Mix toner and developer in bowl or bottle according to manufacturer's directions.

Procedure

Wear gloves for protection throughout the application.

Speed and accuracy of application are crucial for good color results.

Application of low or non-peroxide toners may vary. Your instructor will direct you.

1. Divide hair into four equal sections. Use the end of tail comb or tint brush. Avoid scratching the scalp.
2. At crown of a back quarter, part off ¼" (.625 cm) partings, and apply toner from scalp to porous ends.
3. When the strand test confirms proper color development, gently work toner through ends using brush or fingers.

▶ **NOTE:** Do not bring toner mixture through over-porous ends until the last. If ends tend to absorb too much color, dilute remaining mixture with mild shampoo, conditioner, or distilled water before applying to ends.

4. Apply additional mixture to hair, if needed, and blend. Leave hair loose to permit circulation or cover hair with cap if required.
5. Time according to strand test results. Test frequently until desired shade is reached.
6. Remove toner by wetting hair, and massaging toner to lather.
7. Rinse, shampoo gently, and rinse well.
8. Apply finishing rinse to close cuticle, lower the pH, and prevent fading.
9. Remove any toner stains from the skin, hairline, and neck.
10. Style as desired. Use caution to avoid stretching the hair.
11. Complete record card and file.
12. Clean up in usual manner.

Toner Retouch

A toner retouch requires careful analysis of the hair. The new growth must be pre-lightened to the same stage as the hair was for the first toner application. Based on your analysis and strand test, you will either apply the toner to the entire shaft as in the original application, or you will apply toner to the new growth only. When that area is nearly processed, you can work diluted toner mixture through the remaining hair.

Special Effects Highlighting

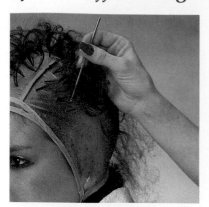

12.33—Draw strands through holes with hook.

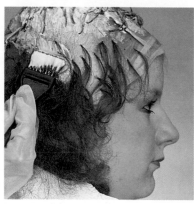

12.34—Apply lightener to strand.

Special effects highlighting involves any technique of partial lightening or coloring. Lightening for special effects is a fashion technique. As styles change, you only need to adapt placement of lightened strands and colors for the trend.

You may create special effects by strategically placing the light and dark colors in the hair. Some colors appear to advance, others appear to recede. Light colors will cause the area to advance toward the eye, appear larger, and make detail more visible. The contrasting dark areas will cause the area to recede, appear smaller, and make detail less visible.

METHODS FOR HIGHLIGHTING

There are three main methods to achieve highlights:

1. Cap technique
2. Foil technique
3. Freehand technique

The *cap technique* involves pulling clean strands of hair through a perforated cap with a hook. (Fig. 12.33) The amount of strands pulled through depends upon the amount of lightness desired. Pull small strands and leave holes empty for a subtle look. The lightening will be greater if all holes are used, and more dramatic if larger strands are pulled through the holes.

The hair is then lightened, usually with a powder or "quick" lightener, or with a tint that can lift a great deal. (Fig. 12.34) The lightener is removed by first rinsing with lukewarm water, then gently cleansing with an acid-balanced shampoo. After towel-blotting and conditioning if necessary, the lightened hair is toned. (Figs. 12.35, 12.36)

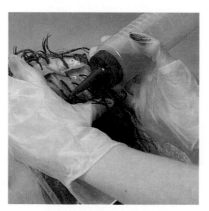

12.35—Apply toner to lightened strand.

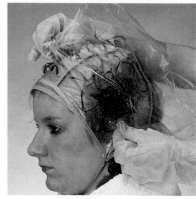

12.36—Cover with a plastic cap.

The *foil technique* involves *weaving* out (taking alternating strands from a subsection) small strands of hair from a subsection. (Fig. 12.37) The selected strands are then placed over foil or plastic wrap, and the appropriate lightener or high-lift tint is applied. The foil is folded to prevent lifting any unwoven hair, and processed as desired. (Fig. 12.38) With this technique, the colorist can strategically place highlights.

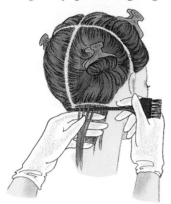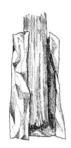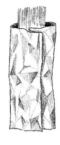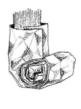

12.37—Weave subsection with tint brush.

12.38—Place hair in foil packet as shown.

Freehand techniques involve the placement of a lightening compound directly onto clean, styled hair. The lightener can be applied with a tint brush, an applicator bottle, or even with gloved fingers. Effects are extremely subtle, and can be used effectively to draw attention to a waveline or an upsweep movement.

Special Problems in Hair Coloring

Each hair coloring service is unique. The colorist must carefully analyze the hair and consult with the client. Strand tests must be taken to ensure good results. But even the most skilled colorist will occasionally have a hair coloring problem. This may be due to the particular structure or condition of the client's hair or to the effects of prior treatments to the hair.

DAMAGED HAIR

Blow drying, wind, harsh shampoos, and chemical services all take their toll on the condition of the hair. Coating compounds such as hairsprays, styling agents, and some conditioners can prevent color penetration. Preventative and corrective steps that you should take include the following:

1. Incorporate reconditioning into any chemical service that you give.
2. Ensure that the client uses high-quality products at home. (Sell the best.)

3. Pre-condition hair if your analysis tells you it is damaged. Use a penetrating conditioner that can deposit protein, oils, and moisture regulators.

4. Complete each chemical service by normalizing the pH with a finishing rinse. This will restore the cuticle's protective capacity.

5. Postpone any further chemical service until the hair is reconditioned.

6. Schedule the client for between-service conditioning.

Hair is considered damaged when the hair has one or more of the following conditions:

Over-porous	Spongy, matted when wet
Brittle and dry	Color fades or absorbs too rapidly
Breakage	Rough texture
No elasticity	

Any of these hair conditions may create problems during a tinting, lightening, permanent waving, or hair relaxing treatment. Therefore, damaged hair should receive reconditioning treatments prior to and after the application of these chemical processes.

Reconditioning Procedure

1. Always thoroughly analyze the hair to determine the problem. Consult with the client until you can discover the source of the damage. You can then correct the problem and avoid its recurrence.

2. Shampoo the hair with a mild shampoo. Use care to keep your hands underneath the hair, and only use gentle massage techniques to avoid tangling the fragile hair.

3. Rinse very well and towel blot gently.

4. Apply the conditioner as the manufacturer directs. If it is liquid, use a spray bottle; if it is a cream, apply with a sanitized spatula or tint brush.

5. Blend the conditioner through the hair with a wide-toothed comb.

6. Cover the hair with a plastic cap if required, and follow the manufacturer's direction in applying heat and timing.

7. Rinse well. Re-examine the hair and proceed with the coloring service only if the hair's condition indicates that the treatment will be successful.

FILLERS

Fillers are specialized preparations that are designed to equalize porosity and deposit a base color in one application. They can be a manufacturer's preparation or a mixture of tint and conditioner that your instructor will assist you in preparing.

Conditioner fillers are used to recondition damaged hair before salon service. Conditioner fillers can be applied in a separate procedure as outlined above, or can be applied immediately prior to color application. The conditioner and the tint are then working at the same time.

Color fillers are recommended if the hair is in a damaged condition and there is doubt that the color result will be an even shade.

Advantages of Using a Color Filler
1. Deposits color to faded ends.
2. Helps hair to hold color.
3. Helps color to develop uniformly from scalp to ends.
4. Prevents streaking.
5. Prevents off-color results.
6. Prevents dullness.
7. Produces more uniform, natural-looking color in a tint.

How to Use Color Fillers
Color fillers may be applied directly from their containers to damaged hair prior to tinting. Color fillers may be added to the tint and applied to damaged ends. They may be used full strength or diluted with distilled water.

Selection of Correct Color Filler
To obtain satisfactory results, select the color filler that will replace the missing primary. Always remember that all three primaries—red, blue, and yellow—must be present for natural-looking hair color. If you have blonde (yellow) hair, for example, that is being tinted back to an ash (yellow and blue) brown, you will need to use a red filler so that the end result will be correct.

TINT REMOVAL

Sometimes it is necessary to remove all or part of the tint from the hair in order to achieve the correct color.

Commercial products are used to remove penetrating tints, and are known as tint or color removers. They may contain ingredients designed to diffuse pigment and are sometimes mixed with hydrogen peroxide.

The removal of a tint is always an advanced technique that requires careful analysis of both condition and color of the hair. Reconditioning is often necessary after tint removal and before corrective coloring.

Procedure

1. Prepare client.
2. Shampoo if required by manufacturer.
3. Section hair into four quarters.
4. Wear gloves to protect your hands.
5. Mix preparation in glass or plastic bowl according to manufacturer's directions.
6. Immediately begin application where hair is darkest.
7. Apply mixture with tint brush. Saturate hair completely. (Fig. 12.39)
8. Work mixture through hair ends.
9. Pile hair loosely on top of head. (Fig. 12.40) Cover with plastic cap if required. (Fig. 12.41)

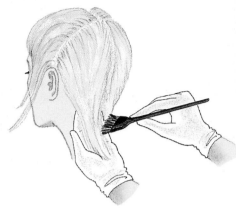

12.39—Apply mixture.

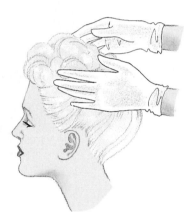

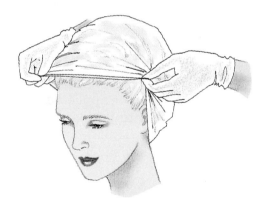

12.40—Pile hair on top of head.

12.41—Cover head with plastic cap if required.

10. Strand test regularly.
11. When color is diffused, rinse thoroughly. (Fig. 12.42)
12. Shampoo gently but thoroughly to ensure all of the chemical is removed from the hair. Any tint remover that remains in the hair will continue to process.
13. Towel dry hair.
14. Analyze hair strength. Condition as required.
15. Perform a strand test.
16. Proceed with the application of desired tint.

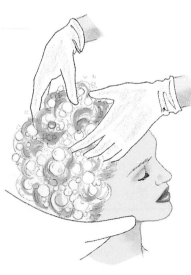

12.42—Shampoo with cool water.

If color cannot be applied, style hair in the usual manner. Schedule reconditioning treatments until the hair can withstand tinting.

TINT BACK TO NATURAL COLOR

Each tint back to natural color must be handled as an individual problem. Check the hair for its natural color next to the scalp. Carefully consult with the client to see if she or he desires a color that dark. You will sometimes need to compromise with a color that has the same color qualities, but is lighter in value. Carefully record all observations and treatments on the client's record card.

Procedure

1. Assemble materials.
2. Prepare client in usual manner.
3. Check results of patch test. Proceed only if results are negative.
4. Shampoo hair as directed. Give conditioning treatments according to your analysis.
5. Perform a strand test. More than one test may be necessary to determine the correct timing for desired results.
6. Section hair into four quarters.
7. Apply filler as directed by your instructor. Remember to replace the missing primary.
8. Process filler according to manufacturer's directions. Proceed directly to tint application.
9. Resection the hair into four quarters.
10. Apply color formula to ¼″ (.625 cm) subsections. Apply the tint as rapidly as possible to both sides of the subsection from the line of demarcation to the porous ends. Process according to your test strand results.
11. When correct color development has been confirmed by strand testing, apply tint to the porous ends. Continue processing.
12. A soap cap may be used after processing time is complete to blend color (optional). For a soap cap add equal amounts of shampoo to the leftover tint and mix it thoroughly. The mixture is applied quickly and worked gently through the ends of the hair.
13. Remove tint from hair with a mild shampoo.
14. Use an acid rinse to close cuticle and prevent fading.
15. Replace moisture with a finishing rinse.
16. Style as desired, using caution to avoid excessive heat or stretching.
17. Offer the client the opportunity to purchase high-quality products to prevent color stripping at home, and schedule the client for conditioning treatments.
18. Complete record card and file.
19. Clean work area in the usual manner.

Hair Coloring Glossary

accelerator: (See *activator*)

accent color: A concentrated color product that can be added to permanent, semi-permanent, or temporary hair color to intensify or tone down the color. Another word for concentrate.

acid: An aqueous (water-based) solution having a pH less than 7.0 on the pH scale.

activator: An additive used to quicken the action or progress of a chemical. Another word for booster, accelerator, protenator, or catalyst.

alkaline: An aqueous (water-based) solution having a pH greater than 7.0 on the pH scale. The opposite of acid.

allergy: A reaction due to extreme sensitivity to certain foods or chemicals.

allergy test: A test to determine the possibility or degree of sensitivity, also known as a patch test, predisposition test, or skin test.

amino acids: The group of molecules which the body uses to synthesize protein. There are some 22 different amino acids found in living protein that serve as units of structure in protein.

ammonia: A colorless pungent gas composed of hydrogen and nitrogen; in water solution it is called ammonia water. Used in hair color to swell the cuticle. When mixed with hydrogen peroxide, activates the oxidation process on melanin and allows the melanin to decolorize.

ammonium hydroxide: An alkali solution of ammonia in water, commonly used in the manufacture of permanent hair color, lightener preparations, and hair relaxers.

analysis (hair): An examination of the hair to determine its condition and natural color. (See *consultation; condition*)

aqueous: Descriptive term for water solution or any medium that is largely composed of water.

ash: A tone or shade dominated by greens, blues, violets, or grays. May be used to counteract unwanted warm tones.

base (alkali): (See *pH; alkaline*)

base color: (See *color base*)

bleeding: Seepage of tint/lightener from foil or cap due to improper application.

blending: A merging of one tint or tone with another.

blonding: A term applied to lightening the hair.

bonds: The means by which atoms are joined together to make molecules.

booster: (See *activator*)

brassy tone: Red, orange, or gold tones in the hair.

breakage: A condition in which hair splits and breaks off.

build-up: Repeated coatings on the hair shaft.

catalyst: A substance used to alter the speed of a chemical reaction.

caustic: Strongly alkaline materials. At very high pH levels, can burn or destroy protein or tissue by chemical action.

certified color: A color which meets certain standards for purity and is certified by the FDA.

cetyl alcohol: Fatty alcohol used as an emollient. It is also used as a stabilizer for emulsion systems and in hair color and cream developer as a thickener.

chelating stabilizer: A molecule that binds metal ions and renders them inactive.

chemical change: Alteration in the chemical composition of a substance.

citric acid: Organic acid derived from citrus fruits and used for pH adjustment. Primarily used to adjust the acid-alkali balance. Has some antioxidant and preservative qualities. Used medicinally as a mild astringent.

coating: Residue left on the outside of the hair shaft.

color: Visual sensation caused by light.

color additive: (See *accent color*)

color base: The combination of dyes which make up the tonal foundation of a specific hair color.

color lift: The amount of change natural or artificial pigment undergoes when lightened by a substance.

color mixing: Combining two or more shades together for a custom color.

color refresher: 1. Color applied to midshaft and ends to give a more uniform color appearance to the hair. 2. Color applied by a shampoo-in method to enhance the natural color. Also called color wash, color enhancer.

color remover: A product designed to remove artificial pigment from the hair.

color test: The process of removing product from a hair strand to monitor the progress of color development during tinting or lightening.

color wheel: The arrangement of primary and secondary and tertiary colors in the order of their relationships to each other. A tool for formulating.

complementary colors: A primary and secondary color positioned opposite each other on the color wheel. When these two colors are combined, they create a neutral color. Combinations are as follows: blue/orange, red/green, yellow/violet.

concentrate: (See *accent color*)

condition: The existing state of the hair; elasticity, strength, texture, porosity, and evidence of previous treatments.

consultation: Verbal communication with a client to determine desired result. [See *analysis (hair)*]

contributing pigment: The current level and tone of the hair; refers to both natural contributing pigment and decolorized (or lightened) contributing pigment. (See *undertone*)

cool tones: (See *ash*)

corrective coloring: The process of correcting an undesirable color.

cortex: The second layer of hair. A fibrous protein core of the hair fiber, containing melanin pigment.

coverage: Reference to the ability of a color product to color gray, white, or other colors of hair.

cuticle: The translucent protein outer layer of the hair fiber.

cysteic acid: A chemical substance in the hair fiber, produced by the interaction of hydrogen peroxide on the disulfide bond (cystine).

cysteine: The disulfide amino acid which joins protein chains together.

D & C colors: Colors selected from a certified list approved by the Food and Drug Administration for use in drug and cosmetic products.

decolorize: A chemical process involving the lightening of the natural color pigment or artificial color from the hair.

degree: Term used to describe various units of measurement.

dense: Thick, compact, or crowded.

deposit: Describes the color product in terms of its ability to add color pigment to the hair. Color added equals deposit.

deposit only color: A category of color products between permanent and semi-permanent colors. Formulated to only deposit color, not lift. They contain oxidation dyes and utilize low volume developer.

depth: The lightness or darkness of a specific hair color. (See *value*; *level*)

developer: An oxidizing agent, usually hydrogen peroxide, that reacts chemically with coloring material to develop color molecules and create a change in natural hair color.

development time (oxidation period): The time required for a permanent color or lightener to completely develop.

diffused: Broken down, scattered; not limited to one spot.

direct dye: A pre-formed color which dyes the fiber directly without the need for oxidation.

discoloration: The development of undesired shades through chemical reaction.

double process: A technique requiring two separate procedures in which the hair is decolorized or pre-lightened with a lightener before the depositing color is applied.

drab: Term used to describe hair color shades containing no red or gold. (See *ash*; *dull*)

drabber: Concentrated color, used to reduce red or gold highlights.

dull: A word used to describe hair or hair color without sheen.

dye: Artificial pigment.

dye intermediate: A material which develops into color only after reaction with developer (hydrogen peroxide). Also known as oxidation dyes.

dye solvents or dye remover: (See *color remover*)

dye stock: (See *color base*)

elasticity: The ability of the hair to stretch and return to normal.

enzyme: A protein molecule found in living cells which initiates a chemical process.

fade: To lose color through exposure to the elements or other factors.

fillers: 1. Color product used as a color refresher or to fill damaged hair in preparation for hair coloring. 2. Any liquid-like substance to help fill a void. (See *color refresher*)

formulas: Mixtures of two or more ingredients.

formulate: The art of mixing to create a blend or balance of two or more ingredients.

gray hair: Hair with decreasing amounts of natural pigment. Hair with no natural pigment is actually white. White hairs look gray when mingled with the still pigmented hair.

hair: A slender thread-like outgrowth of the skin of the head and body.

hair root: That part of the hair contained within the follicle, below the surface of the scalp.

hair shaft: Visible part of each strand of hair. It is made up of an outer layer called the cuticle, an innermost layer called the medulla, and an in-between layer called the cortex. The cortex layer is where color changes are made.

hard water: Water which contains minerals and metallic salts as impurities.

henna: A plant-extracted coloring which produces bright shades of red. The active ingredient is lawsone. Henna permanently colors the hair by coating and penetrating the hair shaft. (See *progressive dye*)

high lift tinting: A single-process color treatment with a higher degree of lightening action and a minimal amount of color deposit.

highlighting: The introduction of a lighter color in small selected sections to increase lightness of hair. Generally not strongly contrasting from the natural color.

hydrogen peroxide: An oxidizing chemical made up of 2 parts hydrogen, 2 parts oxygen (H_2O_2), used to aid the processing of permanent hair color and lighteners. Also referred to as a developer, available in liquid or cream.

level: A unit of measurement, used to evaluate the lightness or darkness of a color, excluding tone.

level system: In hair coloring, a system colorists use to analyze the lightness or darkness of a hair color.

lift: The lightening action of a hair color or lightening product on the hair's natural pigment.

lightener: The chemical compound which lightens the hair by dispersing, dissolving, and decolorizing the natural hair pigment. (See *pre-lighten*)

lightening: (See *decolorize*)

line of demarcation: An obvious difference between two colors on the hair shaft.

litmus paper: A chemically treated paper used to test the acidity or alkalinity of products.

medulla: The center structure of the hair shaft. Very little is known about its actual function.

melanin: The tiny grains of pigment in the hair cortex which create natural hair color.

melanocytes: Cells in the hair bulb that manufacture melanin.

melanoprotein: The protein coating of a melanosome.

melanosome: Protein-coated granule containing melanin.

metallic dyes: Soluble metal salts such as lead, silver, and bismuth which produce colors on the hair fiber by progressive build-up and exposure to air.

modifier: A chemical found as an ingredient in permanent hair colors. Its function is to alter the dye intermediates.

molecule: Two or more atoms chemically joined together; the smallest part of a compound.

neutral: 1. A color balanced between warm and cool, which does not reflect a highlight of any primary or secondary color. 2. Also refers to a pH of 7.

neutralization: The process that counter-balances or cancels the action of an agent or color.

neutralize: Render neutral; counter-balance of action or influence. (See *neutral*)

new growth: The part of the hair shaft which is between previously chemically treated hair and the scalp.

nonalkaline: (See *acid*)

off the scalp lightener: Generally a stronger lightener usually in powder form, not to be used directly on the scalp.

on the scalp lightener: A liquid, cream, or gel form of lightener that can be used directly on the scalp.

opaque: Allowing no light to shine through.

outgrowth: (See *new growth*)

overlap: Occurs when the application of color or lightener goes beyond the line of demarcation.

over-porosity: The condition where hair reaches an undesirable stage of porosity requiring correction.

oxidation: 1. The reaction of dye intermediates with hydrogen peroxide found in hair coloring developers. 2. The interaction of hydrogen peroxide on the natural pigment.

oxidative hair color: A product containing oxidation dyes which require hydrogen peroxide to develop the permanent color.

para tint: A tint made from oxidation dyes.

para-phenylenediamine: An oxidation dye used in most permanent hair colors, often abbreviated as P.P.D.

patch test: A test required by the Food and Drug Act. Made by applying a small amount of the hair coloring preparation to the skin of the arm or behind the ear to determine possible allergies (hypersensitivity). Also called predisposition or skin test.

penetrating color: Color which enters or penetrates the cortex or second layer of the hair shaft.

permanent color: 1. Hair color products which do not wash out by shampooing. 2. A category of hair color products mixed with developer that create a lasting color change.

peroxide: (See *hydrogen peroxide*).

peroxide residue: Traces of peroxide left in the hair after treatment with lightener or tint.

persulfate: In hair coloring, a chemical ingredient commonly used in activators. It increases the speed of the decolorization process. (See *activator*)

pH: The quantity which expresses the acid/alkali balance. A pH of 7 is the neutral value for pure water. Any pH below 7 is acidic; any pH above 7 is alkaline. The skin is mildly acidic and generally in the pH 4.5 to 5.5 range.

pH scale: A numerical scale from 0 (very acid) to 14 (very alkaline), used to describe the degree of acidity or alkalinity.

pigment: Any substance or matter used as coloring: natural or artificial hair color.

porosity: Ability of the hair to absorb water or other liquids.

powder lightener: (See *off the scalp lightener*)

pre-bleaching: (See *pre-lighten*)

predisposition test: (See *patch test*)

pre-lighten: Generally the first step of double-process hair coloring, used to lift or lighten the natural pigment. (See *decolorize*)

pre-soften: The process of treating gray or very resistant hair to allow for better penetration of color.

primary colors: Pigments or colors that are fundamental and cannot be made by mixing colors together. Red, yellow, and blue are the primary colors.

prism: A transparent glass or crystal solid which breaks up white light into its component colors, the spectrum.

processing time: The time required for the chemical treatment to react on the hair.

progressive dyes or progressive dye system: 1. A coloring system which produces increased absorption with each application. 2. Color products that deepen or increase absorption over a period of time during processing.

regrowth: (See *new growth*)

resistant hair: Hair which is difficult to penetrate with moisture or chemical solutions.

retouch: Application of color or lightening mixture to new growth of hair.

salt and pepper: The descriptive term for a mixture of dark and gray or white hair.

secondary color: Colors made by combining two primary colors in equal proportion; green, orange, and violet are secondary colors.

semi-permanent hair coloring: Hair coloring that lasts through several shampoos. It penetrates the hair shaft and stains the cuticle layer, slowly diffusing out with each shampoo.

sensitivity: A skin highly reactive to the presence of a specific chemical. Skin reddens or becomes irritated shortly after application of the chemical. On removal of the chemical, the reaction subsides.

shade: 1. A term used to describe a specific color. 2. The visible difference between two colors.

sheen: The ability of the hair to shine, gleam, or reflect light.

single-process color: Refers to an oxidative tint solution that lifts or lightens while also depositing color in one application. (See *oxidative hair color*)

softening agent: A mild alkaline product applied prior to the color treatment, to increase porosity, swell the cuticle layer of the hair, and increase color absorption. Tint that has not been mixed with developer is frequently used. (See *pre-soften*)

solution: A blended mixture of solid, liquid, or gaseous substances in a liquid medium.

solvent: Carrier liquid in which other components may be dissolved.

specialist: One who concentrates on only one part or branch of a subject or profession.

spectrum: The series of colored bands diffracted and arranged in the order of their wavelengths by the passage of white light through a prism. Shading continuously from red (produced by the longest wave visible) to violet (produced by the shortest): red, orange, yellow, green, blue, indigo, and violet.

spot lightening: Color correcting using a lightening mixture to lighten darker areas.

stabilizer: General name for ingredient which prolongs lifetime, appearance, and performance of a product.

stage: A term used to describe a visible color change that natural hair color goes through while being lightened.

stain remover: Chemical used to remove tint stains from skin.

strand test: Test given before treatment to determine development time, color result, and the ability of the hair to withstand the effects of chemicals.

stripping: (See *color remover*)

surfactant: A short way of saying surface active agent. A molecule which is composed of an oil-loving (oleophilic) part and a water-loving (hydrophilic) part. They act as a bridge to allow oil and water to mix. Wetting agents, emulsifiers, cleansers, solubilizers, dispersing aids, and thickeners are usually surfactants.

tablespoon: ½ of an ounce. 3 teaspoons. 15 milliliters.

teaspoon: ⅙ of an ounce. ⅓ of a tablespoon. 5 milliliters.

temporary coloring or temporary rinses: Color made from pre-formed dyes which are applied to the hair, but are readily removed with shampoo.

terminology: The special words or terms used in science, art, or business.

tertiary colors: The mixture of a primary and an adjacent secondary color on the color wheel. Red-orange, yellow-orange, yellow-green, blue-green, blue-violet, red-violet. Also referred to as intermediary colors.

texture, hair: The diameter of an individual hair strand. Termed: coarse, medium, or fine.

tint: Permanent oxidizing hair color product having the ability to lift and deposit color in the same process.

tint back: To return hair back to its original or natural color.

tone: A term used to describe the warmth or coolness in color.

toner: A pastel color to be used after pre-lightening.

toning: Adding color to modify the end result.

touch-up: (See *retouch*)

translucent: The property of letting diffused light pass through.

tyrosinase: The enzyme (tyrosinase) which reacts together with the amino acid (tyrosine) to form the hair's natural melanin.

tyrosine: The amino acid (tyrosine) which reacts together with the enzyme (tyrosinase) to form the hair's natural melanin.

undertone: The underlying color that emerges during the lifting process of melanin, that contributes to the end result. When lightening hair, a residual warmth in tone always occurs.

urea peroxide: A peroxide compound occasionally used in hair color. When added to an alkaline color mixture, it releases oxygen.

value: (See *level; depth*)

vegetable color: A color derived from plant sources.

virgin hair: Natural hair that has not undergone any chemical or physical abuse.

viscosity: A term referring to the thickness of the solution.

volume: The concentration of hydrogen peroxide in water solution. Expressed as volumes of oxygen liberated per volume of solution. 20 volume peroxide would thus liberate 20 pints (9.4 liters) of oxygen gas for each pint (liter) of solution.

warm: Containing red, orange, yellow, or gold tones.

Review Questions

HAIR COLORING

1. What is the difference between primary, secondary and tertiary colors?
2. What are the classifications of hair color? How do they act on the hair?
3. What is the correct procedure for giving a hair coloring consultation? A strand test?
4. How is temporary hair color applied?
5. What are some advantages of semi-permanent hair coloring?
6. What is the procedure for a single-process tint?
7. How does the procedure vary for a tint retouch?
8. What are the safety precautions to follow during the hair coloring process?
9. What is the activity of hydrogen peroxide during hair coloring?
10. For what two purposes are hair lighteners used?
11. Name the types of lighteners and the uses of each.
12. What methods are available to achieve special effects highlighting?
13. What preventative and corrective steps avoid or solve hair coloring problems?

13

CHEMICAL HAIR RELAXING AND SOFT CURL PERMANENT

LEARNING OBJECTIVES

After completing this chapter, you should be able to:

1. Define the purpose of chemical hair relaxing.

2. List the ingredients of the different products used in chemical hair relaxing.

3. Explain the difference between sodium hydroxide relaxers and thio relaxers.

4. Demonstrate the three basic steps of chemical hair relaxing.

5. Explain client analyzation for a chemical hair relaxing treatment.

6. Demonstrate the procedures used for a sodium hydroxide hair relaxing process, an ammonium thioglycolate hair relaxing process, a chemical blowout, and a soft curl permanent.

Introduction

Chemical hair relaxing is the process of permanently rearranging the basic structure of overly curly hair into a straight form. When done professionally, it leaves the hair straight and in a satisfactory condition, to be set into almost any style.

Chemical Hair Relaxing Products

The basic products that are used in chemical hair relaxing are a chemical hair relaxer, a neutralizer, and a petroleum cream, which is used as a protective base to protect the client's scalp during the sodium hydroxide chemical straightening process.

CHEMICAL HAIR RELAXERS

The two general types of hair relaxers are *sodium hydroxide,* which does not require pre-shampooing, and *ammonium thioglycolate,* which may require pre-shampooing.

Sodium hydroxide (caustic type hair relaxer often called a hair straightener) both softens and swells hair fibers. As the solution penetrates into the cortical layer, the cross-bonds (sulfur and hydrogen) are broken. The action of the comb, the brush, or the hands in smoothing the hair and distributing the chemical straightens the softened hair.

Manufacturers vary the sodium hydroxide content of the solution from 5% to 10%, and the pH factor between 10 and 14. In general, the more sodium hydroxide used and the higher the pH, the quicker the chemical reaction will take place on the hair, and the greater the danger will be of hair damage.

CAUTION

▶ *Because of the high alkaline content of sodium hydroxide, great care must be taken in its use.*

Although ammonium thioglycolate (thio type relaxer often called a relaxer) is less drastic in its action than sodium hydroxide, it softens and relaxes overly curly hair in somewhat the same manner. You may recall that this is the same solution used in permanent waving.

NEUTRALIZER

The *neutralizer* also is called a *stabilizer* or *fixative.* The neutralizer stops the action of any chemical relaxer that may remain in the hair after rinsing. The neutralizer for a thio type relaxer reforms the cysteine (sulfur) cross-bonds in their new position and rehardens the hair.

BASE AND "NO BASE" FORMULAS

When using sodium hydroxide, there are two types of formulas, base and no base. The base formula is a petroleum cream that is designed to protect the client's skin and scalp during the sodium hydroxide chemical straightening process. This protective base also is important during a chemical straightening retouch. It is applied to protect hair that has been straightened previously, and to prevent over-processing and hair breakage.

Petroleum cream has a lighter consistency than petroleum jelly, and is formulated to melt at body temperature. The melting process ensures complete protective coverage of the scalp and other areas with a thin, oily coating. This helps to prevent burning and/or irritation of the scalp and skin. Previously treated hair should be protected with cream conditioner during the straightening process.

"No base" relaxers are also available. These relaxers have the same chemical reaction on the hair, although usually the reaction is milder. The procedure for the application of a "no base" relaxer is the same as for a regular relaxer except that the base cream is not applied. It is advisable to use a protective cream around the hairline and over the ears.

Steps in Chemical Hair Relaxing

All chemical hair relaxing involves three basic steps: *processing, neutralizing,* and *conditioning.*

PROCESSING

As soon as the chemical relaxer is applied, the hair begins to soften so that the chemical can penetrate to loosen and relax the natural curl.

NEUTRALIZING

As soon as the hair has been sufficiently processed, the chemical relaxer is thoroughly rinsed out with warm water, followed by either a built-in shampoo neutralizer or a prescribed shampoo and neutralizer.

CONDITIONING

Depending on the client's needs, the conditioner may be part of a series of hair treatments, or it may be applied to the hair before or after the relaxing treatment.

CAUTION

▶ *Overly curly hair that has been damaged from heat appliances or other chemicals must be reconditioned before a relaxer service is performed.*

Hair treated with lighteners or metallic dyes must not be given a chemical hair relaxer, because it might cause excessive damage or breakage.

RECOMMENDED STRENGTH OF RELAXER

The strength of relaxer used is determined by the strand test. The following guidelines can help in determining which strength relaxer to use for the test.

1. Fine, tinted, or lightened hair—Use mild relaxer.
2. Normal, medium-textured virgin hair—Use regular relaxer.
3. Coarse virgin hair—Use strong or super relaxer.

Analysis of Client's Hair

It is essential that the cosmetologist have a working knowledge of human hair, particularly when giving a relaxing treatment. You will learn to recognize the qualities of hair by visible inspection, feel, and special tests. Before attempting to give a relaxing treatment to overly curly hair, the cosmetologist must judge its texture, porosity, elasticity, and the extent, if any, of damage to the hair. (For more complete information on hair analysis, refer to the chapter on permanent waving.)

CLIENT'S HAIR HISTORY

To help ensure consistent, satisfactory results, records should be kept of each chemical hair relaxing treatment. These records should include the client's hair history, products and conditioners used (see sample form on page 285), and the client's release statement. The release statement is used to protect the cosmetologist, to some extent, from the responsibility for accidents or damages. You should be sure to find out if the client has ever had a hair relaxing. If so, was there any reaction? You must not chemically relax hair that has been treated with a metallic dye. To do so damages or destroys the hair. In addition, it is not advisable to use chemical relaxers on hair that has been bleached lighter.

Before starting to process the hair, you must know how the client will react to the relaxer. Therefore, the client must receive: (1) a thorough scalp and hair examination and (2) a hair strand test.

RELAXER RECORD

Name .... Tel. ....

Address .... City .... State .... Zip ....

DESCRIPTION OF HAIR

Form	Length	Texture		Porosity	
☐ wavy	☐ short	☐ coarse	☐ soft	☐ very porous	☐ less porous
☐ curly	☐ medium	☐ medium	☐ silky	☐ moderately	☐ least porous
☐ extra-curly	☐ long	☐ fine	☐ wiry	porous	☐ resistant
				☐ normal	

Condition

☐ virgin ☐ retouched ☐ dry ☐ oily ☐ lightened

Tinted with ....

Previously relaxed with (name of relaxer) ....

☐ Original sample of hair enclosed ☐ not enclosed

TYPE OF RELAXER OR STRAIGHTENER

☐ whole head ☐ retouch

☐ relaxer .... strength .... ☐ straightener .... strength ....

Results

☐ good ☐ poor ☐ sample of relaxed hair enclosed ☐ not enclosed

Date	Operator	Date	Operator
....	....	....	....
....	....	....	....
....	....	....	....

SCALP EXAMINATION

Inspect the scalp carefully for eruptions, scratches, or abrasions. To obtain a clearer view of the scalp, part the hair into ½" (1.25 cm) sections. Hair parting may be done with the index and middle fingers or with the handle of a rat-tail comb. In either case, you must exercise great care not to scratch the scalp. Such scratches may become seriously infected when aggravated by the chemicals in the relaxer. (Fig. 13.1)

If the client has scalp eruptions or abrasions, do not apply the chemical hair relaxer until the scalp is healthy. If the hair is not in a healthy condition, prescribe a series of conditioning treatments to return it to a more normal condition. Then you may give a strand test.

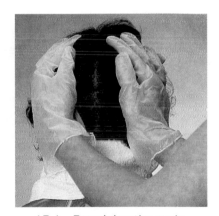

13.1—Examining the scalp.

STRAND TESTS

To help you estimate the results you may expect to get from a chemical relaxing, it is advisable to test the hair for porosity and elasticity. This can be done using one of the following strand tests:

Finger test determines the degree of porosity in the hair. Grasp a strand of hair and run it between the thumb and index finger of the right hand, from the end toward the scalp. If it ruffles or feels bumpy, the hair is porous and can absorb moisture.

Pull test. This test determines the degree of elasticity in the hair. Normally, dry, curly hair will stretch about one-fifth its normal length without breaking. Grasp half a dozen strands from the crown area and pull them gently. If the hair appears to stretch, it has elasticity and can withstand the relaxer. If not, conditioning treatments are recommended prior to a chemical relaxing treatment.

Relaxer test. Application of the relaxer to a hair strand will indicate the reaction of the relaxer on the hair. Take a small section of hair from the crown or another area where the hair is wiry and resistant. Pull it through a slit in a piece of aluminum foil placed as close to the scalp as possible. Apply relaxer to the strand in the same manner as you would apply it to the entire head. Process the strand until it is sufficiently relaxed, checking the strand every 3 to 5 minutes. Make careful note of the timing, the smoothing required, and the hair strength. Shampoo the relaxer from the strand only, towel dry, and cover with protective cream to avoid damage during the relaxing service. If breakage has occurred, you should do another strand test using a milder solution. (Fig. 13.2)

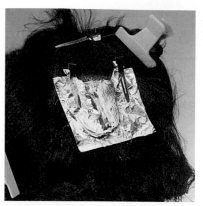

13.2—Relaxer strand test.

Chemical Hair Relaxing Process (with Sodium Hydroxide)

The procedure outlined below is based primarily on products containing sodium hydroxide. For this, or any other kind of product, follow the manufacturer's directions and be guided by your instructor.

EQUIPMENT, IMPLEMENTS, AND MATERIALS

Chemical relaxer	Protective	Conditioner
Neutralizer or	gloves	Absorbent cotton
neutralizing shampoo	Towels	Neck strip
Shampoo and	Rollers	Clips and picks
cream rinse	Comb and	End papers
Shampoo cape	brush	Setting lotion
Protective base	Spatula	Record card
Conditioner-filler	Timer	

PREPARATION

1. Select and arrange the required equipment, implements, and materials.
2. Wash and sanitize your hands.

3. Seat client comfortably. Remove earrings and neck jewelry; adjust towel and shampoo cape.
4. Examine and evaluate the scalp and hair.
5. Give a strand test and check results.
6. Do not shampoo hair. (Hair ends may be trimmed after the application of the chemical relaxer.)
7. Have client sign release card.

PROCEDURE

1. Part hair into four or five sections, as recommended by your instructor. (Figs. 13.3, 13.4)

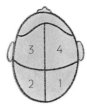

13.3—Part hair into four sections.

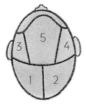

13.4—Part hair into five sections; three sections in front area, two sections in back area.

2. Dry hair. If moisture or perspiration is present on the scalp because of excessive heat or humidity, place the client under a cool dryer for several minutes.
3. Apply protective base. Manufacturers recommend the use of a protective base to protect the scalp from the strong chemicals in the relaxer. To apply it properly, subdivide each of the four or five major sections into ½" to 1" (1.25 to 2.5 cm) partings, to permit thorough scalp coverage. (Fig. 13.5)

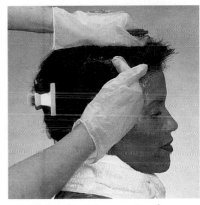

13.5—Applying protective base.

Apply the base freely to the entire scalp with the fingers. The hairline around the forehead, nape of the neck, and area over and around the ears must be completely covered. Complete coverage is important to protect the scalp and hairline from irritation.

▶ **NOTE:** When using a "no base" relaxer, a protective base is not necessary. It is recommended that a protective cream be used on the hairline and around the ears.

APPLYING THE CONDITIONER-FILLER

In many cases a conditioner-filler is required before the chemical relaxer can be used. The conditioner-filler, usually a protein product, is applied to the entire head of hair when dry. It protects over-porous or slightly damaged hair from being over-processed on any part of the hair shaft. It evens out porosity of the hair shaft, and permits uniform distribution and action of the chemical relaxer.

To give complete benefits from the conditioner-filler, rub it gently onto the hair from the scalp to the hair ends, using either the hands or a comb. Then towel dry the hair or use a cool dryer to completely dry the hair.

CAUTION

▶ *Avoid the use of heat, which will open the pores of the scalp and cause irritation or injury to the client's scalp.*
  Protective gloves must be worn by the cosmetologist to prevent damage to hands.

APPLYING THE RELAXER

Divide the head into four or five sections, in the same manner as for the application of the protective base.

The processing cream is applied last to the scalp area and hair ends. The body heat will speed up the processing action at the scalp. The hair is more porous at the ends and may be damaged. In both these areas, less processing time is required, and, therefore, the relaxer is applied last.

There are three methods in general use for the application of the chemical hair relaxer: the comb method, the brush method, and the finger method.

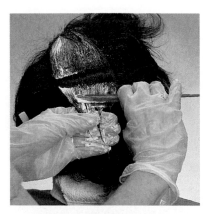
13.6 — Applying relaxer on top of strand.

COMB METHOD

Remove a quantity of relaxing cream from the jar. Beginning in the back right section of the head, carefully part off ¼" to ½" (.66 to 1.25 cm) of hair, depending on its thickness and curliness. Apply the relaxer with the back of the comb, starting ½" to 1" (1.25 to 2.5 cm) from the scalp, and spread to within ½" (1.25 cm) of the hair ends. First apply the relaxer to the top side of the strand. (Fig. 13.6) Then, raise the subsection and apply the relaxer underneath. Gently lay the completed strand up, out of the way. (Fig. 13.7)

Complete the right back area, and moving in a clockwise direction, cover each section of the head in the same manner. Then, go back over the head in the same order, applying additional relaxing cream, if necessary, and spreading the relaxer close to the scalp and up to the hair ends. Avoid excessive pressure or stretching of the hair.

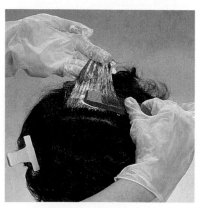
13.7 — Applying relaxer underneath strand.

Smoothing the cream through the hair not only spreads the cream, but also stretches the hair gently into a straight position.

An alternate technique is to begin application at the nape, approximately 1″ (2.5 cm) from the hairline, and continue toward the crown. The last place to apply relaxer is at the hairline. Be guided by your instructor's and the manufacturer's instructions.

BRUSH OR FINGER METHOD

The brush or finger method of applying the relaxer to the hair is the same as the comb method, except the brush or the fingers and palms are used instead of the back of the comb. *Wear protective gloves.*

PERIODIC STRAND TESTING

While spreading the relaxer, inspect its action by stretching the strands to see how fast the natural curls are being removed. Another method of testing is to press the strand to the scalp using the back of the comb or your finger. Examine the strand after your finger is removed. If it lies smoothly, the strand is sufficiently relaxed; if the strand reverts or ''beads'' back away from the scalp, continue processing.

RINSING OUT THE RELAXER

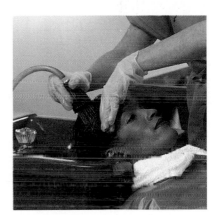

When the hair has been sufficiently straightened, rinse the relaxer out rapidly and thoroughly. The water must be warm, not hot. (Fig. 13.8) If the water is too hot, it may burn the client and cause discomfort because of the very sensitive condition of the scalp. If the water is too cold, it will not stop the processing action. The direct force of the rinse water should be used to remove the relaxer and avoid tangling the hair. Part hair with fingers to make sure no traces of the relaxer remain. Unless the relaxer is completely removed, its chemical action continues on the hair. The stream of water should be directed from the scalp to the hair ends.

13.8—Rinsing out relaxer.

CAUTION

▶ *Do not get relaxer or rinse water into the eyes or on unprotected skin. If the relaxer or rinse water gets into the client's eyes, wash it out immediately, and refer the client to a doctor without delay.*

SHAMPOOING/NEUTRALIZING

When the hair is thoroughly rinsed, neutralize the hair as directed by your instructor. Most manufacturers provide a neutralizing shampoo which is applied to the hair after rinsing. Others prescribe the use of a non-alkaline or a cream shampoo followed by a neutralizer.

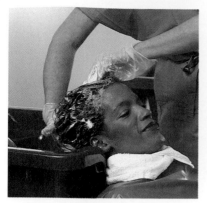

13.9—Shampooing the hair.

Gently work the shampoo into the hair. Use care to avoid tangling the hair or breaking any fragile ends. Manipulate the shampoo by working with the fingers underneath the hair, not on top. Rinse with warm water, making sure to keep the hair straight. Repeat the shampoo until the hair lathers well and all the relaxer is removed. (Fig. 13.9)

After shampooing, completely saturate the hair with the neutralizer if it is required by the manufacturer. Beginning at the nape, carefully comb with a wide-tooth comb, working upward, toward the forehead. Use the comb to:

1.   Keep the hair straight.
2.   Ensure complete saturation with the neutralizer.
3.   Remove any tangles without pulling.

Time the neutralizer as directed and rinse thoroughly. Towel blot gently. Condition hair as necessary and proceed with styling. Discard used supplies. Cleanse and sanitize equipment. Wash and sanitize hands. Complete record of all timings and treatments during the service, and file the record card.

▶ NOTE: Different products used for relaxing require different methods. Always follow the manufacturer's directions.

APPLYING THE CONDITIONER

Many manufacturers recommend that you apply a conditioner before setting the hair, to offset the harshness of the sodium hydroxide in the relaxer and to help restore some of the natural oils to the scalp and hair.

Two types of conditioners available are:

1.   *Cream-type conditioners* are applied to the scalp and hair, then carefully rinsed out. The hair is then towel dried. Apply setting lotion; set the hair on rollers; dry and style the hair in the usual manner.
2.   *Protein-type (liquid) conditioners* are applied to the scalp and hair prior to hairsetting and allowed to remain in the hair to serve as a setting lotion. Set the hair on rollers, dry, and style in the usual manner.

▶ NOTE: Because of the fragile condition of the hair, it is advisable to wind the hair on the roller without extreme tension.

HOT THERMAL IRONS

To avoid hair breakage, excessive heat and excessive stretching should be avoided. Thermal curling with warm heat can be used to curl chemically relaxed hair. Conditioning treatments should be recommended and the hair dried completely before thermal curling. (See chapter on thermal hairstyling for a discussion of thermal irons.)

Success Spotlight

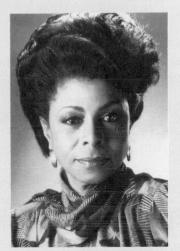

Olive Lee Benson is an international authority on black hair care. Frequently quoted in *Essence, Vogue,* and *Elle* magazines, she has trained salon owners throughout the world.

Born in Cambridge, Massachusetts, Benson was next to the youngest in a family of ten. "From an early age, I loved to do hair," she says. "In fact, under my photo in the high school yearbook, it says, 'Most likely hairdresser.' "

From high school, Benson went on to Wilfred Beauty Academy and has since been inducted into the school's Hall of Fame. When she opened her first salon in 1959, her clients were primarily women with curly hair. Guided by the inspiration of Madame C. J. Walker, the first black woman to become a self-made millionaire through her hair and cosmetology business in the early 1900s, Benson was determined to make an impact on the hair care industry.

"Madame Walker was the founder of the black hair care industry," says Benson. "She developed a product for the black woman's needs when other companies ignored the ethnic market. I admired her because she did it the hard way, selling her products from door to door, and sleeping in cars and trains because at the time, Jim Crow laws wouldn't allow blacks to rent a hotel room."

With advice from competition authorities Bill Wright and Paul Barnes, Benson excelled in hair competitions, capturing many prestigious trophies across the country. An NCA HairAmerica member, she has been a designer and coordinator for that organization, where she set seasonal cutting and styling trends. Benson is also an editorial columnist for *ShopTalk* magazine.

Today, her knowledge is in great demand, both in the United States and in Europe. "Chemical control and the art of hairdressing are my principal areas of instruction," she says.

If you specialize in this area, there's ample room for growth, to which Benson's success is a testament.

SODIUM HYDROXIDE RETOUCH

Hair grows about ¼" to ½" (.66 to 1.25 cm) per month. A retouch should probably be done every 6 weeks to 2 months, depending on how quickly the client's hair grows.

Follow all the steps for a regular chemical hair relaxing treatment, with one exception: *apply the relaxer only to the new growth.* In order to avoid breakage of previously treated hair, apply a cream conditioner over the hair that received the earlier treatment, thus avoiding overlapping and damage.

Chemical Hair Relaxing Process (with Ammonium Thioglycolate)

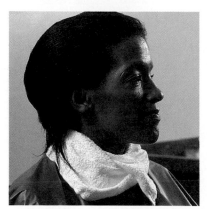

13.10—Relaxed hair.

Ammonium thioglycolate (also called thio relaxer) is the same type of product used in cold waving, with a heavy cream or gel added to the formula in order to keep the hair in a straightened position. (Fig. 13.10)

As in cold waving, the relaxer breaks the sulfur and hydrogen bonds, softening and swelling the hair. The mechanical action of the hands, brush, or fingers smooths the hair and holds it in a straightened position.

Once the hair is straightened, the neutralizer is applied (serving the same purpose as the neutralizer in cold waving). It re-forms the sulfur and hydrogen bonds and rehardens the hair in its newly straightened position.

Manufacturers vary their products according to the texture and condition of the hair. Tinted and lightened hair require a weaker formula than virgin hair.

Thio relaxers have a milder relaxing action on curly hair. You may choose to use them on fine textured hair, or when it is desirable to remove less curl from the hair. Thio relaxers can also be used to reduce excessive curl formed in a permanent wave. Consult your instructor for directions and precautions for this specialized service.

Techniques for thio relaxers vary. The general procedure involves preparing the hair (gently shampooing if required), applying a base if necessary, applying the relaxer in the manner outlined under "Chemical Hair Relaxing Process (with Sodium Hydroxide)," and periodic strand testing. Directions at this point may vary greatly, so follow the manufacturer's directions *carefully.* Remove the relaxer from the hair and neutralize as directed, condition, and proceed with styling of the hair. As with any chemical service, exercise caution so that the hair is not excessively heated or stretched during styling as this may cause damage to both the hair and the desired curl formation.

THIO RETOUCH

As noted earlier, hair grows at the rate of ¼" to ½" (.66 to 1.25 cm) per month. A thio retouch should be given when there is a noticeable regrowth. Follow all steps for a regular thio hair relaxing treatment, with the exception of the relaxer, which is applied only to the new growth. A conditioner should be applied to the previously relaxed hair to protect it from damage.

OTHER RELAXERS

Researchers have also developed acid-based relaxers for the treatment of overly curly hair. Like acid permanent waves, the relaxer works with bisulfites rather than with thioglycolate acid. This type of relaxer is designed as a milder-acting one, much like the thio. Some can also be used as a pre-wrap preparation for performing a permanent wave on excessively curly hair.

Chemical Blowout

To meet the needs of salon clients, great versatility in hairstyling may be achieved with the chemical blowout. This technique removes only a small amount of the curl, leaving the hair in a more manageable condition. A chemical blowout is a combination of chemical hair straightening and hairstyling, which creates a well-groomed style in the Afro-American tradition.

The chemical blowout may be done with either the thio hair relaxer or the sodium hydroxide relaxer. The important consideration with either method is not to over-relax the hair to the point where the blowout process becomes impossible to perform. Usually, when the thio relaxer is used, the hair is shampooed first. When the sodium hydroxide relaxer is used, the hair is shampooed after the hair is relaxed. (Follow the manufacturer's or your instructor's directions.)

EQUIPMENT, IMPLEMENTS, AND MATERIALS

Use the same equipment, implements, and materials as for a regular chemical relaxing, plus a wide-tooth comb (hair lifter or pick), scissors, clippers, and hand blower.

PROCEDURE

1. Prepare and drape client as for a regular hair relaxing treatment.
2. Apply scalp conditioner and/or base to the scalp.
3. Wear protective gloves; apply relaxer in the usual manner.

4. Stop the relaxing procedure by rinsing the relaxer from the hair with warm water before it is straightened and while it still shows a wave or curl formation.
5. Apply neutralizer or neutralizing shampoo.
6. Rinse out neutralizer and towel blot the hair.
7. Apply a conditioner to scalp and hair to help restore the natural oils removed by the relaxer.

If the blowout style is desired, dry the hair with a hand dryer while lifting the hair with a hair lifter or pick. Dry from the scalp out to the ends. Distribute the dry hair evenly around the head and shape with clippers or shears. Continue to lift the hair out from the head to check progress of cut.

The hair can also be shaped while wet, then combed into place to let it dry naturally. For a softer look, the hair can be picked or combed when dry.

Review of Safety Precautions

When giving a chemical relaxing, you can never be too cautious. Here is a review of the safety measures that will ensure a comfortable and safe treatment for your client.

1. Examine the scalp for abrasions; if any are present, do not give a hair relaxing treatment.
2. Analyze the hair; give a strand test.
3. Do not relax damaged hair. Suggest a series of conditioning treatments.
4. Do not shampoo the hair prior to the application of a sodium hydroxide product.
5. Do not apply a sodium hydroxide relaxer over a thio relaxer.
6. Do not apply a thio relaxer over a sodium hydroxide relaxer.
7. Never use a strong relaxer on fine hair, as it may cause breakage.
8. Cool or warm irons may be used on chemically relaxed hair. Do not use excessive heat, as it may cause damage to relaxed hair.
9. Apply a protective base, to avoid burning or irritating the scalp with the sodium hydroxide relaxer.
10. Wear protective gloves.

11. Protect client's eyes.

12. Use extreme care when applying the relaxer to avoid accidentally spreading it on the ears, scalp, or skin.

13. Strand test the action of the relaxer frequently to determine how fast the natural curl is being removed.

14. Be sure to thoroughly rinse the relaxer from the hair. Failure to do so permits the relaxer to continue to process, resulting in hair damage. Direct stream of warm water from scalp to hair ends.

15. Wear protective gloves until all the relaxer has been removed. When rinsing the shampoo from the hair, always work from the scalp to the ends, to prevent tangling the hair.

16. Use a wide-tooth comb and avoid pulling when combing the hair after the relaxation process is complete. Avoid scratching the scalp with comb or fingernails.

17. Apply a conditioner to the scalp and hair before setting the hair.

18. When retouching the new growth, do not allow the relaxer to overlap onto the hair already straightened.

19. Do not give a hair relaxing treatment to hair treated with a metallic dye.

20. At the completion of each treatment, fill out a complete record card.

21. Have the client sign a release statement to protect the salon and the cosmetologist.

22. It is not advisable to use chemical relaxers on lightened hair.

Soft Curl Permanent

Soft curl permanent waving is a method of permanently waving overly curly hair. It is known by various names given by the manufacturers of the products.

CAUTION

▶ *The product used contains ammonium thioglycolate (thio).*
1. *Do not use on hair that has been treated with sodium hydroxide products.*
2. *Do not use on hair that has been treated with metallic dye or compound henna.*

IMPLEMENTS AND MATERIALS

Shampoo cape	Thio gel, cream, or lotion	Plastic cap
Neck strips and towels	Applicators	Neutralizer
Mild shampoo	Curling rods	Styling lotion (curl activator)
Combs	Porous end papers	Finishing rinse
Gloves	Pre-wrap solution	Hair clips
Protective cream	Waving lotion	Scissors or razor
	Cotton or neutralizing bands	Record cards

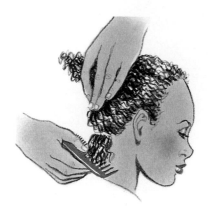

13.11—Remove tangles from hair.

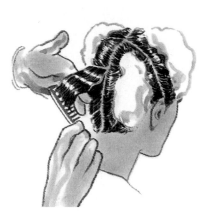

13.12—Part hair into sections and coat with thio gel.

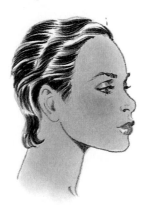

13.13—Comb thio gel through hair.

PROCEDURE

This procedure can be used for both men and women.

1. Examine the client's scalp. Do not use permanent waving gel or cream if the scalp shows signs of abrasions or lesions, or if the client has experienced an allergic reaction to a previous perm.
2. Shampoo and rinse hair thoroughly. Towel dry, leaving hair damp.
3. Remove tangles with a large-tooth comb. (See Fig. 13.11)
4. Part hair into four to five sections, as recommended by your instructor. (If the manufacturer requires it, put a protective cream on the entire scalp, including around the hairline.)
5. Wear protective gloves.
6. Apply thio gel or cream to one section at a time, using the back of a comb, a hair-coloring brush, or fingers. Use a tail comb to part hair and begin the application of thio gel or cream to the hair nearest the scalp, preferably starting at the nape area. Work the thio gel or cream to the ends of the hair.
7. Comb the thio gel or cream through the entire head, first with a wide-tooth comb, then with a smaller-tooth comb. (See Fig. 13.12)
8. When the hair becomes supple and flexible (See Fig. 13.13), rinse with tepid water and towel dry. Do not tangle the hair.

▶ NOTE: Always follow the manufacturer's instructions on the recommended procedure for rinsing off the chemical.

9. Section the hair into eight sections. (See Fig. 13.14) Subsection as you wrap the hair. (See Fig. 13.15)

10. Wrap hair as desired on curling rods. In order to rearrange the curl pattern of the hair, the rod selected must be at least two times larger than the natural curl. In order to achieve a good curl formation, the hair should encircle the rod at least 2½ times.

11. After the wrap has been completed, protect the client's skin by placing cotton around the hairline and neck. (See Fig. 13.16)

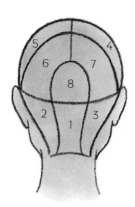

13.14—Divide the hair into eight sections.

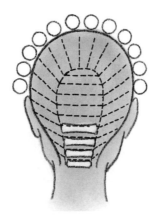

13.15—Subsection as you wrap.

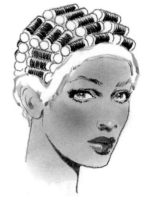

13.16—Protect client's skin with cotton around hairline.

12. Apply thio gel, cream, or lotion to all the curls until they are thoroughly saturated. (See Fig. 13.17) Replace saturated cotton.

13. Cover the client's head with a plastic cap.

14. Have the client sit under a pre-heated dryer for 15 to 25 minutes, or as recommended by the manufacturer. (See Fig. 13.18)

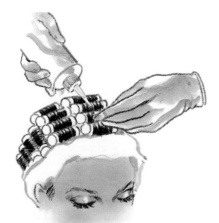

13.17—Apply thio gel to curls.

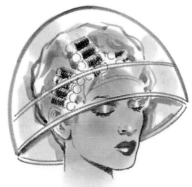

13.18—Process under pre-heated dryer.

15. Take a test curl (See Fig. 13.19), and if the desired curl pattern has not developed, have the client sit under the dryer for another 10 minutes or until a curl pattern develops.

16. When the desired curl pattern has been reached, rinse the hair thoroughly with warm (not hot) water. (See Fig. 13.20) Blot each curl with a towel.

17. Use a prepared neutralizer, or mix neutralizer as directed by the manufacturer, and saturate each curl twice. (See Fig. 13.21) Allow neutralizer to remain on the curls for 5 to 10 minutes, or as directed by the manufacturer.

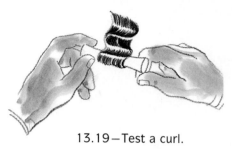

13.19—Test a curl.

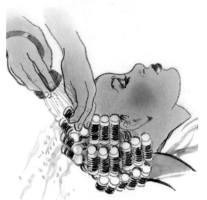

13.20—Rinse the hair.

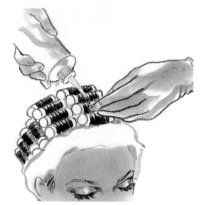

13.21—Apply neutralizer.

18. Carefully remove rods and apply balance of neutralizer to the hair. Work neutralizer through with fingers for thorough distribution (See Fig. 13.22), and allow it to remain on the hair for another 5 minutes.

19. Rinse hair thoroughly with cool water and towel blot.

20. Trim uneven hair ends. (See Fig. 13.23)

21. Apply conditioner as directed by the manufacturer.

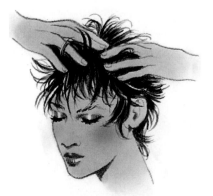

13.22—Work neutralizer through hair.

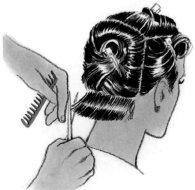

13.23—Trim hair ends.

22. Air dry hair or style as directed. (See Fig. 13.24)

Fig. 13.25 illustrates hairstyle *after* a soft curl permanent was given.

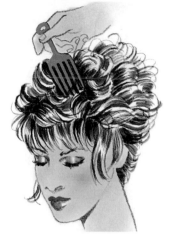 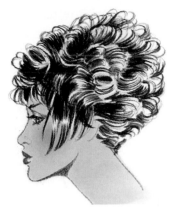

13.24—Style hair.   13.25—Finished hairstyle.

AFTERCARE

1. Do not comb or brush the curls when wet; use a lifting pick instead.
2. Shampoo as often as necessary, using a mild (acid-balanced) shampoo.
3. Conditioner or curl activator should be used daily to maintain flexibility, sheen, and proper moisture balance of the hair.

Review of Safety Precautions

1. Do not give a soft curl permanent to hair treated with sodium hydroxide.
2. Do not give a soft curl permanent to hair that has been colored with a metallic dye or compound henna.
3. Thoroughly analyze the hair and scalp and record the information prior to giving a soft curl permanent.
4. Bleached, tinted, or damaged hair must be reconditioned until the hair is of sufficient strength to ensure that the soft curl service will not cause further damage.
5. If permanent waving lotion or neutralizer accidentally gets into the client's eye, flush the eye immediately with water and refer the client to a doctor.
6. Test curl frequently to ensure proper curl formation without damage.
7. Use protective cream around client's hairline and neck.
8. Complete client's record card carefully and accurately.

Review Questions

CHEMICAL HAIR RELAXING AND SOFT CURL PERMANENT

1. What are the basic products used for chemical hair relaxing?
2. What are the two types of chemical hair relaxers?
3. What are the three steps of chemical hair relaxing?
4. What is the most important point to remember when performing a chemical service?
5. What type of hair relaxing technique achieves the greatest versatility in hairstyling?
6. List the three most important safety precautions for chemical hair relaxing.
7. What is the method of permanently waving overly curly hair?
8. If hair were treated with sodium hydroxide, what service could not be done?
9. If hair is damaged by an appliance or a chemical, what must you do before applying a chemical hair relaxer?

14

THERMAL HAIR STRAIGHTENING (HAIR PRESSING)

LEARNING OBJECTIVES

After completing this chapter, you should be able to:

1. Discuss the purpose served by hair pressing.

2. List the products required for a successful hair pressing.

3. Demonstrate the procedures involved in both soft pressing and hard pressing.

4. Explain the techniques for analyzing the client's hair and scalp prior to a hair pressing.

5. List the safety precautions that must be observed in hair pressing.

Introduction

Hair straightening, pressing, is a profitable service that is popular in the beauty salon. When properly done, hair pressing temporarily straightens overly curly or unruly hair. A pressing generally lasts until the hair is next shampooed. (Permanent hair straightening is covered in the chapter on chemical hair relaxing.)

Hair pressing prepares the hair for additional services, such as thermal roller curling and croquignole thermal curling. A good hair pressing leaves the hair in a natural and lustrous condition and is not harmful to the hair.

There are three types of hair pressing:

1. *Soft press*, which removes about 50% to 60% of the curl and is accomplished by applying the thermal pressing comb once on each side of the hair.

2. *Medium press*, which removes about 60% to 75% of the curl and is accomplished by applying the thermal pressing comb once on each side of the hair using slightly more pressure.

3. *Hard press*, which removes 100% of the curl and is accomplished by applying the thermal pressing comb twice on each side of the hair.

Analysis of Hair and Scalp

Before the cosmetologist undertakes to press the client's hair, there should be an analysis of the condition of the hair and scalp in order to evaluate the client's needs.

CAUTION

▶ *Under no circumstances should hair pressing be given to a client who has a scalp abrasion, contagious scalp condition, scalp injury, or chemically treated hair.*

If the client's hair and scalp are not normal, the cosmetologist should give appropriate advice concerning preliminary corrective treatments. If the hair shows signs of neglect or abuse caused by faulty pressing, lightening, or tinting, the cosmetologist should recommend a series of conditioning treatments. Failure to correct dry and brittle hair can result in hair breakage during hair pressing. *Burnt hair strands cannot be conditioned.*

You should also remember to check the elasticity and porosity of your client's hair. Under normal conditions, if a client's hair has good elasticity, it can be safely stretched about one-fifth of its length. If the ability of the hair to absorb water (porosity) is normal, then the hair returns to its normal curly appearance when it is wet or moistened.

A careful analysis of the client's hair and scalp should cover the following points:

1. Form of hair (curly or overly curly)
2. Length of hair (long, medium, or short)
3. Texture of hair (coarse, medium, fine, or very fine)
4. Feel of hair (wiry, soft, or silky)
5. Elasticity of hair (normal or poor)
6. Shade of hair (natural, faded, streaked, or gray)
7. Condition of hair (normal, brittle, dry, oily, damaged, or chemically treated)
8. Condition of scalp (normal, flexible, or tight)

It is important that the cosmetologist be able to recognize individual differences in hair texture, hair porosity, hair elasticity, and scalp flexibility. Guided by this knowledge, the cosmetologist can determine how much pressure the hair and scalp can tolerate without breakage, hair loss, or burning from a pressing comb that is not adjusted to the right temperature.

HAIR TEXTURE

Variations in hair texture can be traced to the following factors:

1. Diameter of the hair (coarse, medium, or fine). Coarse hair has the greatest diameter. Fine hair has the smallest diameter.
2. Feel of the hair (wiry, soft, or silky).

The client's hair texture also depends on how dry, oily, gray, tinted, lightened, or curly it is. Touching the client's hair and asking specifically about hair characteristics will help you know how to treat the client's hair.

Coarse Hair

Coarse, overly curly hair has qualities that make it difficult to press. Coarse hair has the greatest diameter, and during the pressing process it requires more heat and pressure than medium or fine hair.

Medium Hair

Medium curly hair is the normal type of hair cosmetologists deal with in the beauty salon. No special problem is presented by this type of hair, and it is the least resistant to hair pressing.

Fine Hair

Fine hair requires special care. To avoid hair breakage, less heat and pressure should be applied than for other hair textures. Whereas coarse and medium hair have three layers—cuticle, cortex, and medulla, fine hair has only two layers—cortex and cuticle.

Wiry, Curly Hair

Wiry, curly hair may be coarse, medium, or fine. It feels stiff, hard, and glassy. Because of the compact construction of the cuticle cells, it is very resistant to hair pressing and it requires more heat and pressure than other types of hair.

SCALP CONDITION

The condition of the client's scalp can be classified as normal, tight, or flexible. If the scalp is normal, proceed with an analysis of the texture and elasticity of the hair. If the scalp is tight and the hair coarse, press the hair in the direction in which it grows to avoid injury to the scalp.

The main difficulty with a flexible scalp is that the cosmetologist might not apply enough pressure to press the hair satisfactorily.

RECORD CARD

You should be sure to keep a record of all pressing treatments performed on a client. It also is advisable to question the client about any lightener, tint, color restorer (metallic), or other chemical treatment that was used on his or her hair.

CONDITIONING TREATMENTS

Effective conditioning treatments require special cosmetic preparations for the hair and scalp, thorough brushing, and scalp massage. These treatments usually help get better results from hair pressing. The use of an infrared lamp is optional, depending on the type of treatment being given.

A tight scalp can be rendered more flexible by the systematic use of scalp massage, hair brushing, and direct high-frequency current. The client benefits because there is better circulation of blood to the scalp.

PRESSING COMBS

There are two types of pressing combs: regular and electric. They are both constructed of either good quality stainless steel or brass. The handle is usually made of wood since wood does not readily absorb heat. The space between the teeth of the comb varies with the size and style of the comb. A comb with more space between the teeth produces a coarse looking press. A comb with less space produces a smoother press. Pressing combs vary in size; some are short, to be used with short hair, while long combs are used with long hair. (Fig. 14.1)

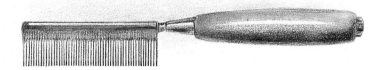

14.1 — Regular pressing comb.

Heating the Comb

Depending on their composition, combs vary in their ability to accept and retain heat. Regular pressing combs may be heated on gas stoves or electric heaters. (Fig. 14.2) While the comb is being heated, its teeth should face upward and the handle should be kept away from the fire. After heating the comb to the proper temperature, test it on a piece of light paper. If the paper becomes scorched, allow the comb to cool slightly before applying it to the hair.

Electric pressing combs are available in two forms: one comes with an "on" and "off" switch; the other is equipped with a thermostat, which has a control switch that indicates high or low degrees of heat.

There is also a straightening comb attachment that fits the nozzle of a standard hand-held dryer and is less damaging than an electric comb or an oven-heated comb.

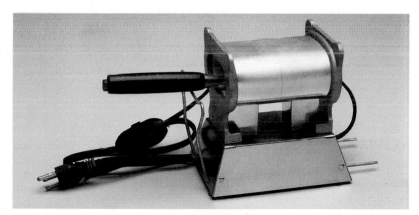

14.2 — Electric heater.

Cleaning the Comb

The pressing comb will perform more efficiently if it is kept clean and free of carbon. Wipe the comb clean of loose hair, grease, and dust before and after each use. The intense heat keeps the comb sterile when all loose hair or clinging dirt is removed. Remove the carbon from the comb by rubbing its outside surface and between its teeth with one of the following: emery board, fine steel wool pad, or fine sandpaper. After using any of these cleaning methods, immerse the metal portion of the comb in a hot baking soda solution for about 1 hour; then rinse and dry. The metal will acquire a smooth and shiny appearance.

PRESSING OIL OR CREAM

Applying pressing oil or cream prior to a hair pressing treatment helps prepare the hair for pressing. Both of these products have the following beneficial effects:

1. Make hair softer
2. Prepare and condition hair for pressing
3. Help prevent hair from burning or scorching
4. Help prevent hair breakage
5. Help condition the hair after pressing
6. Add sheen to pressed hair

HAIR SECTIONING

Divide the head into four main sections. Then subdivide these sections into 1″ to 1½″ (2.5 to 3.75 cm) partings. The size of the subsections depends on the texture and density of the hair.

1. For medium textured hair of average density, use subsections of average size.
2. For coarse hair with greater density, use smaller sections to ensure complete heat penetration and effectiveness.
3. For thin or fine hair with sparse density, use larger sections.

SOFT PRESSING PROCEDURE FOR NORMAL CURLY HAIR

The following procedure is one of several ways to give a hair pressing treatment and can be changed to meet your instructor's method.

Equipment, Implements, and Materials

Pressing comb	Pressing oil	Towels and cape
Heating appliance (gas or electric heater or attachment)	Hairbrush and comb	Spatula
	Grease or pomade	Neck strips
	Shampoo	Thermal irons

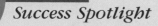

Success Spotlight

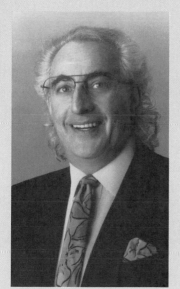

Matrix Essentials's phenomenal rise is a testimonial to the power of Arnie Miller's imagination, determination, and drive. For three decades, Miller has set the highest of professional standards for the beauty industry. As a salon owner, he helped pioneer the full-service concept by offering innovative hairstyling and chemical service techniques, and combining them into hair and skin care retail centers and a fashionable women's boutique. His audacious approach to the large-sized, independent salon business is a model of its kind to this day.

Miller's success as a salon owner motivated him to go on to conquer the world of exclusively distributed, professional salon products. Against all precedents, Matrix Essentials opened the 1980s with a tubed hair-color product. Innovative permanent waving solutions and hair and skin care products followed. Miller built his company believing that "nothing predictable, nothing conventional" was the rule to follow. He also believes that payback to the hairdresser, the industry, and the community is vital. Therefore, Miller has led the fight against non-professional product distribution, winning a landmark case, and created The Professional Beauty Industry Partnership for a Drug-Free America, a grass-roots effort in 160,000 salons to fight the drug war.

Miller has been honored by the American Beauty Association, the National Beauty and Barber Manufacturers Association, and most recently, by the Cosmetology Advancement Foundation, as someone who can attract quality students to the profession.

Preparation

1. Select and arrange required materials.
2. Wash and sanitize hands.
3. Drape client.
4. Shampoo, rinse, and towel dry client's hair.
5. Apply pressing oil or cream. (Note: Some cosmetologists prefer to apply pressing oil or cream to the hair after it has been completely dried.)
6. Dry hair thoroughly.
7. Comb and divide hair into four main sections. Pin up four sections.
8. Place pressing comb in heater.

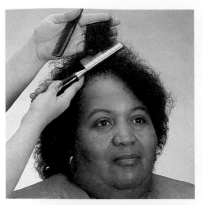

14.3—Proper handling of pressing comb.

Procedure

1. Unpin one section of hair at a time and subdivide into small hair sections. Beginning at the right side of the head, work from front to back. (Some cosmetologists prefer to start at the back of the head and work forward.)

2. If necessary, apply pressing oil evenly and sparingly over the small hair sections.

3. Test the temperature of the heated pressing comb on a white cloth or white paper to determine heat intensity before you place it on the hair.

4. Lift the end of a small hair section with the index finger and thumb of the left hand and hold it upward away from the scalp.

5. Holding the pressing comb in the right hand, insert the teeth of the comb into the top side of the hair section. (Fig. 14.3)

6. Draw out the pressing comb slightly; make a quick turn so that the hair strand wraps itself partly around the comb. The back rod of the comb actually does the pressing.

7. Press the comb slowly through the hair strand until the ends of the hair pass through the teeth of the comb.

8. Bring each completed hair section over to the opposite side of the head.

9. Continue steps 4 to 8 on both sections on the right side of the head; then do the same on both sections on the left side.

Completion

1. Apply a little pomade to the hair near the scalp and brush it through the hair.

2. If desired, thermal roller or croquignole curling can be given at this time. (The procedures and techniques are found in the chapter on thermal hairstyling.)

3. Style and comb the hair according to the client's wishes.

4. Place supplies in their proper places.

5. Sanitize implements and clean equipment.

HARD PRESS

A hard press is recommended when the results of a soft press are not satisfactory. The entire comb press procedure is repeated. Pressing oil may be added to hair strands only if necessary. A hard press is also known as a *double comb press*.

TOUCH-UPS

Touch-ups are sometimes necessary when the hair becomes curly again due to perspiration, dampness, or other conditions. The process is the same as for the original pressing treatment, with the shampoo omitted.

SAFETY PRECAUTIONS

The injuries that can occur in hair pressing are of two types:

1. Injuries that are the immediate results of hair pressing and cause physical damage, such as:
   a) Burnt hair that breaks off
   b) Burnt scalp that causes either temporary or permanent loss of hair
   c) Burns on ears and neck that form scars
2. Injuries that are not immediately evident but can subsequently cause physical damage, such as:
   a) Skin rash if the client is allergic to pressing oil
   b) Progressive breaking and shortening of the hair because of too frequent hair pressings

CAUTION

▶ *In case of a scalp burn, immediately apply 1% gentian violet jelly.*

To avoid damage good judgment should be used, with consideration always given to the texture of the hair and condition of the scalp. The client's safety is assured only when the cosmetologist observes every precaution and is especially careful during the actual hair pressing. The cosmetologist should avoid using the following:

1. Excessive heat or pressure on the hair and scalp
2. Too much pressing oil on the hair
3. Perfumed pressing oil near the scalp if the client is allergic
4. Too frequent hair pressing

RELEASE STATEMENT

A release statement should be used for hair pressing, permanent waving, hair tinting, or any other service that might require the cosmetologist's release from responsibility for accidents or damages.

REMINDERS AND HINTS ON SOFT PRESSING

1. Keep the comb clean and free from carbon at all times.
2. Avoid overheating the pressing comb.
3. Test the temperature of the heated comb on a white cloth or white paper before applying it to the hair.
4. Adjust the temperature of the pressing comb to the texture and condition of the client's hair.
5. Use the heated comb carefully to avoid burning the skin, scalp, or hair.
6. Prevent the smoking or burning of hair during the pressing treatment by:
   a) Drying the hair completely after it is shampooed.
   b) Avoiding excessive application of pressing oil over the hair.
7. Use a moderately warm comb to press short hair on the temples and back of the neck.

Special Problems

PRESSING FINE HAIR

When pressing fine hair, follow the same procedure as for normal hair, being careful not to use a hot pressing comb or too much pressure. To avoid hair breakage, apply less pressure to the hair near the ends. After completely pressing the hair, style it.

PRESSING SHORT, FINE HAIR

When pressing short, fine hair, extra care must be taken at the hairline. When the hair is extra short, the pressing comb should not be too hot because the hair is fine and will burn easily; a hot comb can also cause accidental burns, which are very painful and can cause scars. In the event of an accidental burn, immediately apply 1% gentian violet jelly to the burn.

PRESSING COARSE HAIR

When pressing coarse hair, apply enough pressure so that the hair remains straightened.

PRESSING TINTED, LIGHTENED, OR GRAY HAIR

Tinted, lightened, or gray hair requires special care in hair pressing. Lightened or tinted hair might require conditioning treatments, depending on the extent to which it has been damaged. To obtain good results, use a moderately heated pressing comb applied with light pressure.

▶ NOTE: Avoid excessive heat on tinted, lightened or gray hair as discoloration or breakage can occur.

Review Questions

THERMAL HAIR STRAIGHTENING (HAIR PRESSING)

1. What is another name for hair pressing?
2. What is the purpose of hair pressing?
3. Name the types of hair presses.
4. Under what circumstances should hair not be pressed?
5. How is an accidental scalp burn treated?
6. How do you test implements for your pressing service?
7. What types of hair require moderate heat?

15

THE ARTISTRY OF ARTIFICIAL HAIR

LEARNING OBJECTIVES

After completing this chapter, you should be able to:

1. List the reasons people wear wigs.
2. Identify the different types of wigs, extensions, and hairpieces.
3. Demonstrate the procedure for taking wig measurements.
4. Describe the method used when ordering wigs.
5. Demonstrate the procedures for blocking a wig and fitting a wig.
6. Demonstrate the procedure for cleaning a wig.
7. Demonstrate the procedure for setting and styling a wig.
8. Demonstrate the procedure for coloring a wig.

Introduction

Throughout history, people have used wigs to beautify their appearance. The ancient Egyptians first wore wigs in 4000 B.C. for a very practical reason: to protect their hair from the sun. The wearing of wigs spread from Asia and Europe to America, where their use has become increasingly popular.

The use of wigs and hairpieces in hairstyling worldwide is a significant and exciting part of the beauty industry. The sale, styling, and servicing of artificial hair can be a source of increased salon income.

To offer the best possible service, the stylist must learn the following:

1. How wigs and hairpieces can improve the client's appearance.
2. How wigs and hairpieces are made and fitted.
3. How to select and style wigs and hairpieces to best benefit the client.
4. How to clean and service wigs and hairpieces.

Why People Wear Wigs

People wear wigs for several reasons:

1. Personal choice—to cover up baldness due to heredity, and sparse or damaged hair.
2. Medical—to cover hair loss due to a health problem. Wigs have become popular hair replacements for use by people who have had hair loss due to illness, injury, or shock to the nervous system. Both men and women use wigs in these instances to replace lost hair and maintain their usual hairstyle.
3. Fashion—for changes in everyday hairstyles, to increase length and volume, and for decorative purposes and special occasions.
4. Practicality—for flexibility and ease of style change. For example, black clients might want to wear a straight style without chemically relaxing their hair, and a wig provides the flexibility to do so.

Types of Wigs

Wigs can be made from human hair, synthetic hair (*modacrylic* is the general term used to describe synthetic wig fibers), animal hair, or a blend of two or three types.

You can use a simple test to tell the difference between human hair and synthetic hair. Cut a small piece of hair from the back of the wig. With a lighted match, burn this hair and observe the following:

1. Human hair burns slowly and gives off a strong odor.
2. Synthetic hair burns quickly and gives off little or no odor. You can feel small, hard beads in the burnt ash of synthetic hair.

HUMAN HAIR WIGS

The quality of a wig depends largely on whether it is constructed by hand or by machine. Expensive, custom-made wigs are hand knotted into a fine mesh foundation. (See Figs. 15.1, 15.2) In cheaper wigs, hair is sewn by machine into a net cap in circular rows. (See Figs. 15.3–15.5)

The quality of a wig also depends on the kind of hair it contains (human or synthetic), and how it is fitted to the client's measurements.

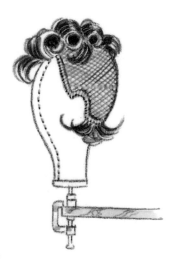

15.1—Hand-knotted wig.

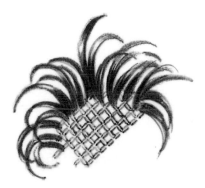

15.2—Hair crocheted and hand knotted into mesh foundation.

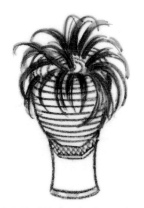

15.3—Weft wig (top view).

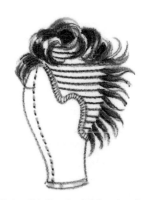

15.4—Weft wig (side view).

15.5—Hair sewn by machine into net cap or weft in circular rows.

SYNTHETIC WIGS AND HAIRPIECES

The manufacture of synthetic fibers has greatly improved. Mod-acrylic fibers, such as dynel, kanekalon, venicelon, and others, have eliminated most of the disadvantages of synthetic hair. Synthetic hair now closely resembles human hair in texture, resiliency, porosity, pliability, durability, sheen, and feel. These fibers can retain curl well, are nonflammable, and do not oxidize and change color in sunlight. In fact, some synthetic fibers appear so much like human hair that it is difficult to distinguish between them.

The many advantages of synthetic hair have led manufacturers to accept its use in wigs and hairpieces. Synthetically produced hair costs less than human hair and its supply is unlimited. It is also easier for the cosmetologist to use since synthetic hair is rolled on spools. Manufacturers weave synthetic wigs and hairpieces from long threads drawn from these spools.

You can find handmade synthetic stretch wigs, machine-made synthetic stretch wigs, and handmade synthetic fitted wigs. (See Fig. 15.6) You must carefully select any type of wig for quality, proper fit, and good workmanship in order to satisfy your clients in terms of wear, comfort, and style.

Also available is the **no-cap wig,** composed of rows of wefting sewn to elastic bands. No-cap wigs are lighter and cooler to wear than other types of wigs. (See Fig. 15.7)

Wig caps and hairpieces can be made of cotton, synthetic and cotton, all synthetic, or reinforced elastic. Hairpieces are generally made with a synthetic base that does not shrink when shampooed. Synthetic hairpieces come in wiglets, demi-wigs, braids, chignons, cascades, and falls.

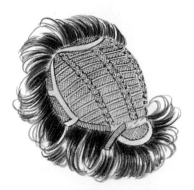

15.6—Synthetic, handmade stretch wig.

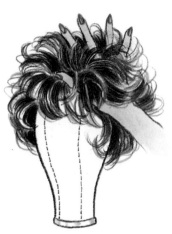

15.7—No-cap wig.

HAIR EXTENSIONS

Hair extensions are permanent additions of hair that can make hair look longer, add thickness and volume, or vary an existing hairstyle. Extensions can be made from either human or synthetic hair, and can be affixed by gluing, fusing or braiding the additional hair.

MEN'S WIGS

Many men now use wigs or toupees to compensate for hair loss. A toupee has adhesive applied to the base of the hairpiece so that the hairpiece sticks to the scalp.

To make men's hair appear fuller, many clients are using hair extensions. These extensions are interwoven or braided onto the existing hair, giving sparse areas the appearance of added thickness.

Once added, the extensions are styled to complement the client's hair type and facial features.

Taking Wig Measurements

To ensure a comfortable and secure fit, you must accurately measure the client's head. First, brush the hair down smoothly and pin it as flatly and tightly to the scalp as possible. Then, keeping close to the head without pressure, measure the head with a tape measure.

PROCEDURE

1. Measure the circumference of the head. Place the tape completely around the head, starting at the hairline at the middle of the forehead; place the tape above the ears, around the back of the head, and return to the starting point. (See Fig. 15.8)

2. Measure from the hairline at the middle of the forehead, over the top, to the nape of the neck. Bend the head back and measure to the point where the wig will ride on the base of the skull at the nape. (See Fig. 15.9)

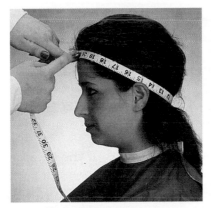

15.8—Measure circumference of head.

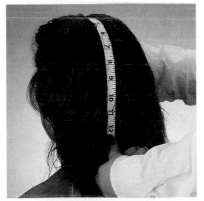

15.9—Measure from hairline at middle of forehead to nape.

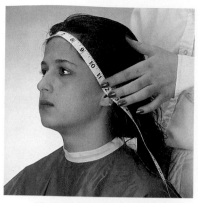

15.10—Measure across forehead.

3. Measure from ear to ear, across the forehead. (See Fig. 15.10)
4. Measure from ear to ear, over the top of the head. (See Fig. 15.11)
5. Place the tape across the crown and measure from temple to temple. (See Fig. 15.12)
6. Measure the width of the napeline, across the nape of the neck. (See Fig. 15.13)

▶ NOTE: Always check to make certain your measurements are accurate.

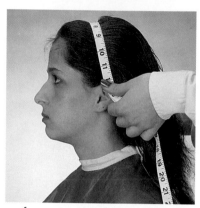

15.11—Measure top of head.

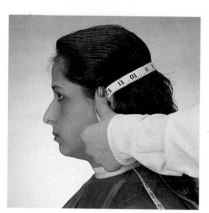

15.12—Measure from temple to temple.

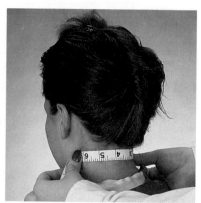

15.13—Measure width of napeline.

Ordering the Wig

When ordering the wig, keep a written record of the client's head measurements and forward a copy to the wig dealer or manufacturer. Also specify what you desire as to:

1. Hair shade. If necessary, submit samples of the client's hair to the manufacturer. When you submit hair samples, you should use hair that has been freshly shampooed, tinted, or rinsed.
2. Quality of hair.
3. Length of hair.
4. Type of hair part and pattern.

Blocking the Wig

A block is a head-shaped form usually made of canvas covered cork or styrofoam, to which a wig is secured for fitting, cleaning, and styling. Use properly protected canvas blocks for all professional wig services, because they stand up under continuous pinning and rough handling. T-pins ("T" shaped pins) are used to attach a hairpiece to a block. There are six sizes of canvas blocks available: 20", 20½", 21", 21½", 22", and 22½" (50, 51.25, 52.5, 53.75, 55, and 56.25 cm). A swivel clamp is used for better block control.

Good blocking gives you professional results when shaping, setting, and combing out a wig. It also reduces the possibility of disturbing the comb-out when you remove the T-pins.

Fit the wig comfortably on the right size block. Do not stretch a wig onto a block that is too big or let it hang too loosely on a block that is too small. If you stretch and pin a wig, it can expand if you wet the cap; when you hang a wig too loosely, it can shrink if you wet the cap (if made of cotton).

Mount the wig on the correct head size block and pin as follows:

1. At the center of the forehead.
2. At each side of the temple. (See Fig. 15.14)
3. At the center of the nape.
4. At each corner of the nape. (See Fig. 15.15)
   (These illustrations show the proper placement of T-pins.)

Styrofoam blocks are used for storing or displaying the wig.

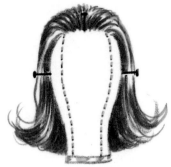
15.14—Place one T-pin at center of forehead and one at each side.

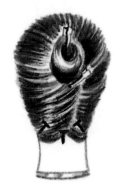
15.15—Place one T-pin at center of nape and one at each corner.

Fitting the Wig

After the wig has been made according to specific measurements, you might have to adjust it to fit your client's head comfortably.

ADJUSTING THE WIG TO A LARGER SIZE

If the wig is too tight, you might have to stretch it. Turn the wig inside out and wet its foundation with hot water. Stretch the wig carefully (without ripping) onto a larger size block and pin it securely. Then allow the wig to dry naturally. (This process may have to be repeated more than once if the wig has to be enlarged more than one size.)

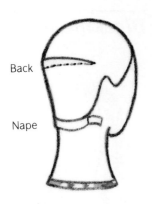

15.16—Horizontal tuck.

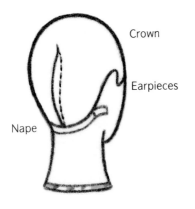

15.17—Vertical tuck.

ADJUSTING THE WIG TO A SMALLER SIZE

If the wig is too loose, you must adjust it to fit properly.

Tucking

You can sew tucks to improve the fit of a wig that is too big.

1. *Horizontal tucks* shorten the wig from front to nape. They are made across the back of the wig to remove excess bulk, and shorten the length of the crown area of the wig. (See Fig. 15.16)
2. *Vertical tucks* remove width at the back of the wig from ear to ear. (See Fig. 15.17)

Check the cap fit after each tuck. Too much tucking can cause the wig to ride up and create new fitting problems.

Check both earpieces to be certain they are directly across from each other and do not touch the ears. If the wig touches the ear, make a small horizontal tuck over the ear to raise the wig. If the wig rubs or touches the side of the ear, make a small vertical tuck behind the ear to pull the wig back and eliminate the problem.

If a wig is too long from forehead to nape, make a tuck approximately ¼" (.625 cm) deep on the weft. Always sew a tuck toward the crown, never away from it, or hair will stand away from the wig when you comb it out. When tacking a tuck, be certain that you take out as much hair as possible before you complete the stitching process. The same applies if a wig is too large from the crown to the ear and it leans on the client's ears. You can correct this by stitching horizontally along the wefting.

▶ NOTE: When you adjust a ventilated or hand-tied wig, you should sew the tucks on the inside of the foundation. However, when you adjust a machine-made or wefted wig, you can sew horizontal tucks either inside or outside the wig.

THE ELASTIC BAND

In the final step of the wig adjustment process, you must adjust the elastic band at the back of the wig. Pull the elastic band at the back of the wig to make the wig fit evenly and snugly at the back of the head and then fasten it. Some stylists favor pinning the ends of the elastic band with a small safety pin to allow for more convenience when making later adjustments or replacements. The elastic band does require periodic adjustment or replacement, because these bands stretch or deteriorate when exposed to body heat and cleaning fluids over a period of time. Other stylists believe that the band should be stitched securely and the stitches broken when adjustment or replacement is needed. (Fig. 15.18)

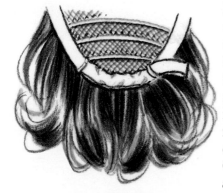

15.18—Elastic band.

Cleaning Wigs

HUMAN HAIR WIGS

You should clean a human hair wig every 2 to 4 weeks, depending on how often it is worn or when you are ready to restyle it, using a non-flammable liquid cleanser. Refer to the manufacturer's suggestions and cleaning instructions.

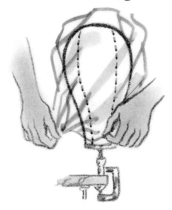

15.19—Covering block.

Procedure

1. Cover the block with a plastic cover to protect the canvas. (See Fig. 15.19)
2. Block the wig. Remove back-combing, if necessary. Direct the hair off the hairline. Brush the hair to loosen dirt and hair spray.
3. Before you take the wig off the block to clean it, mark the size of the wig on the block so you can keep the wig the same size after you have finished cleaning it. You do this by placing a T-pin into the block on an angle next to the edge of the cap and directly in front of the six T-pins securing the wig. (See Figs. 15.20, 15.21) Remove the wig and proceed with the cleaning.

15.20—Front view.

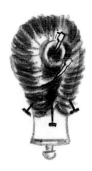

15.21—Back view.

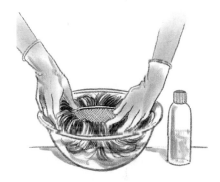

15.22—Wash wig with non-flammable liquid cleanser.

4. Wear rubber gloves to protect your hands. Saturate the wig in 3 ounces (90 ml) of nonflammable liquid cleanser in a large glass or porcelain bowl. With the hair side down, dip the wig up and down until it is clean. (See Fig. 15.22)

    Alternate method: Swirl the wig around in the liquid cleanser. If necessary, clean the edges and inside foundation with a cotton ball or toothbrush.

5. Gently shake the wig to remove excess fluid. Place the wet wig immediately on the canvas block. Stretch the wig lightly and pin it securely to the block. (See Fig. 15.23)
6. When the wig is dry, set and style it.

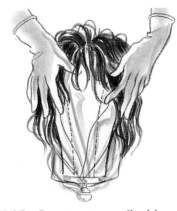

15.23—Remove excess liquid.

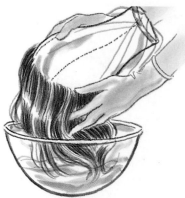

15.24—Saturate wig and work solution through hair.

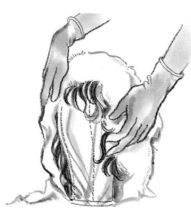

15.25—Towel dry hair.

HAND-TIED WIGS

Since hand-tied wigs have a more delicate structure than machine-made wigs and cost much more, you should clean them on a block.

Procedure

1. Cover the canvas block with plastic to protect the canvas.
2. Clean the edges and inside foundation with a cotton ball or toothbrush.
3. Block the wig.
4. Saturate the wig in a large glass or plastic bowl containing liquid cleaner. (See Fig. 15.24)
5. Soak the wig for 3 to 4 minutes.
6. Comb the cleaning solution through the length of hair with a wide-tooth comb.
7. Work the solution into the entire wig.
8. Carefully towel blot. (See Fig. 15.25)
9. Allow to dry naturally on the block for about ½ hour.
10. Give a conditioning treatment, if necessary.
11. Set and style the wig.

SYNTHETIC WIGS

Synthetic wigs and hairpieces need not be cleaned as often as human hair wigs. Synthetic fibers are nonabsorbent (lack porosity) and do not attract dust and dirt.

Clean and style synthetic wigs and hairpieces about every 3 months, depending on the amount of wear and styling. Use tepid or cool water to clean the wig; hot water takes the curl out of synthetic wigs. Do not comb or brush while wet.

Procedure

1. Cover the block with plastic to protect the canvas.
2. Mount the wig on the block and outline the size (as described earlier).
3. Brush the wig free of tangles and spray before cleaning.
4. Fill a container with mild shampoo or a specially formulated cleaner, according to the manufacturer's directions. Use tepid or cool water.
5. Remove the wig from the block. Swish the wig through cleaning solution for a few minutes. Rinse thoroughly in cool water.
6. Use a small brush or cotton to clean the mesh foundation.
7. Squeeze out excess water and towel blot. (Do not wring or twist wig.)
8. T-pin the wig on the proper size block and let dry naturally.

9. Do not brush a synthetic wig when it is wet; this can take out the curl.
10. Do not expose a synthetic wig to the excess heat of a hairdryer. This concentrated heat can cause the synthetic hair strands to stick together and lose their curl.
11. When the wig dries completely, brush out the hair and spray with conditioner to add luster.

▶ **NOTE:** If you must reduce drying time, place the wig in a cool dryer using only the fan. Since most synthetic wigs are pre-styled, they require no further styling.

CONDITIONING THE WIG

A wig differs from natural human hair in that it does not have its own supply of natural oils for self-lubrication. Since wig cleaners usually dry the hair excessively, use a conditioning treatment after each cleaning to keep the wig hair from drying and looking dull. This also keeps the wig in good condition. (See Fig. 15.26)

Procedure

1. Cover the block with plastic and block the wig properly.
2. Apply conditioner. Distribute the conditioner evenly on clean, damp hair using a wide-tooth comb. Rinse conditioner out of hair according to product's instructions.
3. Set and style the wig.

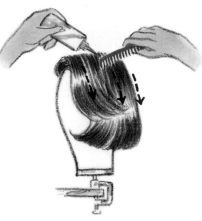

15.26—Condition wig after cleaning.

Shaping Wigs

HUMAN HAIR WIGS

You can shape (cut) a wig in the same way you cut natural hair on the head. However, you must consider the fact that a wig holds about twice as much hair as a human head. Thus, if you do not thin and taper the wig properly, it will look bulky and artificial. You can thin the wig with either a razor or thinning shears. Concentrate on removing bulk from the top hairline, in back of the ears, and around the face. You do not usually have to thin these areas on natural hair.

Cut as close to the wig foundation as possible, without damaging the cap itself. Thin hair close to the cap to remove additional bulk and to make sure you have not left hair spurs that will stick out when you style the wig later. Special care must be taken so that knots on the hand-knotted wig remain tight. Take equal care to not cut any of the wefts or sewing threads on the wefted wig. When you cut a wig, keep in mind that the hair will not grow back to cover an error in judgment. Proceed cautiously. Although it is more convenient to shape the wig on a canvas block, it is a good idea to cut the wig while it is on the client's head in order to suit the client's natural hair and facial features.

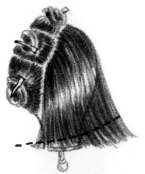

15.27—Part off a 2″ (5 cm) guideline and cut to desired length.

Thus, you might find that the best technique is to cut a guideline on the client's head and then transfer the wig to the block. This ensures you that the wig is being cut to the proper length. Then, you can move the wig to the block, secure it firmly, and avoid slippage during the rest of the shaping process. When you place the wig on the canvas block to cut it, set it carefully at the correct hairline distance and continue cutting the remaining hair evenly. Continue the shaping process, section by section, until the entire wig has been shaped. (Figs. 15.27–15.33)

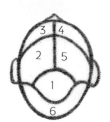

15.28—Top front.

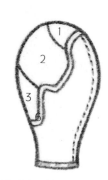

15.29—Right side.

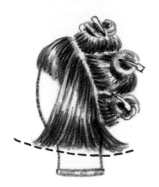

15.30—Left side of head. This illustrates a completely cut guideline.

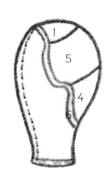

15.31—Left side.

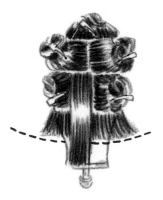

15.32—Back of head. Let down center back hair. Cut to the same length as guideline.

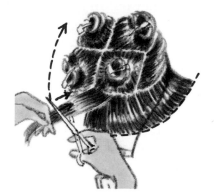

15.33—Back of head. Pick up a strand of the guideline. With hands arched at a 45° (.785 rad.) angle, cut into longer hair. Proceed with a sweeping upward motion.

SYNTHETIC HAIR WIGS

Always cut synthetic wigs when dry, because the fibers can stretch out of shape if pulled when wet. Use only scissors and thinning shears on synthetic fiber or on a mixture of synthetic and human hair. Because synthetic fibers do not have the resiliency or flexibility of human hair, they can dull a razor badly. As a result, a razor can cause permanent damage to the wig.

Setting wig hair resembles setting hair on the human head, except for hairline coverage and the need for a tight curl at the nape area. You must also consider the added fullness of the client's hair, plus the hair and foundation of the wig when setting and styling the wig. Wigs are always set and styled on the blocking. (Figs. 15.34, 15.35)

Setting and Styling Wigs

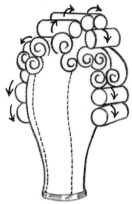

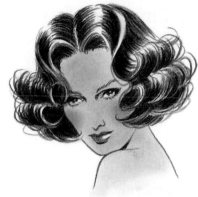

15.34—Setting on block.

15.35—Finished style.

Pin curls replace rollers in the front hairline, temple, and nape to keep the style close to the head. (Fig. 15.36) Use T-pins instead of clippies or bobby pins to hold both rollers and curls more securely. Set, dry, and style hair in the usual manner. (Fig. 15.37)

Cutting and styling synthetic wigs differs from cutting and styling human hair wigs in the following ways:

You may only tease or back comb wigs at the base of their fibers. Otherwise, you will damage the fibers that should be kept perfectly smooth at the wig surface. Damage to the hair shaft (by thinning) leaves you with a frizzy, fuzzy-looking wig.

Synthetic wigs are pre-cut into definite styles by their manufacturers. If the client desires a change, a good quality synthetic wig can be combed into different styles by a skilled stylist. These comb-out styles are all based on the basic pre-cut factory-created style. However, a stylist must be guided by the client's wishes.

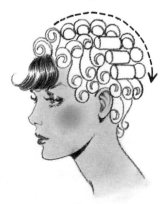

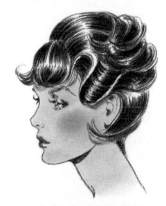

15.36—How the setting would look on the head.

15.37—Finished style.

Putting on and Taking Off a Wig

A simple but very important procedure is the way you remove a wig from a block and place it on the client's head. (Fig. 15.38) (It is a good idea to show the client the proper way to put on and take off the wig.)

COMBING CLIENT'S HAIR INTO A WIG

Depending on the style, set the client's hair that is to be blended with the wig in pin curls. When the wig is ready to be combined with the client's own hair, secure the wig starting either at the top or bottom depending on where you set the pin curls. When the wig is comfortably adjusted, comb and blend the client's hair into the style of the wig. (Fig. 15.39)

REMOVING A WIG

To remove a wig, place only your thumb under the cap at the nape. *Do not put your fingers into the hair.* Have the client bend down his or her head. Then, slide the wig off.

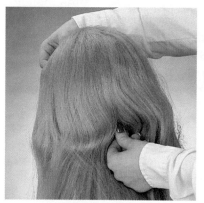

15.38—Place wig on front of client's head. While holding wig securely on top, glide it back to nape. Pull securely over sides, front, and back.

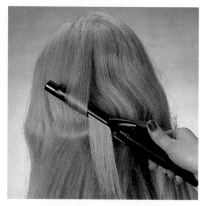

15.39—Recomb, adjust and style to suit client.

Wig Coloring

COLOR RINSES

Color rinses temporarily color human hair wigs and must be re-applied whenever you clean the hair. Color rinses can only darken the hair; if the client desires a lighter color, a different wig must be worn.

Here is one way to apply a color rinse. (Your instructor's method may be equally correct.)

Procedure

1. Pin the wig securely on a plastic-covered block.
2. Dampen the clean hair, using a spray applicator bottle.
3. If you are unsure about which color to use, strand test the color rinse on the back of the wig.
4. Spray hair with the color rinse. Distribute it evenly with a downward motion, using a small brush and wide-tooth comb. (See Fig. 15.40)
5. Apply setting lotion in the usual manner. (See Fig. 15.41)
6. Set, dry, (See Fig. 15.42) and comb out the hair to the desired style.

▶ NOTE: In addition to color rinses, you can color human hair wigs with a semi-permanent tint. However, you should never attempt to lighten (bleach) any wig or hairpiece.

SEMI-PERMANENT TINTS

Semi-permanent tints are referred to as 6-week tints. They are self-penetrating and require no peroxide. They do not change the basic structure of the hair.

Here is one way to apply semi-permanent tints to machine-made wigs:

Procedure

1. Mount the wig on the appropriate plastic-covered block and outline the size with T-pins.
2. Remove all teasing, tangles, and snarls.
3. Clean the wig and comb the hair smooth.
4. Remove the wig from the block.
5. Immerse the wig in a glass bowl of hot water and semi-permanent tint solution.
6. Leave it completely immersed for 10 minutes.
7. Remove it and rinse with cold water.
8. Apply conditioner.
9. Block, set, dry, and comb out in the usual manner.

PERMANENT TINTS

Since 100% human hair wigs and hairpieces have been subjected to extensive processing, applying a permanent tint to this kind of hair can be very risky and will result in uneven coloring.

CAUTION

▶ *When tinting wigs, be sure to follow the manufacturer's directions.*

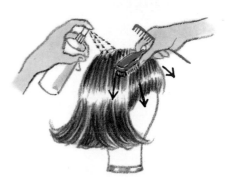

15.40—Spray hair with color rinse.

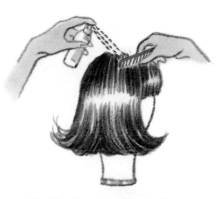

15.41—Apply setting lotion.

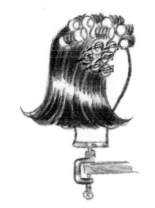

15.42—Set, dry, and comb out.

Hairpieces

You can create a variety of hairstyles with hairpieces, fashioning them for either daytime or evening wear. Hairpieces come in various forms, such as:

1. *Switches.* These are long wefts of hair mounted with a loop at the end. They are constructed with one to two stems of hair. Better switches are constructed with three stems to provide greater flexibility in styling and braiding. They can be worked into the hair or braided to create special styling effects. (See Fig. 15.43)

2. *Wiglets.* These are hairpieces with a flat base that are used in special areas of the head. They are used primarily to blend with the client's own hair in order to extend the range of hair in a particular section of the head. Wiglets can be worked into the top of the hair in curls or under the hair to give height and body. They can also be used to create special effects. (See Fig. 15.44)

3. *Bandeau.* This is a hairpiece that is sewn to a headband. The headband, which is replaceable and comes in different colors, serves as an excellent disguise for the hairline. The bandeau hairpiece is usually worn over the hair and dressed casually. (See Fig. 15.45)

4. *Fall.* This is a section of hair, machine wefted on a round base, running across the back of the head and available in various lengths. Falls have a thick, plushy look. *Short falls* range from 12″ to 14″ (30 to 35 cm) in length (See Fig. 15.46); *demi-falls* from 15″ to 20″ (37.5 to 50 cm); and *long falls* from 18″ to 24″ (45 to 60 cm).

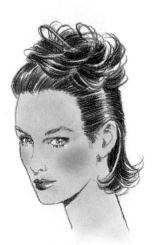

15.43—Switch.

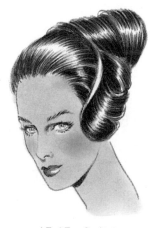

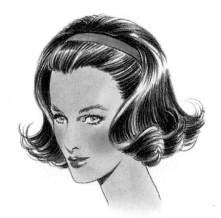

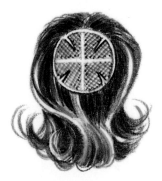

15.44—Wiglet.   15.45—Bandeau.   15.46—Short fall.

5. *Demi-fall* or *demi-wig.* This is a large-base hairpiece designed to fit the shape of the head. The demi-fall or demi-wig generally ranges in length from 15″ to 20″ (37.5 to 50 cm).

6. *Cascade.* This is a hairpiece on an oblong base that offers an endless variety of styling possibilities. Cascades can be styled in curls, braids, a pageboy, or used as a filler with the client's own hair. (See Fig. 15.47)

7. *Braid.* This is a switch whose strands are woven, interlaced, or entwined. Some are prepared with a thin wire inside so that they can be formed into various shapes. Wireless braids hang loose on the head.

8. *Chignon.* This is a knot or coil of hair, created from synthetic hair, that is worn at the nape or crown of the head. A chignon works best when worn in combination with another hairpiece.

9. *Crown curls.* These are a group of light curls worn on top of the head.

10. *Frosting curls.* These are segments of frosted or blended hair pinned into natural hair to simulate frosted or streaked hair.

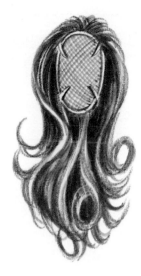

15.47—Cascade.

Safety Precautions

1. Take great care when combing or brushing wigs to avoid matting.
2. When cleaning a wig or hairpiece, never rub or wring out the fluid.
3. When you shape (cut) a wig or hairpiece, use great care; once the hair has been cut, it cannot grow back.
4. When you comb a freshly set wig, use a wide-tooth comb to help you gain greater control and to avoid damaging the wig's foundation.
5. When you clean or work with a wet wig, always mount it on a block of the same head size as the wig to avoid stretching.
6. Take accurate measurements of the client's head to ensure a comfortable and secure fit.
7. Recondition wigs as often as necessary to prevent dry or brittle hair.
8. If needed, clean wigs before setting and styling.
9. Brush and comb wigs and hairpieces with a downward movement.
10. Never lighten (bleach) a wig or hairpiece.
11. Never give a permanent to a wig or hairpiece.

Business Tips

Preparing for a successful career involves examining all your opportunities.

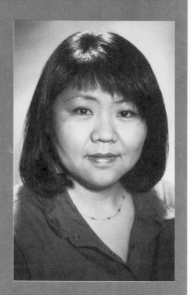

Keiko Shino, a stylist in Southern California since 1970, increases her income by combining all of her professional skills in human hair extension services. This specialized area of service has a higher price structure than most salon services, and reflects the heightened level of professional skills involved. "If I do two hair extension clients in a 2-day week, my income is equal to what I would earn if I worked 7 days just doing cut, color, and perm," says Shino.

When you consider adding human hair extensions to your service menu, remember to keep professionalism first and foremost in your mind. Human hair extensions require that you service the client's own hair and scalp as well as the human hair wefts, and that you use safe, professional attachment techniques that maintain the health and condition of the client's natural hair.

While educational videos and books get you started in the extension business, nothing replaces practice and patience. And, once you become a specialist in extensions, there are opportunities beyond the salon. Shino's talents led to a position as technical director and top educator for Garland Drake International, the major supplier of human hair for use in extensions.

When you are planning your financial future, consider all your service options and areas of specialization, and you'll find the sky's the limit.

Review Questions

THE ARTISTRY OF ARTIFICIAL HAIR

1. List some of the reasons people wear wigs.
2. Name the different types of wigs, extensions, and hairpieces.
3. What is the purpose of a hair extension?
4. What is the purpose of blocking a wig?
5. How often should a human hair wig be cleaned?
6. Where should a wig be set and styled?
7. What effect does a color rinse have on a human hair wig?

16

MANICURING AND PEDICURING

LEARNING OBJECTIVES

After completing this chapter, you should be able to:

1. List the abilities of a good manicurist.
2. Identify the four natural nail shapes.
3. Demonstrate the proper use of implements, cosmetics, and materials used in manicuring.
4. Demonstrate the proper procedure and sanitary precautions for a manicure.
5. Demonstrate massage techniques used when giving a manicure.
6. Define and demonstrate the different types of manicures.
7. Explain and demonstrate advanced nail techniques.
8. List the safety precautions for manicuring.
9. Demonstrate the procedure for a pedicure.

Introduction

The ancients regarded long, polished, and colored fingernails as a mark of distinction between aristocrats and common laborers. Manicuring, once considered a luxury for the few, is now a service used by many. In fact, many well-groomed women and men regularly use the services of a professional manicurist or nail technician. The services provided by a nail technician include the application of artificial nails as well as pedicures.

The word *manicure* (**MAN**-i-kyoor) is derived from the Latin "manus" (hand) and "cura" (care), which means the care of the hands and nails. The purpose of a manicure is to improve the appearance of the hands and nails.

A client pleased with a professional manicure or other more advanced nail technique is more likely to become a regular client for these services, as well as for other beauty services.

A manicurist should have:

1. Knowledge of the structure of hands, arms, and nails.
2. Knowledge of the composition of the cosmetics used in manicuring.
3. The ability to give a good manicure efficiently.
4. The ability to care for the client's manicuring problems.
5. The ability to distinguish between disorders that may be treated in the salon and diseases that must be treated by a physician.
6. Knowledge of the structure of the foot and the ability to give a good pedicure.

A nail technician should possess the above qualifications *and* be able to execute advanced nail techniques safely and professionally.

Shape of Nails

Nails naturally vary greatly in shape, but are usually classified into four general shapes: square, round, oval, and pointed. (Fig. 16.1)

Before you begin to work on a client's nails, both you and the client should agree on the best nail shape. The shape of the nail should conform to that of the fingertips for a more natural effect. In general the oval-shaped nail, nicely rounded at the base, and slightly pointed at the tips, fits most hands. Only an attractive hand can afford to direct attention to itself by exaggeration of shape and color. People who perform work with their hands usually require shorter, more round-shaped nails in order to avoid nail breakage and injury.

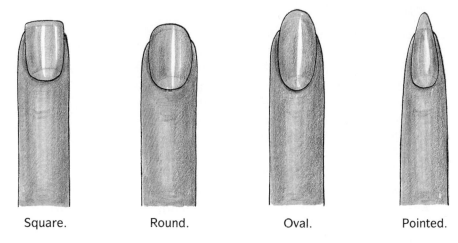

Square.   Round.   Oval.   Pointed.

16.1—Shapes of nails.

Equipment, Implements, Cosmetics, and Materials

The articles used in manicuring that are durable are referred to as equipment and implements. (Fig. 16.2) Cosmetics and materials refer to the supplies that are consumed and must be replaced.

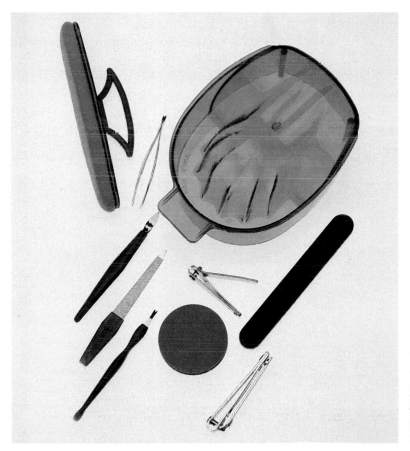

16.2—Manicuring implements— clockwise, from top left: nail buffer; tweezers; finger bowl; fingernail clippers; emery board; toenail clippers; filing disk; cuticle pusher; large nail file; steel pusher.

EQUIPMENT

Manicuring table and *adjustable lamp.*

Client's chair and *manicurist's chair* or *stool.*

Cushion (8" × 12" [20 × 30 cm]), covered with a washable slip-cover or sanitized towel, on which the client rests his or her arm. A towel, folded and covered by a small sanitized towel, may be used instead of the cushion.

Supply tray for holding cosmetics.

Finger bowl (plastic, china, or glass) with removable paper cup for holding warm, soapy water.

Container for clean absorbent cotton.

Electric heater for heating oil when giving a hot oil manicure.

Wet sanitizer container with sterile cotton and 70% alcohol.

Glass containers for cosmetics and accessories.

IMPLEMENTS

Orangewood sticks (2) for loosening cuticle, for working around nail, and for applying oil, cream, bleach, or solvent to the nail and cuticle. (Fig. 16.3)

Nail file (7" or 8" [17.5 or 20 cm] long, thin and flexible) for shaping and smoothing the free edge of the nail. (Fig. 16.4)

Cuticle pusher for loosening and pushing back the cuticle. (Fig. 16.5)

Cuticle nippers or *cuticle scissors* for trimming the cuticle. (Fig. 16.6)

Nail brush for cleansing the nails and fingertips with the aid of warm, soapy water.

Emery boards (2) for shaping the free edge of the nail with the coarse side, and for smoothing the nail with the finer side. (Fig. 16.7)

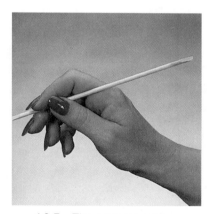

16.3—The orangewood stick is held in the same manner as in writing with a pencil.

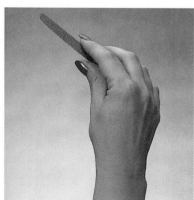

16.4—Hold nail file in the right hand, with the thumb underneath it for support and the other four fingers on its upper surface.

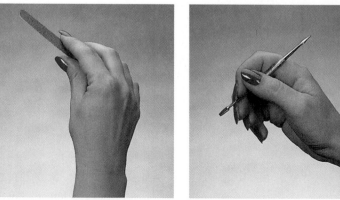

16.5—The steel pusher is held in the same manner as in writing with a pencil. The dull side is used to push back and loosen the cuticle.

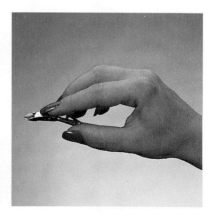

16.6—Use cuticle nippers to trim cuticles.

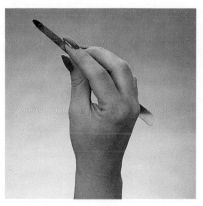

16.7—The emery board is held in the same manner as the nail file.

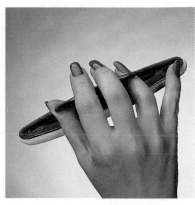

16.8—Holding a nail buffer.

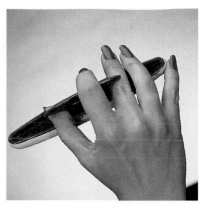

16.9—Alternate way to hold a nail buffer.

Nail buffer (with removable frame to permit replacement of the chamois cover) for buffing and polishing the nails. (Figs. 16.8, 16.9) (Some states do not permit the use of a nail buffer.)

Fine camel's hair brush for applying lacquer or liquid nail polish. (Camel's hair brush is usually attached to the top of the nail polish bottle.)

Tweezers for lifting small bits of cuticle.

COSMETICS

Nail and hand cosmetics vary in their composition and usage according to the purpose they serve.

Nail cleansers consist of detergent, usually cake, liquid, or flakes.

Nail polish removers contain organic solvents and are used to dissolve old polish on nails. To offset the drying action of the solvent, oil may be present in the nail polish remover.

Cuticle oil softens and lubricates the skin around the nails.

Cuticle creams are usually lanolin, petroleum or beeswax based. They are used to prevent or correct brittle nails and dry cuticle.

Cuticle removers or *solvents* may contain 2% to 5% sodium or potassium hydroxide plus glycerine. Milder solutions may instead contain **trisodium phosphate** and **triethanolamine** or **alkanolamines**. After the cuticle is softened with this liquid, it can be removed easily.

Nail bleaches contain hydrogen peroxide or diluted organic acids in a liquid form, or they can be mixed with other ingredients to form a white paste. When applied over nails, under the free edges, and on fingertips, they remove stains.

Nail whiteners are applied as a paste, cream, or coated string. They consist mainly of white pigments (zinc oxide or titanium dioxide). When applied under the free edges of the nails, they keep the tips looking white.

Dry nail polish usually is prepared in the form of powder or paste. The main ingredient is a mild abrasive, such as tin oxide, talc, silica, or kaolin. It smooths the nail and gives it a gloss during buffing (where permitted).

An *abrasive* is available as a pumice powder and used with a buffer to smooth irregular nail ridges.

Liquid nail polish or *lacquer* is used to color or gloss the nail. It is a solution of nitro cellulose in **volatile solvents**, such as **amyl acetate**, together with a **platiciser** (castor oil), which prevents too rapid drying. Also present are resin and color.

Nail polish thinner, containing **acetone** or other solvent, is used to thin out nail polish when it has thickened.

A *base coat* is a liquid product applied before the liquid nail polish. It allows the nail polish to adhere readily to the nail surface. It also forms a hard gloss, which prevents the color in the nail polish from staining the nail tissue.

A *top coat*, or *sealer*, is a liquid applied over the nail polish. This product protects the polish and minimizes its chipping or cracking.

Nail hardeners or *strengtheners* are designed to prevent nails from splitting or peeling. Some are applied only to the tips of the nails, and others are applied over the entire nail. The nails must be thoroughly clean, free of oils or creams, and dry. Hardeners are applied before the base coat. They are never applied over polish. There are four types of hardeners: protein hardeners, formaldehyde hardeners, nylon fiber hardeners, and nail conditioners. Protein hardeners are a combination of clear polish and a protein such as collagen. Formaldehyde hardeners utilize keratin fibers to strengthen and contain no more than 5% formaldehyde, because the ingredient can cause damage to the nail. Nylon fiber hardeners are a mixture of clear polish and nylon fibers applied first vertically, then horizontally over the entire nail. Nail conditioners are used independently of a manicure, usually overnight, on clean, dry nails. They contain moisturizing ingredients to combat dryness and brittleness.

A *nail dryer* is a solution that protects the nail polish against stickiness and dulling. It can be used either as a spray or brush-on, and it is applied over the top coat or directly on the nail polish.

Powdered alum or *alum solution* is used to stop the bleeding of minor cuts.

Hand creams and *hand lotions* are recommended for dry, chapped, or irritated skin. Hand creams are made up of emollients, **humectants** (such as glycerine or propylene glycol), which promote the retention of water, emulsifiers, and preservatives. Hand lotions are similar in composition to hand creams, although they are a thinner consistency due to a higher oil content.

MATERIALS

Absorbent cotton for application of cosmetics to the nails.

Cleanser (liquid or other form) for finger bath.

Warm water for finger bath.

Sanitized towel for each client.

Cleansing tissue for use whenever necessary.

Chamois for replacing soiled chamois on buffer.

Paper cups for replacing used paper cups in finger bowl.

Antiseptic for use in finger bath and to avoid infection when minor injuries to tissues surrounding the nails occur.

Disinfectant for sanitizing implements and for disinfecting the manicuring table.

Spatula for removing creams from jars.

Mending tissue, silk, linen, or *liquid nail wrap,* and *mending adhesive* for repairing or covering broken, split, torn, or weak nails.

70% alcohol is used in a jar sanitizer where implements are kept during a manicure. It is also used to sanitize a client's fingers before a manicure.

Preparation of the Manicuring Table

To give a professional manicure, all rules of sanitation must be followed. The table and the manicurist's hands must be perfectly clean. Everything, including containers, bowls, instruments, and materials, must be in perfect order. Sanitize manicuring implements after each use. Do not ask the client to sit at the table with the remains of the previous manicure in sight. Always clean the table immediately upon completion of a manicure so that it will be ready for the next client. This will make the manicure more pleasant for the client, and will put him or her in a more receptive mood for your advice and suggestions.

PROCEDURE

1. Sponge the manicuring tabletop with a disinfectant.
2. Place a clean towel over the armrest or cushion.
3. Place a bowl of warm, soapy water to the left of the client.
4. Place the metal implements and orangewood sticks in a jar sanitizer containing cotton saturated with alcohol.
5. Arrange cream jars, lotion bottles, and nail polishes in the order to be used and place them to the left of the manicurist.
6. Place the nail file (which has been sponged with alcohol) and fresh emery boards to the right of the manicurist.
7. Attach a small plastic bag to the table with scotch tape, on either the right or left side, for waste materials.

MANICURING TABLE SETUP

(Your instructor's manicuring table setup is equally correct.)

1. Towel wrapped armrest
2. Nail file
3. Emery board
4. Alcohol
5. Cotton container
6. Finger bowl
7. Nail brush
8. Wet sanitizer containing manicuring implements
9. Tray with nail polishes
10. Plastic bag
11. The drawer may be used for the following items:
    - Nail whitener
    - Instant dry enamel
    - Peroxide
    - Dry polish (powder or paste)
    - Pumice stone
    - Thinner
    - Antiseptic
    - Buffer

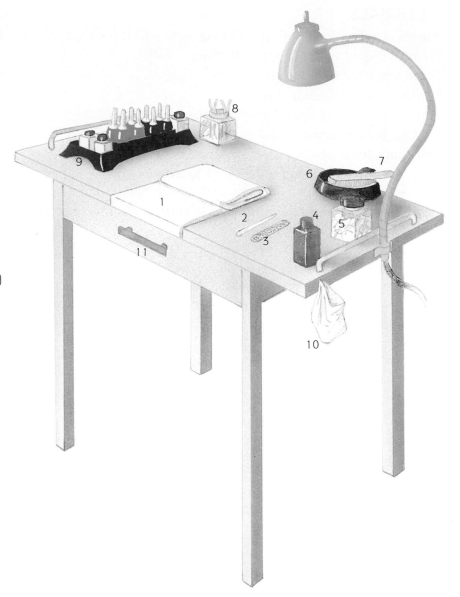

16.10 — Manicuring table setup.

The manicuring table drawer always should be clean and neat. Do not use it for waste materials; use the plastic bag. (Fig. 16.10)

Plain Manicure

PREPARATION

The routine outlined in this text is one of several ways in which to give a manicure. Whatever routine your instructor outlines for you is equally correct.

1. Prepare manicuring table as previously outlined.
2. Seat client.
3. Wash your hands.
4. Examine client's hands.
5. Sanitize client's hands.

CAUTION

▶ *Be extremely careful to avoid cutting the client's skin. However, if this occurs administer 3% hydrogen peroxide or powdered alum.*

PROCEDURE

1. Remove old polish. (Start with the little finger of left hand.) Moisten cotton with nail polish remover and press over the nail for a few moments to soften the polish. With a firm movement, bring the cotton from the base of the nail to the tip. Do not smear the old polish into the cuticle or surrounding tissues. (An alternate method of removing nail polish is to moisten small pledgets of cotton with nail polish remover and press over old polish on each nail. Then moisten another pledget of cotton with nail polish remover and use it for removing the small pledgets on the nails. The pressed-on pledget acts as a blotter and does not leave a polish smear on the cuticle.) (Fig. 16.11)

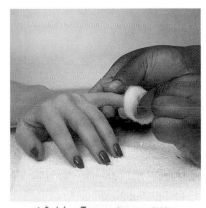

16.11—Removing polish.

2. Shape nails. Discuss with the client the nail shape best suited for him or her. File the nails of the left hand, starting with the little finger and working toward the thumb, in the following manner:

    a) Hold the client's finger between the thumb and the first two fingers of the left hand.

    b) Hold the file or emery board in the right hand and tilt it slightly so that filing is confined mainly to the underside of the free edge.

    c) Shape nails as agreed with the client. Use the file or emery board to shape the nails. File each nail from corner to center, going from right to left and then from left to right. Filing nails according to the way the nail grows avoids splitting. Use two short, quick strokes and one long, sweeping stroke on each side of the nail. (Fig. 16.12)

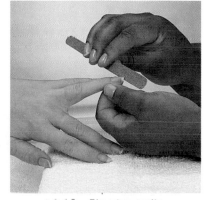

16.12—Shaping nails.

▶ **NOTE:** Avoid filing deep into the corners of the nails. They will look longer and be stronger if permitted to grow out at the sides.

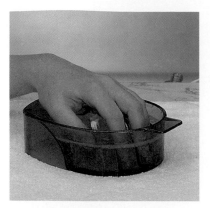

16.13—Softening cuticle.

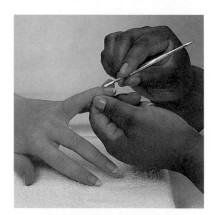

16.14—Towel-drying fingertips.

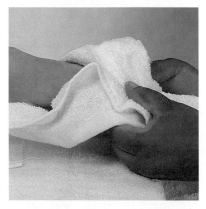

16.15—Loosening dead cuticle with pusher.

3. Soften cuticle. After filing the nails of the left hand, file two nails of the right hand. Then, immerse the left hand into the finger bowl (soap bath) to permit softening of the cuticle. Finish filing the nails of the right hand. Remove the left hand from the finger bowl. (Fig. 16.13)

4. Dry fingertips. Holding a towel with both hands, carefully dry the left hand, including the area between the fingers. With the towel, gently loosen and push back the cuticle and adhering skin on each nail. (Fig. 16.14)

5. Apply cuticle remover (solvent). Wind a thin layer of cotton around the blunt edge of an orangewood stick for use as an applicator. Apply cuticle solvent around the cuticle of the left hand.

6. Loosen cuticle. Use the spoon end of the cuticle pusher to gently loosen the cuticle. Keep the cuticle moist while working. Use the cuticle pusher, in a flat position, to remove dead cuticle adhering to the nail without scratching the nail plate. (Fig. 16.15) Push the cuticle back with a towel over the index finger.

▶ NOTE: Use light pressure when using a cuticle pusher or orangewood stick so the tissue at the root of the nail will not be injured.

7. Clean under free edge. Use a cotton-tipped orangewood stick, dipped in soapy water, to clean under free edge, working from the center toward each side, employing gentle pressure. (Fig. 16.16)

8. Trim cuticle. If necessary, use cuticle nippers to remove dead cuticle, uneven cuticle, or hangnails. In cutting the cuticle, be careful to remove it as a single segment. (Fig. 16.17)

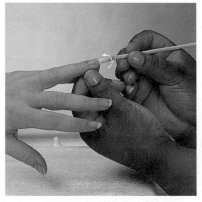

16.16—Clean under free edge with cotton-tipped orangewood stick.

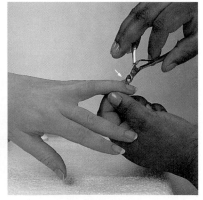

16.17—Trimming cuticle with nippers.

9. When cutting the cuticle of the middle finger of the left hand, immerse fingers of the right hand into finger bowl, while continuing to manicure the left hand.

10. Bleach under free edge (optional). With a cotton-tipped orangewood stick, apply hydrogen peroxide or other bleaching preparation under the free edge of each nail.

11. Apply nail whitener under free edge of nails (optional). Use orangewood stick as applicator to apply chalk paste, or use a string treated with nail whitener.

12. Apply cuticle oil or cream around the sides and base of the nail and massage with the thumb in a rotary movement.

13. Remove right hand from finger bowl. Manicure the nails and cuticles of right hand as described in steps 4 through 12.

14. Cleanse nails. Brush the nails over the finger bowl, using a downward movement, to clean the nails of both hands. (Fig. 16.18)

15. Dry hands and nails thoroughly.

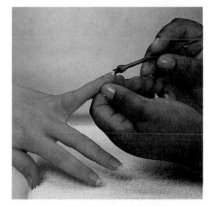
16.18—Clean under nails with downward stroke.

NAIL PROBLEMS

A fringe of loose skin left around the nail after a manicure is caused by trimming the cuticle closer than necessary and then rolling back the epidermis. To prevent the occurrence of such loose skin, trim the cuticle only enough to allow a tiny margin of cuticle to remain.

Callus growth at the fingertips can be softened by the application of creams and lotions, and by removing the constant pressure that is causing it. Gentle rubbing with pumice powder also is helpful to start the removing process.

Stains on fingernails may be bleached with prepared nail bleach or peroxide. Slightly damp pumice powder also may be applied and the nails buffed to help remove stains.

COMPLETION

1. Re-examine nails and cuticles. Carefully re-examine the nails for defects. Use the fine side of an emery board to give the nails a smooth beveled edge. Remove remaining pieces of cuticle.

2. If required, repair split or broken nails.

3. As an added service, a hand massage or a hand and arm massage may be given at this time.

4. Apply base coat. Apply base coat to the left hand with long strokes, starting with the little finger and working toward the thumb. Allow it to dry until "slick to a light touch." (Fig. 16.19)

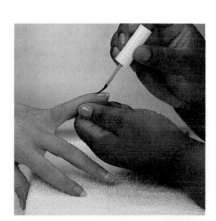
16.19—Applying base coat.

5. Apply liquid polish. Dip the camel's hair brush into the polish and wipe off excess by pressing it gently against the sides of the bottle.

    Apply the polish lightly and quickly, using sweeping strokes, from the base to the free edge of the nail, as shown in the illustrations. (Figs. 16.20–16.22) Always keep the polish thin enough to flow freely. If the polish is thick, add a little polish solvent and shake well.

6. Remove excess polish. Dip a cotton-tipped orangewood stick into nail polish remover. Apply it carefully around the cuticles and nail edges to remove excess polish.

7. Apply top or seal coat. Apply top coat to the left hand with long strokes, and then apply it to the right hand in the same manner. Brush around and under tips of nails for added support and protection.

8. Apply hand lotion. As an additional service, after the top coat is completely dry, apply hand lotion with light manipulations over the hands, from wrists to fingertips.

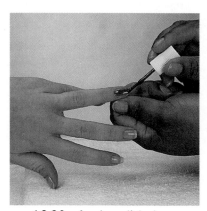

16.20—Apply polish down center of nail.

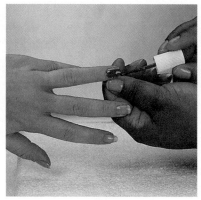

16.21—Apply polish to right side of nail.

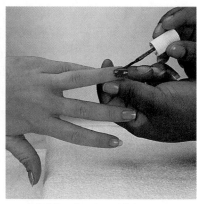

16.22—Apply polish to left side of nail.

FINAL CLEANUP

1. Sanitize used manicuring implements; place them in a cabinet sanitizer.
2. Place used materials (tissues, cotton, emery board, etc.) into closed containers or plastic bag attached to manicuring table.
3. Wipe manicuring table with disinfectant; put everything in order.
4. Clean the tops of nail polish bottles with polish remover.
5. Inspect the manicuring table drawer for cleanliness and order.
6. Wash and dry your hands.

> ### Business Tips

Nail technician Barbara Griggs goes to great lengths to satisfy her nail clients. According to her, the key to a full book is knowing how to match a service with what your client wants.

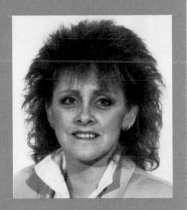

"All your client knows is that she wants a nail that lasts and that looks natural," says Griggs. "It is up to you to decide if tips, wraps, freeform sculpting, or a liquid and powder system will suit her needs. If your client has a nicely curved nail plate and a bit of length, sculptured nails will give her all the strength she needs. On the other hand, if she has small, short nail plates, she needs the extra strength of a tip with an overlay.

"Knowing your product lines also helps you to make a smart service decision. Some products form a hard ridged nail, others may offer more flexibility. Both are strong but in different ways. Some systems require a primer and some do not. You must know which product works best for each client. A proper diagnosis will result in a long-term service and a happy client."

Griggs's final business-building tip: Clients will blame *you* for a bad job if *they* ruin their nails, so always teach proper home care and nail sanitation as you work.

Safety Rules in Manicuring

Observing safety rules in manicuring can be of great help in preventing accidents and injury to the client or nail technician. The following safety rules will guide the nail technician:

1. Keep all containers covered and labeled.
2. Hold or move containers with dry hands.
3. Handle sharp-pointed implements carefully and avoid dropping them.
4. Dull oversharpened cutting edges of sharp implements with an emery board.
5. Bevel a sharp nail edge with an emery board.
6. Do not file too deeply into nail corners.
7. Do not use a sharp, pointed implement to cleanse under the nail.
8. Avoid excessive friction in nail buffing (where permitted).
9. Apply an antiseptic immediately if the skin is accidentally cut.
10. Apply styptic powder or alum solution to stop the bleeding from a small cut. Never use a styptic pencil.
11. Avoid pushing the cuticle back too far.
12. Avoid too much pressure at the base of the nail.
13. Do not work on a nail when the surrounding skin is inflamed or is infected.

Individual Nail Styling

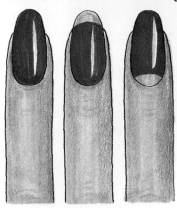

16.23—Correct nail styling for oval nail.

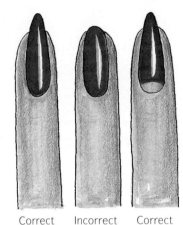

Correct   Incorrect   Correct

16.24—Nail styling for slender nail.

For a more natural effect, the shape of the nail should conform to that of the fingertip. A gracefully shaped nail adds beauty to the hands.

Nail shapes can be divided into four types:

1. Oval
2. Slender tapering (pointed)
3. Square or rectangular
4. Clubbed (round)

The oval nail is the ideal nail shape and can be styled by either covering the entire nail with polish, leaving the free edge white, or leaving the half moon white at the base of the nail. (Fig. 16.23)

The slender tapering nail is well suited for the thin, delicate hand. The nail should be tapered somewhat longer than usual to enhance the slender appearance of the hand. The nail can be completely polished, or a half moon can be left at the base. (Fig. 16.24)

The square or rectangular nail should extend only slightly past the tip of the finger with the nail tip rounded off. The entire nail may be polished with a slight half moon left at the base and a white margin left at the sides of the nail. (Fig. 16.25)

The clubbed nail should be slightly tapered and extend just a bit past the tip of the finger. The entire nail should be polished with a thin white margin left at the sides. (Fig. 16.26)

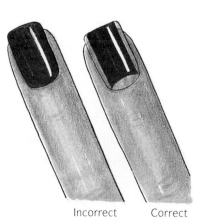

Incorrect   Correct

16.25—Nail styling for square or rectangular nail.

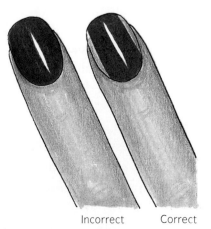

Incorrect   Correct

16.26—Nail styling for clubbed nail.

Hand Massage

Include a hand massage with each manicure. It keeps the hands flexible, well-groomed, and smooth.

PROCEDURE

1. Hold the client's hand in your hand. Place a dab of hand lotion on the back of the client's hand and spread it to the fingers and wrist.
2. Hold the client's hand firmly. Bend the hand slowly with a forward and backward movement to limber the wrist. Repeat three times. (See Fig. 16.27)
3. Grasp each finger. Gently bend each finger, one at a time, to limber the top of the hand and finger joints. As the fingers and thumb are bent, slide your thumb down toward the fingertips. (See Fig. 16.28)
4. With the client's elbow resting on the table, hold the hand upright. Massage the palm of the hand with the cushions of your thumbs, using a circular movement in alternate directions. This movement will completely relax the client's hand. (See Fig. 16.29)
5. Rest client's arm on the table. Grasp each finger at the base, and rotate it gently in large circles, ending with a gentle squeeze of the fingertips. Repeat three times. (See Fig. 16.30)

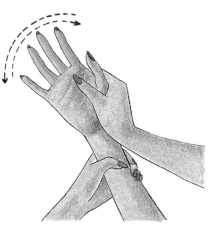

16.27—Movement to limber the wrist.

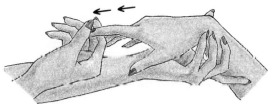

16.28—Movement to limber the top of hand and finger joints.

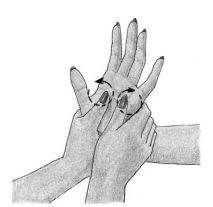

16.29—Movement to relax the client's hand.

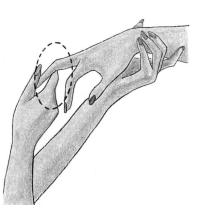

16.30—Grasp each finger at base and rotate gently.

6. Hold the client's hand. Massage the wrist, then top of the hand with a circular movement. Slide back and with both hands wring wrist in opposite direction three times. Repeat movements three times. (See Fig. 16.31)

7. Finish massage by tapering each finger. Beginning at the base of each finger, rotate, pause, and squeeze with gentle pressure. Then, pull lightly with pressure until tip is reached. Repeat three times. (See Fig. 16.32)

8. Repeat steps 1 to 7 on other hand.

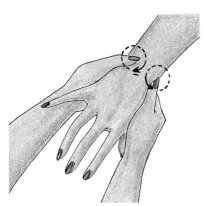

16.31 — Massage wrist and top of hand with a circular movement.

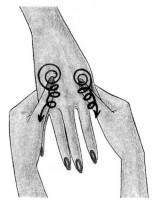

16.32 — Finish massage by tapering each finger.

Hand and Arm Massage

The hand and arm massage is a special service that may be added to the plain manicure. The procedure used is similar to the manicure with hand massage. However, all applications are extended to the forearm, including the elbow.

PROCEDURE

1. Complete hand massage as outlined.

2. Place client's arm on table, palm turned downward. Massage the arm from wrist to elbow, using a slow, circular motion in alternate directions. Repeat three times. Turn client's palm upward and repeat the same movements three times. (See Fig. 16.33)

3. Firmly massage the underpart of the arm to the elbow, using fingers of each hand in alternate crosswise directions. Repeat three times. (See Fig. 16.34)

4. Massage the top of the arm from the wrist to the elbow. Apply thumbs in opposite directions with a squeezing motion. Repeat three times. (See Fig. 16.35)

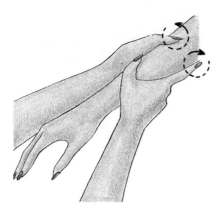

16.33—Massage the arm from wrist to elbow.

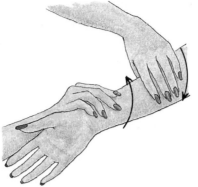

16.34—Massage the under-part of the arm to the elbow.

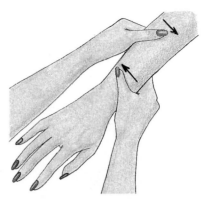

16.35—Massage the top of the arm from wrist to elbow.

5. Cup elbow joint in your hand. Massage the elbow with a circular motion. Repeat three times. (See Fig. 16.36)

6. Stroke the arm firmly in opposite directions, from the elbow to wrist. (See Fig. 16.37) Finally, stroke each finger, ending with a gentle squeeze of the fingertips.

7. Repeat steps 1 to 6 on the other arm.

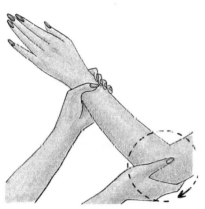

16.36—Massage elbow with circular motion.

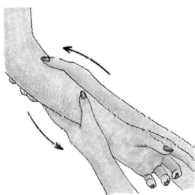

16.37—Stroke arm firmly in opposite directions.

Other Types of Manicures

ELECTRIC MANICURE

The electric manicure is given with a portable device operated by a small motor. It uses a variety of attachments, including an emery wheel, cuticle pusher, cuticle brush, and buffer. Before using an electric manicure machine, read the manufacturer's instructions carefully. State regulations on this procedure may vary.

OIL MANICURE

An oil manicure is beneficial for ridged and brittle nails and for dry cuticles. It also improves the hands by leaving the skin soft and pliable.

Procedure

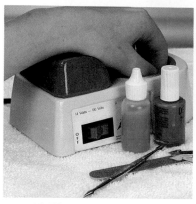

16.38—Hot oil manicure heater.

1. Heat vegetable (olive) oil or commercial preparation to a comfortable temperature in an electric heater. (Fig. 16.38)
2. Perform a plain manicure to the point where you place the hand in the finger bowl; at that point, have client place his or her fingers in the heated oil.
3. Massage the hands and wrists with the oil; then treat the cuticles in the usual manner. Cuticle remover, cuticle oil, or cream is not needed.
4. Remove oil from the hands with a warm, damp towel.
5. Wipe each nail carefully with polish remover to remove all traces of the oil before applying the base coat.
6. Complete as you would a plain manicure.

MEN'S MANICURE

Men usually prefer a conservative manicure. File the nails either round or square. Apply a dry polish instead of a liquid polish.

Implements, materials, and supplies are the same as those used for a plain manicure. Follow the same procedure for a plain manicure up to the application of a base coat.

Buff nails (where permitted). Apply a small dab of paste polish over the buffer. Then buff the nails with downward strokes, from the base to the free edge of each nail, until a smooth, clear gloss has been obtained. To prevent a heating or burning sensation, lift the buffer from the nail after each stroke. Buffing the nails increases the circulation of the blood to the fingertips, smooths the nails, and gives them a natural gloss or sheen.

Remove all residue from the nails by washing and drying the fingertips. If a clear liquid polish is used, buffing is not required. Apply polish in the same manner as for a plain manicure.

BOOTH MANICURE

A booth manicure is one that is given in the booth and not at the manicuring table. It is usually given while the client is receiving another service—for example, while a man is having his hair cut or styled.

Advanced Nail Techniques

Clean, attractive hands and nails are an admirable part of anyone's top-to-toe grooming. When a person cannot grow natural nails of the desired length and strength, he or she could solve the problem with the help of advanced nail techniques, which include nail wrapping, sculptured nails, nail tipping, dipping, press-on nail caps, or acrylic overlays. When performed properly, these advanced nail techniques yield natural-looking artificial nails.

Artificial nails may be used for the following purposes:

1. To mend or conceal broken or damaged nails.
2. To improve the appearance of very short or badly shaped nails.
3. To help overcome the habit of nail biting.
4. To protect a nail or nails against splitting or breakage.

NAIL WRAPPING

Nail wrapping is done to mend torn, broken or split nails, and to fortify weak or fragile nails. Mending tissue, silk, linen, or acrylic fiber are among the materials available for use in this procedure. Bolstering nails with silk will give a smooth, even appearance to the nail. Linen gives a more durable wrap; however, the coarseness of the material requires a colored polish to cover the completed nail.

The following two procedures are for use with materials which must be cut to fit the nail or nail fissure. Several manufacturers have recently made available pre-cut swatches of material which are adhesive backed and are attached only to the front of the nail.

Mending the Nail

1. Lightly file the split or chipped portion of the nail with the fine side of the emery board to help the mending material adhere to the nail.
2. Tear a small piece of mending material and saturate it with mending adhesive.
3. Place saturated mending material over the split or chipped area.
4. Tuck the material under the nail with an orangewood stick. The surface of the patch must be smoothed away from the nail edge with an orangewood stick dipped in polish remover.
5. If the split is deep, add a second patch for reinforcement.
6. Dry patch thoroughly before applying the base coat and polish.

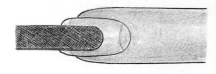

16.39—Roughen nail surface and cut wrap to fit nail.

Fortifying the Nail

1. Roughen the nail surface with the fine side of an emery board.
2. Tear or cut the wrapping material to fit the nail. If using mending tissue, tear into strips making sure edges of the tissue are feathered. (See Fig. 16.39)
3. If using mending tissue, saturate each strip with mending adhesive. If using other material, place a line of mending adhesive down the center of the nail. (See Fig. 16.40)
4. Using two fingers, place the wrapping material over the nail and hold until it adheres. Starting at the middle of the nail, use the orangewood stick to push the material in all directions, toward the edges and tip of the nail. Keep dipping the orangewood stick into the polish remover and patting the material until it is smooth. (See Fig. 16.41)

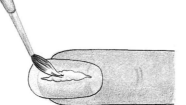

16.40—Apply adhesive.

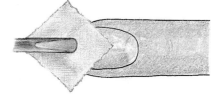

16.41—Apply mending tissue.

5. Trim excess material extending past the free edge and sides of the nails. (See Fig. 16.42)
6. If using mending tissue, turn the finger over and apply adhesive to the underside of the nail. Then, using the fingertips, fold the tissue over the nail edge and smooth out the tissue under the free edge with a pusher. If using other material, take the fine side of an emery board and lightly file the entire nail, top sides, and free edge until smooth. (See Fig. 16.43)

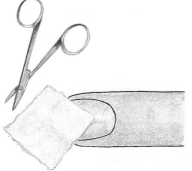

16.42—Trim excess.

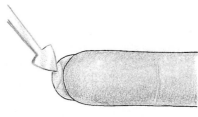

16.43—Tuck tissue under free edge.

7. Apply one or two coats of adhesive on the top and underside of the free edge of the nail. (See Fig. 16.44)

8. Apply a protective base coat to the top and underside of the free edge of the nail, and allow it to dry. Apply nail enamel and top coat or sealer, the same as for a plain manicure.

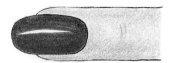

16.44—Apply base and top coats.

Alternative Method

In step 3, when applying mending tissue, coat entire nail bed with adhesive and apply tissue.

Removing Nail Wraps

Remove polish from the client's right hand. To loosen the nail wrap, have the client place her fingertips in an approved type of solvent specified by the manufacturer's directions or recommended by your instructor.

After removing the polish from the left hand, have the client remove her right hand from the bowl, and ask her to place the fingertips of her left hand in the bowl of solvent. Gently remove the loosened wrap with an orangewood stick or metal pusher, and then place the fingertips in warm oil. Repeat the same procedure for the left hand.

Liquid Nail Wrap

Liquid nail wrap is a polish made of tiny fibers designed to strengthen and preserve the natural nail as it grows. It is brushed on to the nail in several directions to create a network that once hardened protects the nail. It is similar to nail hardener, though it is of a thicker consistency and contains more fiber.

SCULPTURED NAILS

Scupltured nails, also known as build-on nails, are used when one or more nails are to be lengthened. The manicurist should build the type of nail that best conforms to the shape of the client's fingers and hands.

Implements and Materials

Use all of the regular implements for manicuring plus the following:

Nail forms	Nail lengthener powder
Measuring spoon	Special liquid to dilute powder
Mixing cup	Brushes for application
Acrylic nippers	

Procedure

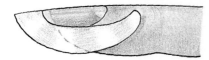

16.45—Apply nail form.

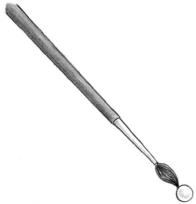

16.46—Form a smooth ball of acrylic.

16.47—Place ball of acrylic on tip of free edge.

1. Give plain manicure up to but not including hand and arm massage. Scrub nails to remove oil from area.
2. Roughen nail slightly with emery board.
3. Dust the nail bed with a cosmetic brush or cotton swab.
4. Apply approved nail primer to the surface of the nail with a brush, according to the manufacturer's instructions.
5. Peel a nail form from its paper backing, and using the thumb and index finger of each hand, bend the tip to the desired nail shape. The adhesive tabs of the nail form grip the sides of the fingers when pressed with the thumb and index finger. Check to see that the form is snug under the free edge of the nail. (See Fig. 16.45)
6. Dip the brush into the liquid mixture, wipe excess material on the side of the bowl and then immediately dip tip of brush into the powder, rotating it slightly as you draw it toward yourself to form a smooth ball of acrylic. (See Fig. 16.46)
7. Place the ball of acrylic on the tip of the free edge of the nail. Form the new acrylic tip of the nail by dabbing and pressing material with the base of the brush. (See Fig. 16.47)
8. Pick up additional acrylic material as in step 6 and place at the center of the nail and shape with the brush, making sure to avoid touching the cuticle. (See Fig. 16.48)
9. Make an extremely wet acrylic mixture (very little powder) and place at the center of the lower half of the nail bed. Spread mixture to the sides of the nail bed, being careful not to touch the cuticle. (See Fig. 16.49)

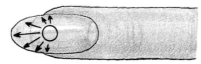

16.48—Use additional acrylic material and shape with brush.

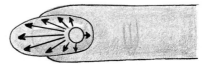

16.49—Apply wet acrylic mixture.

10. Allow nails to dry and remove nail forms.
11. File new nail to desired shape and then buff nails until entire surface is smooth.
12. Wash the nail or nails thoroughly. Allow them to dry.
13. Apply a base coat, polish, and top coat sealer.

Removing Sculptured Nails

Soak nails in an approved solvent specified by the manufacturer or your instructor. When acrylic nails are sufficiently softened, remove them with acrylic nippers using a rolling technique. *Do not pry acrylic material from nail bed.*

Repairs and Fill-ins for Sculptured Nails

1. Remove nail polish with non-acetone polish remover.
2. Using acrylic nippers, clip any loose material on the nail bed, rolling the broken material toward you. (See Fig. 16.50)

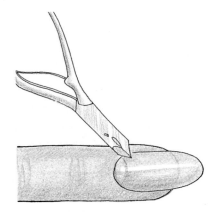

16.50 — Clip any loose material on the nail bed.

3. Roughen newly exposed area with an emery board, then dust area with a cosmetic brush or cotton swab.
4. Brush exposed area with primer, following the manufacturer's instructions.
5. Dip tip of brush into liquid, then into powder to form a small acrylic ball.
6. Place acrylic material on exposed area, pressing and shaping it with the base of the brush until it blends into the existing sculptured nail. Let area dry. Reshape nail with emery board and buff for a smooth appearance.

If an acrylic nail is badly chipped or cracked, it will probably have to be clipped back. A new nail form is then attached and acrylic material added to the free edge of the nail. A new tip is then formed and blended into the old material still adhering to the nail.

Acrylic Overlays

Acrylic overlays can strengthen weak nails or repair damaged ones. The acrylic material is used on sculptured nails, except that nails are reinforced on the top surface instead of extended.

Safety Precautions

1. Clean brush by dipping it into polish remover and wiping it clean.
2. Clean mixing dish by lifting hardened content out with pusher.
3. Make sure bottles are tightly capped when not in use.
4. Do not store product near heat, or use near open flame.
5. Do not apply to injured or inflamed skin.
6. Make sure work area is well ventilated.

When sculptured nails lift, crack, or grow out and are not attended to immediately, moisture and dirt become trapped under the nail, and fungus begins to grow. The spread of fungus can lead to nail injury or loss. Do not attempt to treat the condition yourself. It is very contagious and should be referred to a physician.

A change in the color of the natural nail after sculptured nails have been applied usually means that fungus has become trapped under the acrylic. Most primers have aseptic ingredients which sterilize the nail before acrylic is applied. To help ensure that contamination does not occur, *do not touch the nail after primer is applied*.

PRESS-ON ARTIFICIAL NAILS

Press-on nails are a convenient way to lengthen and beautify nails. They can be worn every day or on special occasions. Press-on nails are constructed of either plastic or nylon, and the manufacturer's instructions must be followed carefully.

Implements and Materials

Use all the regular implements and materials for manicuring, plus artificial press-on nails, nail adhesive, and adhesive remover.

Preparation

1. Remove polish from client's nails, and give a manicure up to, but not including, the application of polish.
2. Roughen the client's nails by going over them with an emery board.
3. Select the proper nail size for each finger. With sharp manicuring scissors, trim and then file the artificial nail at the cuticle end so that it fits to the shape of the natural nail. Artificial nails can be flattened by being firmly pressed down before application. They also can be reshaped by being held in warm water for a few seconds and molded to the desired shape.

Procedure

1. Apply a small amount of adhesive evenly on the edges of the client's nails. Do not apply adhesive on the center of the nails.
2. Apply adhesive on the inside of the artificial nail, excluding tip.
3. Allow the adhesive to dry thoroughly (about 2 minutes).
4. Press artificial nail gently onto the natural nail, with the base touching the cuticle or under it. As each nail is applied, hold it firmly in place for about a minute.
5. Carefully wipe away any excess adhesive from tips and around nails.
6. Allow the artificial nails to dry thoroughly. Advise the client to avoid disturbing the nails while they are drying.
7. Finish the manicure by applying base coat, polish, and top coat.

Removing Polish

To remove nail polish from nails constructed of plastic, use only nail polish remover that has an oily base and is non-acetone.

Reminder: Polish remover containing acetone will damage plastic artificial nails.

If nylon-constructed nails have been used, an acetone type of polish remover will not damage them.

Removing Press-on Artificial Nails

Apply a few drops of oily nail polish remover around the edge of the nail; then gently lift from the side with an orangewood stick. Do not attempt to pull or twist off the nail, as this could damage or injure the natural nail. Adhesive solvent can be used to remove press-on nails. It also can be used to remove any surplus adhesive from artificial nails and from natural nails. Press-on nails should be dried carefully and stored in a box. With proper care, they can be reused.

Reminders and Hints on Press-on Artificial Nails

1. Never apply artificial nails over sore or infected areas.
2. Most manufacturers suggest that artificial nails not be worn for more than 2 weeks at a time, in order to allow for natural growth of the nail.
3. Most artificial nail adhesives are flammable; be cautious with cigarettes, matches, and lighters.
4. When wearing artificial nails, do not subject them to a long period of immersion in water as they might tend to loosen.
5. Do not contaminate the adhesive with oil, cream, or powder.

Other Advanced Techniques

Following are several other advanced nail techniques you should be familiar with.

DIPPED NAILS

Dipped nails are artificial nail tips which are sprayed with an adhesive and then applied with glue to the ends of the natural nails. After filing and sanitizing, glue is applied down the center of the nail. The nail is then dipped for a short period of time into an acrylic mixture. When the acrylic dries, the nail is filed, buffed, and coated with adhesive. Dipped nails are removed with an adhesive solvent recommended by the manufacturer or your instructor.

NAIL TIPPING

Anyone can have long-looking nails by simply extending the natural nail artificially.

Procedure

1. Give manicure up to but not including polish.
2. Select proper sized tip to fit client's natural nail.
3. Slightly roughen the free edge of the nail.
4. File tip to fit the shape of the free edge of the nail only. (See Fig. 16.51)
5. Hold nail tip with thumb and index finger and apply half a drop of glue to the free edge of the nail.
6. Press tip onto the free edge of the nail, and then hold until dry. (See Fig. 16.52)

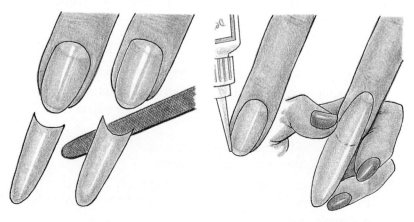

16.51 — Select size and shape nail.

16.52 — Apply glue and affix nail.

7. Buff the nail where the free edge of the nail and the tip form a seam. Leave resulting dust on the nail. (See Fig. 16.53)

8. Apply nail glue to seam where nail tip and free edge of nail meet. (See Fig. 16.54) Glue placed over the nail dust will act as a bond and filler. Repeat glue application twice.

9. File sides of tip to blend with the natural nail. (See Fig. 16.55) Cut nail to desired shape.

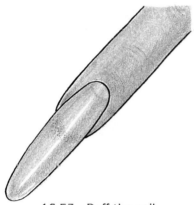

16.53—Buff the nail.

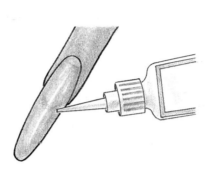

16.54—Apply glue to seam.

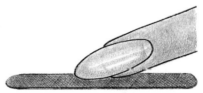

16.55—File sides.

10. Apply glue from seam to the free edge of the nail tip. (See Fig. 16.56) Buff seam and repeat procedure.

11. Apply nail polish as in a regular manicure. (See Fig. 16.57)

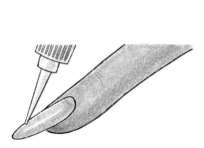

16.56—Apply glue from seam to nail tip.

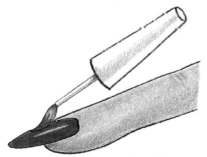

16.57—Apply nail polish.

Removing Nail Tips

To remove nail tips, fill a small container with adhesive solvent recommended by the manufacturer or by your instructor. Soak nail tips until softened, and gently wipe fingers with a tissue. (See Fig. 16.58)

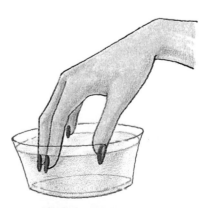

16.58—Soak nail tips.

Pedicure

Pedicuring is the care of the feet, toes, and toenails. It has become an important salon service because of the shoe styles that expose various parts of the heel and toes. Neglected toenails and rough, harsh heels detract from the finest of footwear. Foot care not only improves personal appearance, it also adds to the comfort of the feet.

Abnormal foot conditions, such as corns, calluses, and ingrown nails, are best treated by a qualified podiatrist.

Ringworm of the foot (athlete's foot) is an infectious condition which can spread from one person to another. For an in-depth explanation of this disease, see the chapter on the nail and its disorders.

CAUTION

▶ *Do not administer a manicure or pedicure on hands or feet with a contagious disease (for example, ringworm, or athlete's foot). Clients with such a condition should be referred to a physician.*

EQUIPMENT, IMPLEMENTS, AND MATERIALS

The equipment, implements, and materials required for pedicuring are the same as those for manicuring, with the following additions:

Low stool for cosmetologist or pedicurist.

Ottoman on which to rest client's foot.

Two basins of warm water, each large enough for foot bath and rinse.

Waterproof apron, or an extra towel, to place over the lap to protect the uniform.

Two towels for drying client's feet.

Special toenail clippers.

Witch hazel or other *astringent.*

Antiseptic solution.

Cotton pledgets and *foot powder.*

Paper towels.

PREPARATION

1. Arrange required equipment, implements, and materials.
2. Seat client in chair; have client remove shoes and stockings.
3. Place client's feet on a clean paper towel on footrest.
4. Wash your hands.
5. Fill the two basins with enough warm water to cover the ankles.
6. Add antiseptic to one basin. Place both feet in bath for 3 to 5 minutes.
7. Remove feet from basin, rinse feet in second basin, and wipe dry.

PROCEDURE

1. Remove old polish from the nails of both feet. (See Fig. 16.59)
2. File toenails of the left foot with an emery board. File the toenails straight across, rounding them slightly at the corners to conform to the shape of the toes. To avoid ingrown nails, do not file into the corners of the nails. Smooth rough edges with the fine side of an emery board. (See Fig. 16.60)
3. Place the left foot in warm, soapy water. (See Fig. 16.61)

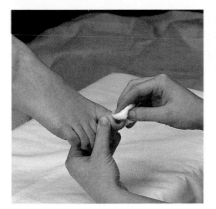

16.59—Remove old polish.

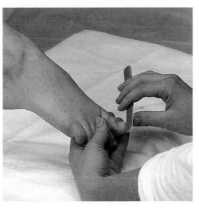

16.60—File toenails.

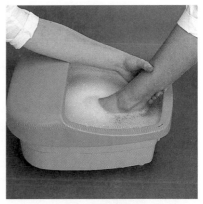

16.61—Soak foot.

4. Shape the nails of the right foot.
5. Remove the left foot from the basin and dry. (See Fig. 16.62)
6. With a cotton-tipped orangewood stick, apply cuticle solvent to the cuticle and under the free edge of each toenail. (See Fig. 16.63)
7. Place the right foot in the bath.
8. Loosen the cuticle gently on the left foot with a cotton-tipped orangewood stick. Keep the cuticle moist with additional lotion or water. Do not use excessive pressure. Avoid the use of the metal pusher.
9. Do not cut the cuticle. Only nip a large, ragged hangnail.
10. Rinse the left foot and dry. Massage each toe with cuticle cream or oil.
11. Repeat steps 5 to 10 on right foot.
12. Scrub both feet in warm, soapy water, rinse, and dry thoroughly.

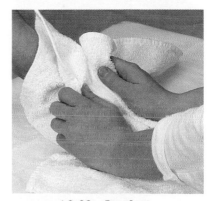

16.62—Dry foot.

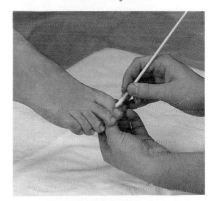

16.63—Apply cuticle solvent.

Foot Massage

PROCEDURE

1. Apply lotion or cream over the foot to just above the ankle.
2. Start at the instep of the left foot and apply firm, rotary movements down to the center of the toes. (See Fig. 16.64)
3. Slide the thumbs firmly back to the instep, and repeat same movement.
4. Slide the thumbs back to the hollow of the heel, and repeat same movement.
5. Slide the thumbs back to the base of the foot, and repeat same movement.
6. Start at the heel and work down to the center of the toes. (See Fig. 16.65)
7. Slide firmly back to the heel, and repeat same movement up each side of the foot.
8. Hold one toe in one hand and the heel in the other hand, and apply three rotary movements; do the same with the other toes. (See Fig. 16.66)
9. Slide the right hand to the ankle and the heel of your left hand to the ball of the foot, and apply six firm, rotary movements. (See Fig. 16.67)
10. Repeat steps 2 to 9 with the right foot.

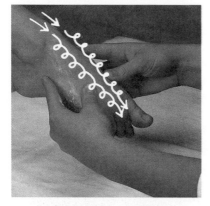

16.64—Massage from instep to the center of the toes.

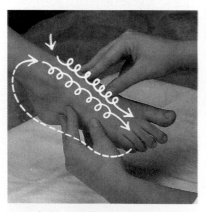

16.65—Massage from heel down to the center of the toes.

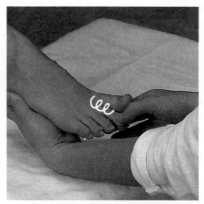

16.66—Rotary movement of the toes.

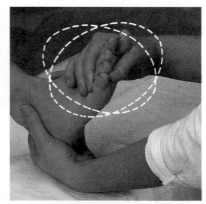

16.67—Rotary movement of the foot.

COMPLETION

1. Remove lotion or cream from both feet with a warm towel.
2. Apply witch hazel or astringent to the feet with a large cotton pledget.
3. Dust lightly with talcum powder.
4. Wipe each toenail with polish remover to remove lotion or cream.
5. Apply a base coat, polish, and seal coat in the same manner as for a manicure. (See Fig. 16.68)
6. Cleanup. Clean and sanitize implements, and place in dry sanitizer. Discard used materials. Wash your hands.

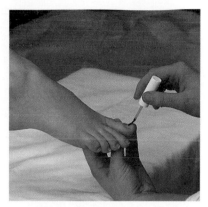

16.68—Applying base coat.

LEG MASSAGE

The foot massage may be extended up to and above the knee. When massaging from the ankle to the knee, do not massage over the shinbone and above the knee. It is advisable to keep the pressure to the muscular tissue on either side of the shinbone. On the calf area of the leg, you may use kneading upward movements up to the underpart of the knee.

People Skills

As you start working with clients, you'll discover that it pays to keep your sense of humor. Damien Miano, co-owner of La Dolce Vita in New York, recalls that the funniest thing that ever happened in his salon was a result of a write-up in *Elle* magazine.

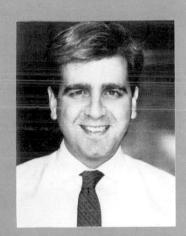

Elle ran a feature on natural treatments and, for photographic drama, had the salon prepare a full fruit salad "conditioning treatment," which was photographed on top of a model's head. The intent was to get attention, and get attention it did. Several months after the feature ran, a client came into the salon demanding the fruit salad treatment. Since so much time had passed, the salon had difficulty understanding what the client wanted, and the client got the photograph confused with a second article on pedicures and insisted that she get the fruit salad pedicure.

Always willing to please a client, the staff dutifully hiked to the corner deli, selected a fine mixture of fresh fruit, and gave the client her pre-pedicure fruit soak, for which she now returns on a regular basis.

"We call this the ultimate illustration that the customer is always right," said Miano.

Review Questions

MANICURING

1. What is the Latin word and definition for manicure?
2. What are the four general natural nail shapes?
3. What are some of the implements used in manicuring?
4. How do you file nails?
5. Why should a hand massage be included with a manicure?
6. List the different types of manicures.
7. List some of the advanced nail techniques available.
8. What is pedicuring and why is it an important client service?

17

THE NAIL AND ITS DISORDERS

LEARNING OBJECTIVES

After completing this chapter, you should be able to:

1. Describe the structure and composition of nails.
2. Describe the structures adjoining and affecting nails.
3. Discuss how nails grow.
4. List the various disorders and irregularities of clients' nails.
5. Recognize diseases of the nails that should not be treated in the beauty salon.

Introduction

The *nail*, an appendage of the skin, is a horny, translucent plate that protects the tips of the fingers and toes. *Onyx* (**ON**-iks) is the technical term for the nail.

The condition of the nail, like that of the skin, reflects the general health of the body. The normal, healthy nail is firm and flexible and appears to be slightly pink in color. Its surface is smooth, curved, and unspotted, without any hollows or wavy ridges.

The Nail

The nail is composed mainly of *keratin* (**KER**-a-tin), a protein substance that forms the base of all horny tissue. The nail is whitish and translucent in appearance and allows the pinkish color of the nail bed to be seen. The horny nail plate contains no nerves or blood vessels.

NAIL STRUCTURE

The nails consist of three parts: nail body, nail root, and free edge. The *nail body*, or *plate*, is the visible portion of the nail that rests upon, and is attached to, the *nail bed*. The nail body extends from the *root* to the *free edge*.

Although the nail plate seems to be one piece, it is actually constructed in layers. This structure can be seen readily, in both length and thickness, when nails split.

The *nail root* is at the base of the nail and is embedded underneath the skin. It is attached to an actively growing tissue known as the *matrix* (**MAY**-triks).

The *free edge* is the end portion of the nail plate that reaches over the tip of finger or toe. (Figs. 17.1, 17.2)

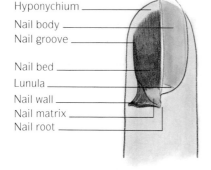

Hyponychium
Nail body
Nail groove

Nail bed
Lunula
Nail wall
Nail matrix
Nail root

17.1 — Diagram of a nail.

NAIL BED

The *nail bed* is the portion of the skin upon which the nail body rests. It has many blood vessels that provide the nourishment necessary for the continued growth of the nail. The nail bed also is abundantly supplied with nerves. (Figs. 17.1, 17.2)

MATRIX

The *matrix* is the part of the nail bed that extends beneath the nail root and contains nerves, lymph, and blood vessels to nourish the nail. The matrix produces cells that generate and harden the nail. The matrix will continue to grow as long as it receives nutrition and remains in a healthy condition.

Growth of the nails can be retarded if an individual is in poor health, if a nail disorder or disease is present, or if there is an injury to the nail matrix. (Figs. 17.1, 17.2)

Free edge

Nail body

Nail bed

Eponychium
Nail root

Nail matrix

17.2 — Cross section of a nail.

LUNULA

The *lunula* (lu-**NOO**-lah), or *half-moon*, is located at the base of the nail. The light color of the lunula is caused by the reflection of light where the matrix and the connective tissue of the nail bed join. (Figs. 17.1, 17.2)

Structures Surrounding the Nail

The *cuticle* (**KYOO**-ti-kel) is the overlapping skin around the nail. A normal cuticle should be loose and pliable.

The *eponychium* (ep-o-**NIK**-ee-um) is the extension of the cuticle at the base of the nail body that partly overlaps the lunula.

The *hyponychium* (heye-poh-**NIK**-ee-um) is that portion of the epidermis under the free edge of the nail.

The *perionychium* (**PER**-i-o-nik-ee-um) is that portion of the epidermis surrounding the entire nail border.

The *nail walls* are the folds of skin overlapping the sides of the nail.

The *nail grooves* are slits, or tracks, at either side of the nail upon which the nail moves as it grows.

The *mantle* (**MAN**-tl) is the deep fold of skin in which the nail root is embedded. (Figs. 17.1, 17.2)

Nail Growth

The growth of the nail is influenced by nutrition, general health, and disease. A normal nail grows forward, starting at the matrix and extending over the tip of the finger. Normal, healthy nails can grow in a variety of shapes, according to the individual. (Fig. 17.3) The average rate of growth in the normal adult is about ⅛″ (.3125 cm) per month. Nails grow faster in the summer than they do in the winter. Children's nails grow more rapidly, whereas those of elderly persons grow more slowly. The nail of the middle finger grows fastest and the thumbnail grows slowest. Although toenails grow more slowly than fingernails, they are thicker and harder.

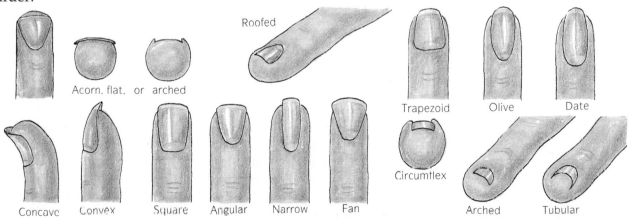

17.3—Various shapes of nails.

NAIL MALFORMATION

If the nail is separated from the nail bed through injury, it becomes distorted or discolored. Should the nail bed be injured after the loss of a nail, the new nail will be badly formed.

Nails are shed neither automatically nor periodically, as is hair. They may be torn off accidentally or lost because of infection or disease. Nails lost under these conditions are frequently badly shaped when they grow back. This is due to interference at the base of the nail. A nail is replaced as long as the matrix remains in good condition. Ordinarily, replacement of the nail takes about four months.

NAIL DISORDERS

Diseases of the nail should never be treated by a nail technician. However, the technician should recognize normal and abnormal nail conditions, and understand the reasons for them. Simple nail irregularities and blemishes come within the province of cosmetology and can be treated by the technician. A client with an infection, soreness, or irritation should be referred to a physician.

NAIL IRREGULARITIES

Corrugations, or *wavy ridges*, are caused by uneven growth of the nails, usually the result of illness or injury. When manicuring a client with this condition, carefully buff the nails slightly with pumice powder. This helps to remove or minimize the ridges. Ridge filler used with colored polish can give a smooth look to the nail.

Furrows (depressions) in the nails can run either lengthwise or across the nail. These are usually the result of illness or an injury to the nail cells in or near the matrix. They can also be caused by pregnancy or stress. Since these nails are exceedingly fragile, great care must be exercised when giving a manicure. Avoid the use of the metal pusher; use a cotton-tipped orangewood stick around the cuticle. (Fig. 17.4)

Leuconychia (loo-ko-**NIK**-ee-ah), or white spots, appear frequently in the nails, but do not indicate disease. They can be caused by injury to the base of the nail. As the nail continues to grow, these white spots eventually disappear. (Fig. 17.5)

Onychauxis (on-i-**KOK**-sis), or *hypertrophy* (heye-**PUR**-tro-fee), is an overgrowth of the nail, usually in thickness rather than length. It is usually caused by a local infection and can also be hereditary. If infection is present, the nail is not to be manicured. If infection is not present, the nail may be included in the manicure. File the nail smooth and buff with pumice powder. (Fig. 17.6)

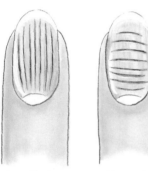

Lengthwise   Crosswise
depressions   depressions

17.4 — Furrows.

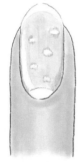

17.5 — Leuconychia.

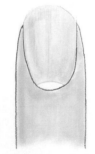

17.6 — Onychauxis or hypertrophy.

Onychatrophia (on-i-kah-**TROH**-fee-ah), *atrophy*, or *wasting away*, of the nail causes the nail to lose its luster, become smaller, and sometimes be shed entirely. Injury or disease might account for this nail irregularity. File the nail smooth with the fine side of the emery board. Advise the client to protect it from further injury or from exposure to strong soaps and washing powders. (Fig. 17.7)

Pterygium (te-**RIJ**-e-um) is a forward growth of the cuticle that adheres to the base of the nail. It can be caused by circulatory problems. Use the cuticle nippers carefully to remove the growth. (If nipping is permitted by your state board.) Suggest oil manicures. (Fig. 17.8)

Onychophagy (on-i-**KOH**-fa-jee), or bitten nails, is a result of an acquired nervous habit that prompts the individual to chew the nail or the hardened cuticle. Advise the client that frequent manicures and care of the hardened cuticle often help to overcome this habit. (Fig. 17.9)

Onychorrhexis (on-i-koh-**REK**-sis) refers to *split* or *brittle nails*. Among the causes of split nails are injury to the finger, careless filing of the nails, vitamin deficiencies, illness, frequent exposure to strong soap and water, and excessive use of cuticle solvents and nail polish removers. Suggest oil manicures. (Fig. 17.10)

Hangnail (agnail) is a condition in which the cuticle splits around the nail. Dryness of the cuticle, cutting off too much cuticle, or carelessness in removing the cuticle can result in hangnails. Advise the client that proper nail care, such as hot oil manicures, will aid in correcting such a condition. If not properly cared for, a hangnail can become infected. (Fig. 17.11)

Eggshell nails are nails that have a noticeably thin, white nail plate and are more flexible than normal. The nail plate separates from the nail bed and curves at the free edge. This disorder can be caused by a chronic illness of systemic or nervous origin. (Fig. 17.12)

Blue nails can be caused by poor blood circulation or a heart disorder. However, a client with this condition may receive a regular manicure. (Fig. 17.13)

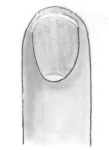

17.7—Onychatrophia.

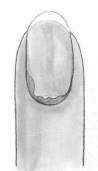

17.8—Pterygium.

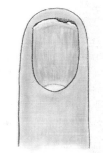

17.9—Onychophagy.

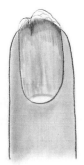

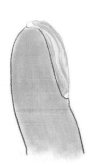

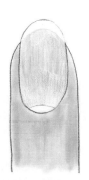

17.10—Onychorrhexis.   17.11—Hangnails.   17.12—Eggshell nail.   17.13—Blue nail.

A *bruised nail* will have dark, purplish (almost black or brown) spots, usually due to injury and bleeding in the nail bed. The dried blood attaches itself to the nail and grows out with it. Treat this injured nail gently. Avoid pressure.

Treating cuts. If a client is accidentally cut during a manicure, apply an antiseptic immediately. Do not buff or apply nail polish to the injured finger. To protect against infection, apply a sterile band-aid.

Infected finger. In the case of an infected finger, the client should be referred to a physician.

Nail Diseases

There are several nail diseases that you may encounter. Any nail disease that shows signs of infection or inflammation (redness, pain, swelling, or pus) must not be treated in a beauty salon. Medical treatment is required for all nail diseases.

A person's occupation plays an important role in the cause of many nail infections. Infections develop more readily in people who immerse their hands regularly in alkaline solutions. Natural oils are removed from the skin by frequent exposure to soaps, solvents, and other substances. The cosmetologist's hands are exposed daily to chemical materials. Many of these are harmless, but some are potentially dangerous. A cosmetologist's hands and nails should be protected with gloves when working with chemicals.

Onychosis (on-i-**KOH**-sis) is a technical term applied to nail disease.

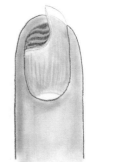

17.14—Onychomycosis.

Onychomycosis (on-i-koh-meye-**KOH**-sis), *tinea unguium* (**TIN**-ee-ah **UN**-gwee-um), or *ringworm* of the nails is an infectious disease caused by a fungus (vegetable parasite). A common form is whitish patches that can be scraped off the surface. A second form is long, yellowish streaks within the nail substance. The disease invades the free edge and spreads toward the root. The infected portion is thick and discolored. In a third form, the deeper layers of the nail are invaded, causing the superficial layers to appear irregularly thin. These infected layers peel off and expose the diseased parts of the nail bed. (Fig. 17.14)

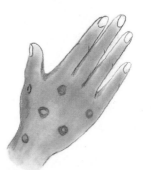

17.15—Ringworm of the hand.

Ringworm (tinea) of the hands is a highly contagious disease caused by a fungus. The principal symptoms are red lesions occurring in patches or rings over the hands. Itching may be slight or severe. (Fig. 17.15)

Most cases of dermatitis of the hands resemble tinea but are actually a contact dermatitis, plus a staphylococcic infection. Only a physician can determine this condition.

Ringworm of the foot (athlete's foot). In acute conditions, deep, itchy, colorless *vesicles* (blisters) appear. These appear singly, in groups, and sometimes on only one foot. They spread over the sole and between the toes, perhaps involving the nail fold and

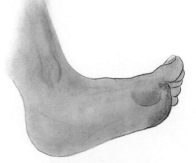

17.16—Athlete's foot.

infecting the nail. When the vesicles rupture, the skin becomes red and oozes. The lesions dry as they heal. Fungus infection of the feet is likely to become chronic. (Fig. 17.16)

Both the prevention of infection and beneficial treatment are accomplished by keeping the skin cool, dry, and clean.

Paronychia (par-oh-**NIK**-ee-ah), or *felon* (**FEL**-un), is an infectious and inflammatory condition of the tissues surrounding the nails. It is also characterized by gradual thickening and brownish discoloration of the nail plate. This condition can be traced to a bacterial infection. (Fig. 17.17)

Onychia (on-**NIK**-ee-ah) is an inflammation of the nail matrix, accompanied by pus formation. Improperly sanitized nail implements and bacterial infection can cause this disease.

Onychocryptosis (on-i-koh-krip-**TOH**-sis), or ingrown nails, can affect either the finger or toe. In this condition, the nail grows into the sides of the flesh and can cause an infection. Filing the nails too much in the corners and failing to correct hangnails are often responsible for ingrown nails. Ill-fitting shoes can also cause hangnails. (Fig. 17.18)

Onychoptosis (on-i-kop-**TOH**-sis) is the periodic shedding of one or more nails, either in whole or in part. This condition might follow certain diseases, such as syphilis. (Fig. 17.19)

Onycholysis (on-i-**KOL**-i-sis) is a loosening of the nail, without shedding. It is frequently associated with an internal disorder. (Fig. 17.20)

Onychophyma (on-i-koh-**FEE**-mah) denotes a swelling of the nail. (Fig. 17.21)

Onychophosis (on-i-**KOH**-foh-sis) refers to a growth of horny epithelium in the nail bed. (Fig. 17.22)

Onychogryposis (on-i-koh-greye-**POH**-sis) pertains to enlarged and increased curvature of the nails. (Fig. 17.23)

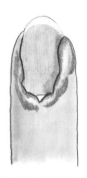

17.17 — Paronychia.

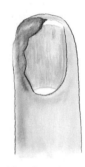

17.18 — Onychocryptosis.

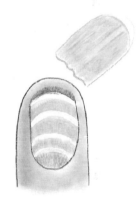

17.19 — Onychoptosis.

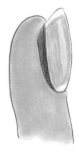

17.20 — Onycholysis.

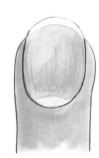

17.21 — Onychophyma.

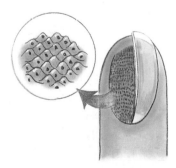

17.22 — Onychophosis.

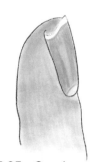

17.23 — Onychogryposis.

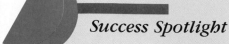

Success Spotlight

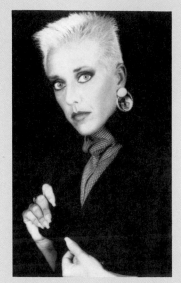

Jan Bragulla, president of Creative Nail Design, was always fascinated with the pace, excitement, creativity, and financial opportunities in the beauty and fashion business. Bragulla is the daughter of Dr. Stuart Nordstrom, who discovered that certain theories and products related to dental cosmetic bonding could be adapted to sculptured nails and nail extensions. Bragulla began her career in retail fashion, but soon discovered that the salon industry offered faster growth and greater opportunity.

Says Bragulla, "I'll never forget the enthusiastic reception my father received from cosmetology students when he made a special presentation to them. It was an important part of the encouragement he needed to put his theories to work and form Creative Nail Design, a company that has been devoted from day one to the advancement of the professional nail artist."

Excited by the endless choices she saw ahead, Bragulla helped start the family business and concentrated on developing one of the most comprehensive educational programs in the nail industry today.

Explains Bragulla, "Quality products are vital, but it is also essential that you take your education seriously. Education and learning to be the best that you can be are processes that never end.

"Career choices in this business are endless," she continues. "You can work for a manufacturer in sales, marketing, or product research and development. If you're entrepreneurial, you can own a salon. Don't settle for simply earning a living. Set a goal and go for it.

"While you're wrapping perms, mixing color, mastering nail artistry, and burying your head in textbooks, never forget that what awaits you is an industry that needs your talent and dedication. It's also an industry you can feel proud to be part of. I know that I do."

Review Questions

THE NAIL AND ITS DISORDERS

1. Describe a normal healthy nail.
2. What is the technical term for nail?
3. What is the composition of a nail?
4. Describe the structure of the nail.
5. List the structures surrounding the nail.
6. What part of the nail contains the nerve and blood supply?
7. What are the diseases of the nails that should not be treated in the beauty salon?

18

THEORY OF MASSAGE

LEARNING OBJECTIVES

After completing this chapter, you should be able to:

1. Describe the purpose of massage.

2. Describe the manipulations used in massage, and their benefits.

3. Identify the various types of massage movements and how they are applied.

4. Identify the motor nerve points of the face and neck.

5. List the physiological effects of massage.

Introduction

Massage is used to exercise facial muscles, maintain muscle tone, and stimulate circulation. Cosmetologists give massages to their clients to help them keep their skin healthy and muscles firm.

To master massage techniques, you must have a knowledge of anatomy and physiology, and considerable practice in performing the various movements.

Massage involves the application of external manipulations to the head and body. This is accomplished manually or with the use of electrical appliances, such as therapeutic lamps, high-frequency current, facial steamers, heating caps, scalp steamers, and vibrators.

Your services are limited to only certain areas of the body: scalp, face, neck, and shoulders; upper chest and back; hands and arms; and feet and lower legs.

To inspire confidence in a client it is important that you give a massage with a firm, sure touch. To do this, you must develop strong flexible hands, a quiet temperament, self-control, and the use of psychology.

Keep your hands soft by using creams, oils, and lotions. File and shape nails smooth so that you do not scratch the client's skin. Your wrists and fingers should be flexible, your palms firm, and warm.

Cream or oil should be applied to your hands to permit smoother and gentler hand movements and prevent drag or damage to the client's skin.

Basic Manipulations Used in Massage

HOW MANIPULATIVE MOVEMENTS ARE ACCOMPLISHED

Every massage treatment combines one or more of the basic movements. Each manipulation is applied in a definite way for a particular purpose. It is used according to the client's condition and the desired results. The result of a massage treatment depends on the amount of pressure, the direction of movement, and the duration of each type of manipulation. Direction of movement is generally from the insertion of a muscle toward its origin. Massaging a muscle in the wrong direction (from its origin to its insertion) could result in loss of resiliency and the sagging of the skin and muscles.

The origin of a muscle is the fixed attachment of one end of that muscle to a bone or tissue.

The insertion is the attachment of the opposite end of the muscle to another muscle, or to a movable bone or joint.

EFFLEURAGE

Effleurage (ef-**LOO**-rahzh) is a light, continuous stroking movement applied with the fingers (digital) and palms (palmar) in a slow and rhythmic manner. No pressure is used. The palms work over large surfaces, while the cushions of the fingertips work over small surfaces (around the eyes). Effleurage is frequently applied to the forehead, face, scalp, back, shoulders, neck, chest, arms, and hands for its soothing and relaxing effects.

Position of Fingers for Stroking

Curve your fingers slightly, with just the cushions of the fingertips touching the skin. Do not use the ends of the fingertips for these massage movements. Since the tips of the fingers are pointier than the cushions, the effleurage will be less smooth, and the free edges of your fingernails are likely to scratch the client's skin. (Figs. 18.1 and 18.3)

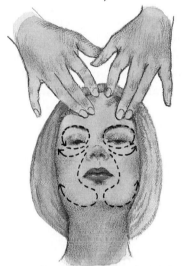

18.1—Digital stroking of face.

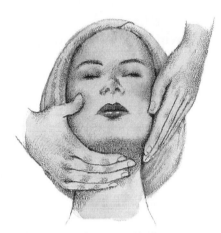

18.2—Palmar stroking of face.

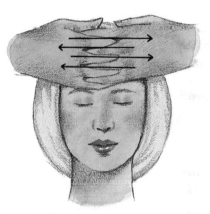

18.3—Digital stroking of forehead.

Position of Palms for Stroking

Hold your whole hand loosely, keep your wrist and fingers flexible, and curve your fingers to conform to the shape of the area being massaged. (Fig. 18.2)

PETRISSAGE

Petrissage (**PE**-tre-sahzh) is a kneading movement. Grasp the skin and underlying flesh between your fingers and palm of the hand. As you lift the tissues from their underlying structures, squeeze, roll, or pinch with a light, firm pressure. This movement invigorates the part being treated and is usually limited to back, shoulder, and arm massage.

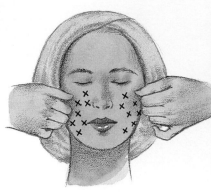

18.4—Digital kneading of cheeks.

Purpose of Kneading

Kneading movements give deeper stimulation to the muscles, nerves, and skin glands, and improve the circulation. Digital kneading of the cheeks can be achieved by light pinching movements. (Fig. 18.4) The pressure should be light but firm. When grasping and releasing the fleshy parts, the movements must be rhythmic, never jerky.

Fulling

Fulling is a form of petrissage used mainly for massaging the arms. With the fingers of both hands grasping the arm, apply a kneading movement across the flesh. The kneading movement must be used with light pressure on the underside of the client's forearm, and between the shoulder and elbow.

FRICTION

Friction (**FRIK**-shun) is a deep rubbing movement requiring pressure on the skin while moving it over the underlying structures. Use your fingers or palms. Friction has a marked influence on the circulation and glandular activity of the skin. Circular friction movements are usually used on the scalp, arms, and hands. Light circular friction movements are usually used on the face and neck. (Fig. 18.5) Chucking, rolling, and wringing are variations of friction and are used principally to massage the arms and legs.

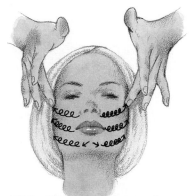

18.5—Circular friction on face.

The chucking movement is accomplished by grasping the flesh firmly in one hand and moving the hand up and down along the bone, while your other hand keeps the arm or leg in a steady position.

The rolling movement requires that the tissues be compressed firmly against the bone and twisted around the arm or leg. Both of your hands are active as you twist the flesh down the arm in the same direction.

Wringing is a vigorous movement in which your hands are placed a little distance apart on both sides of the client's arm or leg. While working your hands downward, apply a twisting motion against the bones in the opposite direction. (Fig. 18.6)

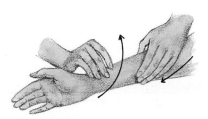

18.6—Wringing movement of arm.

PERCUSSION OR TAPOTEMENT MOVEMENT

Percussion (per-**KUSH**-un), or *tapotement* (tah-**POT**-mant), consists of tapping, slapping, and hacking movements. This form of massage is the most stimulating. It should be applied with care and discretion.

In facial massage, use only light digital tapping. In tapping, bring the fingertips down against the skin in rapid succession. Your fingers must be flexible, to create an even force over the area being massaged. (Fig. 18.7)

In slapping movements, flexible wrists permit your palms to come in contact with the skin in light, firm, and rapid slapping movements. One hand follows the other. With each slapping stroke (which must be nothing more than a firm, light, and quick contact with the skin) lift the flesh slightly.

For hacking movements, use the wrists and outer edges of the hands. Both the wrists and fingers must move in fast, light, firm, flexible motions against the skin in alternate succession. Hacking and slapping movements are used mainly to massage the back, shoulders, and arms.

Percussion movements tone the muscles and impart a healthy glow to the part being massaged.

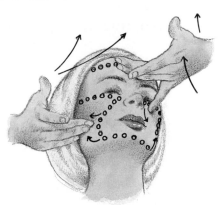

18.7—Digital tapping on face.

VIBRATION

Vibration (vi-**BRA**-shun) is a shaking movement accomplished by rapid muscular contractions in your arms, while the balls of the fingertips are pressed firmly on the point of application. It is a highly stimulating movement, and should be limited to only a few seconds duration on any one spot. Muscular contractions also can be produced by the use of a mechanical vibrator. (Fig. 18.8)

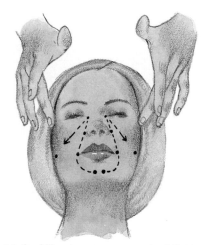

18.8—Vibratory movement of face.

JOINT MOVEMENTS

Joint movements are restricted to the massage of the arm, hand, and foot. These movements are applied either with or without resistance. (Fig. 18.9) (For information on joint movements, see the chapter on manicuring.)

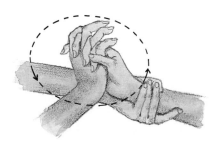

18.9—Joint movement.

Physiological Effects of Massage

To obtain proper results from a scalp or facial massage, you must have a thorough knowledge of all the structures involved: muscles, nerves, and blood vessels. Every muscle and nerve has a **motor point**. Some examples are illustrated here. (Figs. 18.10, 18.11) In order to obtain the maximum benefits from a facial massage you must consider the motor nerve points which affect the underlying muscles of the face and neck. The location of motor points varies among individuals due to differences in body structures. However, a few manipulations on the proper motor points will relax the client early in the massage treatment.

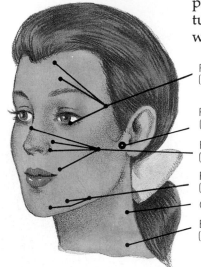

Facial nerve
(temporal branch)

Facial nerve.
(main trunk)

Facial nerve
(buccal branch)

Facial nerve
(mandibular branch)

Cervical nerve

Brachial Plexus
(Erb's point)

18.10—Motor nerve points of the face.

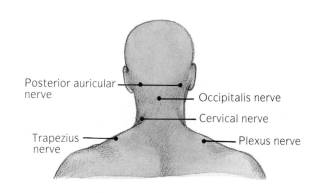

Posterior auricular
nerve

Occipitalis nerve

Cervical nerve

Trapezius
nerve

Plexus nerve

18.11—Motor nerve points of the neck.

Skillfully applied massage directly or indirectly influences the structures and functions of the body. The immediate effects of massage are first noticed on the skin. The part being massaged responds by increased circulation, secretion, nutrition, and excretion. The following beneficial results may be obtained by proper facial and scalp massage:

1. The skin and all its structures are nourished.
2. The skin is rendered soft and pliable.
3. The circulation of the blood is increased.
4. The activity of the skin glands is stimulated.
5. The muscle fiber is stimulated and strengthened.
6. The nerves are soothed and rested.
7. Pain is sometimes relieved.

Relaxation is achieved through light but firm, slow rhythmic movements, or very slow, light hand vibrations over the motor points for a short time. Another technique is to pause briefly over the motor points, using light pressure.

Body tissues are stimulated by movements of moderate pressure, speed, and time, or by light hand vibrations of moderate speed and time.

Body contours or fatty tissues are reduced by firm kneading, or by fast, firm, and light slapping movements over a fairly long period of time. Moderately fast hand vibrations with firm pressure also will accomplish this reduction.

The frequency of facial or scalp massage depends on the condition of the skin or scalp, the age of the client, and the condition to be treated. As a general rule, normal skin or scalp can be kept in excellent condition with the help of a weekly massage, accompanied by proper home care.

People Skills

Skin care is an intimate business. Not only must your client feel that she is in a clean environment, she must feel at ease when taking off her clothes for a body treatment and totally comfortable discussing her cellulite or acne with you. It is no wonder that skin care demands finely tuned people skills.

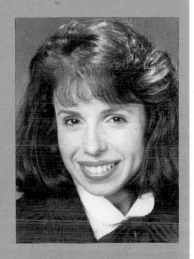

According to Lynn Parentini, vice president of Esthetic Research Group (a private label skin care company), almost every woman tries a facial at least once. Whether or not your client will return a second time depends on how great you make her feel and on how well you can educate her.

"The key to success is in developing the perfect formula for approaching clients," says Parentini. "First, always keep your facial room completely clean. As soon as you meet your client, make her feel comfortable and welcome. Gather as much information about her as you can through the consultation and skin analysis. Then, explain the service in detail before you begin it.

"As you work, have a definite procedure and method so that everything flows smoothly and seems perfectly natural to the client. Answer all her questions when she asks them by providing specific information on your services and products. Try not to leave the room and never leave a first-time client alone—especially when giving body treatments, which make the client feel vulnerable.

"When the service is over, review the client's home care program with her, make future treatment recommendations and again, answer any questions. Don't forget to write all her information on your consultation card.

"A warm, personalized, professional approach that is also well organized and executed takes a little practice, but it will help you to build a highly successful career in esthetics."

Review Questions

THEORY OF MASSAGE

1. Describe the purpose of massage.
2. What is meant by massage?
3. Describe the origin of a muscle.
4. Describe the insertion of a muscle.
5. In which direction should a muscle be massaged?
6. What are some beneficial results of a proper facial and scalp massage?
7. Name the five types of massage manipulations.

19

FACIALS

LEARNING OBJECTIVES

After completing this chapter, you should be able to:

1. Describe the physical and psychological effects of a facial.

2. List the materials and equipment required for facial treatments.

3. Describe the beneficial effects of a facial.

4. Demonstrate the procedure and manipulative skills required to give a facial.

5. Identify the various types of corrective facials given in the beauty salon.

Introduction

A professional facial is one of the most enjoyable and relaxing services available to the salon client. Those individuals who have engaged in this very restful or stimulating experience do not hesitate to return for repeat facials. When taken regularly, facials result in very noticeable improvement in the client's skin tone, texture, and appearance.

Facial Treatments

The cosmetologist does not treat skin diseases. However, you must be able to recognize the various skin ailments and you must also know when to advise the client to see a physician for treatment.

Facial treatments fall under two categories:

1. *Preservative*—maintaining the health of the facial skin by using correct cleansing methods, increasing circulation, relaxing the nerves, and activating the skin glands and metabolism through massage.
2. *Corrective*—correcting some facial skin conditions, such as dryness, oiliness, blackheads, aging lines, and minor conditions of acne.

Facial treatments are beneficial for:

1. Cleansing the skin.
2. Increasing circulation.
3. Activating glandular activity.
4. Relaxing the nerves.
5. Maintaining muscle tone.
6. Strengthening weak muscle tissue.
7. Correcting certain skin disorders.
8. Helping prevent the formation of wrinkles and aging lines.
9. Softening and improving skin texture and complexion.
10. Adding to the client's confidence.

Facial Massage

PREPARATION FOR FACIAL MASSAGE

1. Help the client to relax by speaking in a quiet and professional manner. Explain the benefits of the products and service, and answer any questions the client may have.

2. Provide a quiet atmosphere; work quietly and efficiently.

3. Maintain neat, clean, sanitary conditions in the facial work area and an orderly arrangement of supplies.

4. For sanitary reasons you should never remove products from their containers with your fingers. Always use a *spatula.* Obtain and arrange in an orderly manner all the items you will be using for the facial before the client arrives.

5. Follow systematic procedures.

6. If your hands are cold, warm them before touching the client's face.

7. Keep your nails smooth so as not to scratch the client's skin.

EQUIPMENT, IMPLEMENTS, AND MATERIALS

The following is a basic list of items you will need to give a facial to a client. You can add other items that are beneficial to the client. (Also see chapter on electricity and light therapy for an explanation of light and electrical equipment used in facials.)

Cleansing cream/lotion

Moisturizer and protective lotion

Mask

Gauze (for mask)

Astringent

Freshening lotion (mild astringent)

Antiseptic lotion

Lubricating oil

Cleansing tissues

Absorbent cotton

Cotton swabs and pledgets

Cotton pads

Sponges

Tissue strips

Headband or head covering

Towels

Clean sheet or other covering

Salon gown

Safety and bobby pins

Spatulas

Facial steamer

Makeup tray

High-frequency machine

Infrared lamp

Magnifying lamp

PROCEDURE

The information given here may be changed to conform with your instructor's routine.

1. Prepare the client.
   a) Greet the client and say something complimentary. This puts the client at ease.
   b) Ask the client to remove any jewelry (such as necklace and earrings) and store it in a safe place. Clients might want to keep their handbags nearby during the facial.

c) Show the client to the dressing room and offer assistance if needed.

d) Place a clean towel across the back of the facial chair to prevent the client's bare shoulders from coming in contact with the chair.

e) Seat the client in the facial chair (offer assistance, if needed). Then place a towel across the client's chest. Next, place the coverlet (or sheet) over the client's body and fold the top edge of the towel over the coverlet. Remove the client's shoes and tuck the coverlet around the feet. Some salons provide booties for the feet. These are worn to and from the dressing room.

f) Fasten a headband lined with tissue, a towel, or other head covering around the client's head to protect the hair. There are several types of head coverings on the market. Some types are of a turban design; others are designed with elastic, similar to a shower cap. They are generally made of either cloth or paper towels. Draping the head with a towel is done in the following manner (for paper towel procedure, be guided by your instructor):

1. Fold the towel lengthwise from one of the top corners to the opposite lower corner, and place it over the headrest with the fold facing down. Place the towel on the headrest before the client enters the facial area. When the client is in a reclining position, the back of the head should rest on the towel, so that one side of the towel can be brought up to the center of the forehead to cover the hairline. (See Fig. 19.1)

2. With the other hand, bring the other side of the towel over the center and cross it over. (See Fig. 19.2)

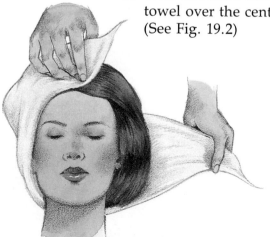

19.1—Place towel around client's head.

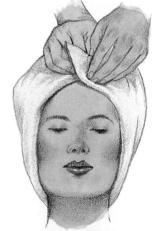

19.2—Join towel at center of client's head.

3. Use a regular bobby pin to hold the towel in place. Check to be sure that all strands of hair are tucked under the towel, earlobes are not bent, and the towel is not wrapped too tightly. (See Fig. 19.3)

g) Remove lingerie straps from the client's shoulders. (*Alternate method:* If client is given a strapless gown to wear, tuck the shoulder lingerie straps into the top of the gown.)

h) Adjust the headrest, then lower the facial chair to a reclining position. (Fig. 19.4)

i) Wash your hands.

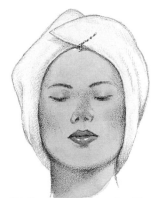

19.3—Secure towel with a bobby pin.

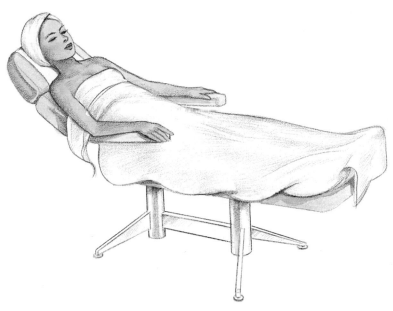

19.4—Client is prepared for facial.

2. Analyze the client's skin.
  a) Remove makeup to determine:
    1. If the skin is dry, normal, or oily.
    2. If fine lines or creases exist.
    3. If blackheads (*comedones*) or acne are present.
    4. If broken capillaries are visible.
    5. If the skin texture is smooth or rough.
    6. If the skin's color is even.
  b) This analysis will determine:
    1. The choice of products to use for the massage.
    2. The areas of the face that need special attention.

3. The amount of pressure to use when giving the massage.

4. If lubricating oil or cream is needed around the eyes.

5. Equipment or apparatus to use.

3. Apply cleansing cream.

a) Remove about a teaspoon of cleansing cream or lotion from the container with a spatula. Blend the cream or lotion with your fingers to soften it. If the client is wearing heavy eye and lip makeup, use a small amount of cleanser and moist cotton pads or soft tissue to remove the excess makeup. Be very gentle when working around the eyes and on the mouth.

b) Starting at the neck, use both hands in a sweeping movement to spread the cleansing product upward on the chin, jaws, cheeks, base of nose to temples, and along the sides and the bridge of the nose. (See Fig. 19.5) Make small circular movements with your fingertips around the nostrils and sides of the nose. Continue the sweeping upward movements between the brows and across the forehead to the temples.

c) Take additional cleansing cream or lotion from the container with a spatula and blend. Smooth down the neck, chest, and back with long, even strokes.

d) Starting at the center of the forehead, move your fingertips in a circle lightly around the eyes to the temples and back to the center of the forehead.

e) Slide your fingers down the nose to the upper lip, to the temples and forehead, lightly down to the chin, then firmly up the jawline to the temples and forehead.

4. Remove the cleansing cream.

a) Remove the cleansing cream or lotion with tissues; warm, moist towels; moist cotton pads; or facial sponges. Start at the forehead and follow the contours of the face. Remove all the cream from one area of the face before proceeding to the next. Finish with the neck, chest, and back. (See Fig. 19.6) (If eyebrows are to be arched, they should be done at this time.)

5. Steam the face (optional).

a) Steam the face mildly with warm, moist towels or with a facial steamer to open the pores so they can be cleansed of oil, blackheads, makeup, and other debris. Steam also helps to soften superficial lines and increases blood circulation to the surface of the skin.

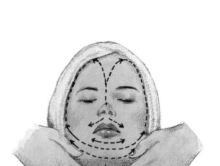

19.5—Spreading cream over the face, neck, chest, and back.

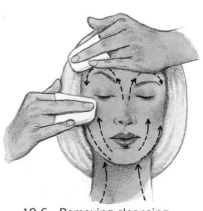

19.6—Removing cleansing cream with tissues or with a warm, moist towel.

6. Apply massage cream.
   a) Select a massage cream for the client's skin type. Using the same procedure employed to apply cleansing cream, apply massage cream to face, neck, shoulders, chest, and back.
   b) If needed, apply lubrication oil or cream around the eyes and on the neck.
7. Give facial manipulations.
   a) Cover the client's eyes with cotton pads moistened with a mild astringent.
   b) Massage the face using the facial manipulations described in this chapter.
8. Expose the face to infrared light. (See Fig. 19.7) Infrared lamp may be given during or after facial manipulations.
   a) Cover the client's eyes with cotton pads moistened with a mild astringent.
   b) Place the lamp at a comfortable distance from the face.
   c) Expose the face to infrared rays for 3 to 5 minutes.
9. Remove massage cream.
   a) Remove cream with tissues; warm, moist towels; moist cleansing pads; or sponges. Follow the same procedure as for removing cleansing cream.
10. Apply astringent or mild skin freshening lotion.
    a) Sponge the face with cotton pledgets moistened with the lotion.
11. Apply a treatment mask formulated for the client's skin condition. Leave on the face for about 7 to 10 minutes.
12. Remove the mask with wet cotton pledgets or towels.
13. Wipe the face with pledgets saturated with a mild astringent.
14. Apply a moisturizer or protective lotion.
15. Completion.
    a) Discard all disposable supplies and materials.
    b) Close product containers tightly, clean them, and put them in their proper places. Return unused cosmetics and other items to the dispensary.
    c) Place used towels, coverlets, head covers, and like items in appropriate containers
    d) Tidy up the work area.
    e) Wash and sanitize your hands.

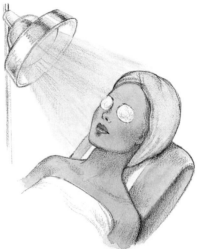

19.7 — Exposing the face to an infrared lamp.

Facial Manipulations

In giving facial manipulations, you must remember that an even tempo, or rhythm, induces relaxation. Do not remove your hands from the client's face once the manipulations have been started. Should it become necessary to remove your hands, feather them off, and then gently replace them with feather-like movements.

(*Note*: Each instructor may have developed her own routine in giving manipulations. The following illustrations merely show the different movements that may be used on the various parts of the face, chest, and back. Follow your instructor's routine.)

Massage movements are usually directed toward the origin of a muscle, in order to avoid damage to muscular tissues.

1. Chin movement. Lift the chin, using a slight pressure. (See Fig. 19.8)
2. Lower cheeks. Using a circular movement, rotate from chin to ears. (See Fig. 19.9)
3. Follow diagram for mouth, nose, and cheek movements. (See Fig. 19.10)

▶ NOTE: Many facial specialists prefer to start massage manipulations at the chin, while others prefer to start at the forehead. Both are correct. Be guided by your instructor.

4. Linear movement over forehead. Slide fingers to temples; rotate with pressure on upward stroke; slide to left eyebrow; then stroke up to hairline gradually moving hands across forehead to right eyebrow. (See Fig. 19.11)

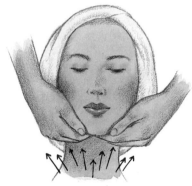

19.8—Chin movement.

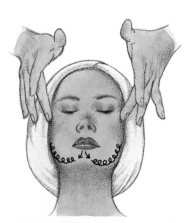

19.9—Circular movement of lower cheeks.

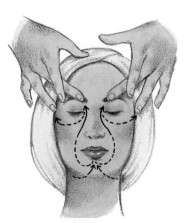

19.10—Mouth, nose, and cheek movements.

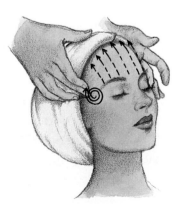

19.11—Linear movement over forehead.

5. Circular movement over forehead. Starting at eyebrow line, work across middle of forehead, and then toward the hairline. (See Fig. 19.12)

6. Criss-cross movement. Start at one side of forehead and work back. (See Fig. 19.13)

7. Stroking (headache) movement. Slide fingers to center of forehead; then draw fingers, with slight pressure, toward temples, and rotate. (See Fig. 19.14)

8. Brow and eye movement. Place middle fingers at inner corners of eyes and index fingers over brows. Slide to outer corners of eyes, under eyes, and back to inner corners. (See Fig. 19.15)

9. Nose and upper cheek movement. Slide fingers down nose. Apply rotary movement across cheeks to temples, and rotate gently. Slide fingers under eyes and back to bridge of nose. (See Fig. 19.16)

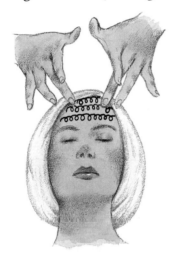

19.12—Circular movement over forehead.

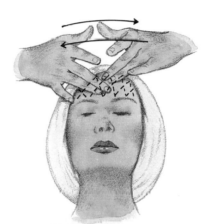

19.13—Criss-cross movement.

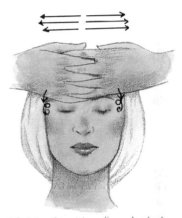

19.14—Stroking (headache) movement.

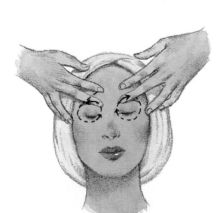

19.15—Brow and eye movement.

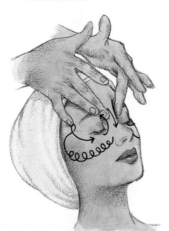

19.16—Nose and upper cheek movement.

10. Mouth and nose movement. Apply circular movement from corners of mouth up sides of nose. Slide fingers over brows and down to corners of mouth. (See Fig. 19.17)

11. Lip and chin movement. Draw fingers from center of upper lip, around mouth, going under lower lip and chin. (See Fig. 19.18)

12. Optional movement. Hold head with left hand; draw fingers of right hand from under the lower lip, around mouth, to center of upper lip. (See Fig. 19.19)

13. Lifting movement of cheeks. Proceed from the mouth to ears, and then from nose to top part of ears. (See Fig. 19.20)

14. Rotary movement of cheeks. Massage from chin to ear lobes, from mouth to middle of ears, and from nose to top of ears. (See Fig. 19.21)

15. Light tapping movement. Work from chin to earlobe, mouth to ear, nose to top of ear, and then across forehead. Repeat on other side. (See Fig. 19.22)

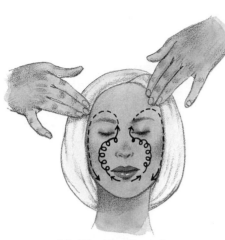

19.17—Mouth and nose movement.

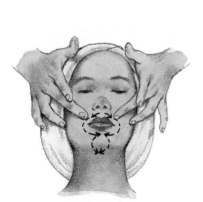

19.18—Lip and chin movement.

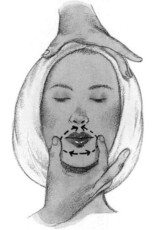

19.19—Optional movement.

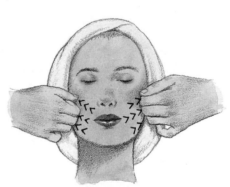

19.20—Lifting movement of cheeks.

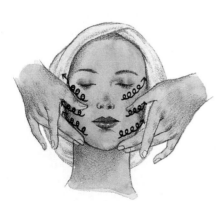

19.21—Rotary movement of cheeks.

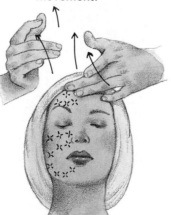

19.22—Light tapping movement.

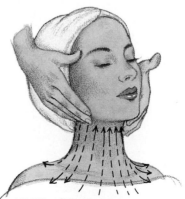

19.23—Stroking movement of neck.

16. Stroking movement of neck. Apply light upward strokes over front of neck. Use heavier pressure on sides of neck in downward strokes. (See Fig. 19.23)

17. Circular movement over neck and chest. Starting at back of ears, apply circular movement down side of neck, over shoulders, and across chest. (See Fig. 19.24).

18. Infrared lamp (optional). Protect eyes with eye pads; adjust lamp over client's face; leave on for about 5 minutes. (See Fig. 19.25)

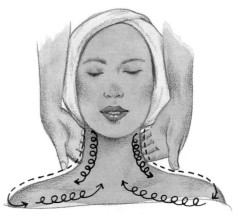

19.24—Circular movement over neck and chest.

CHEST, BACK, AND NECK MANIPULATIONS (OPTIONAL)

Some instructors prefer to treat these areas first before starting the regular facial. A suggested procedure is as follows:

1. Apply and remove cleansing cream.
2. Apply massage cream.
3. Give manipulations as outlined below.
4. Chest and back movement. Use rotary movement across chest and shoulders, then to spine. Slide fingers to base of neck. Rotate three times. (See Fig. 19.26)
5. Shoulders and back movement. Rotate shoulders three times. Glide fingers to spine, then to base of neck. Apply circular movement up to back of ear, and then slide fingers to front of earlobe. Rotate three times. (See Fig. 19.27)
6. Back massage (optional). To stimulate and relax client, use thumbs and bent index fingers to grasp the tissue at the back of the neck. Rotate six times. Repeat over shoulders and back to the spine. (See Fig. 19.28)
7. Remove cream with tissues or warm, moist towel.
8. Dust the back lightly with talcum powder and smooth.

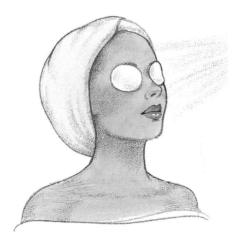

19.25—Infrared lamp (optional).

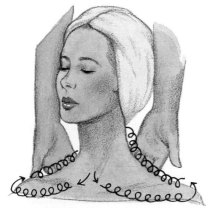

19.26—Chest and back movement.

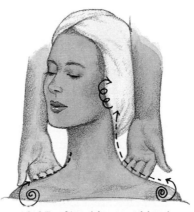

19.27—Shoulders and back movement.

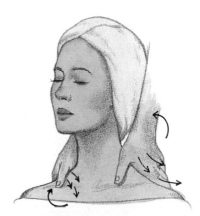

19.28—Back massage (optional).

Special Problems

FACIAL FOR DRY SKIN

A dry skin is caused by an insufficient flow of sebum (oil) from the sebaceous glands. The facial for dry skin helps correct the dry condition of the skin. It may be given with or without an electrical current. For more effective results, the use of electrical current is recommended.

Procedure with Infrared Rays

1. Prepare the client as for a plain facial.
2. Apply cleansing cream; remove with tissues or with a warm, moist towel.
3. Sponge the face with cleansing lotion (for dry skin).
4. Apply massage cream.
5. Apply lubricating oil, or eye cream, over and under the eyes.
6. Apply lubricating oil over the neck.
7. Cover the client's eyes with cotton pads moistened with witch hazel and boric acid solution.
8. Expose the face and neck to infrared rays for not more than 5 minutes.
9. Give manipulation three to five times.
10. Remove massage cream and oil with tissues or with a warm, moist towel.
11. Apply skin lotion suitable for dry skin.
12. Blot face with tissues or towel.
13. Apply a base foundation suitable for the client's skin.
14. Complete and clean up as for a plain facial.

CAUTION

▶ *For dry skin, avoid using lotions that contain a large percentage of alcohol. Read the manufacturer's directions.*

Procedure with Galvanic Current

The procedure for giving a dry skin facial with galvanic current is similar to the procedure for giving a dry skin facial with infrared rays, with a few changes:

1. Repeat steps 1 to 3 of the procedure with infrared rays.
2. Apply negative galvanic current for 3 to 5 minutes, to open the pores.
3. Repeat steps 4 to 11 of the procedure with infrared rays.

4. Apply positive galvanic current 3 to 5 minutes, to close the pores.
5. Repeat steps 12 to 14 of the procedure with infrared rays.

Procedure with Indirect High-Frequency Current

1. Follow steps 1 through 8 of the procedure for a facial with infrared rays.
2. Give manipulations, using the indirect method of applying high-frequency current, for not more than 7 minutes. (See Fig. 19.29)
3. Apply two to three cold towels to the face and neck.
4. Sponge the face and neck with skin freshener.
5. Apply a moisturizer of protective fluid.

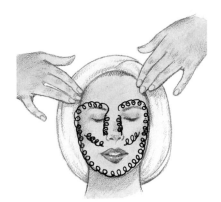

19.29—High-frequency indirect method. (Client holds electrode.)

FACIAL FOR OILY SKIN AND BLACKHEADS (COMEDONES)

An oily skin and/or blackheads (comedones) are caused by a hardened mass of sebum formed in the ducts of the sebaceous glands. Sometimes the client's diet may be a factor in the condition. For an appropriate diet to help minimize oily skin and blackheads, the client should see a physician.

Procedure

1. Prepare the client as for a plain facial. Sanitize your hands.
2. Apply cleansing lotion and remove it with a warm, moist towel, moist cotton pads, or facial sponges.
3. Place the moistened eyepads on the client's eyes, then analyze the skin under a magnifying lamp.
4. Steam the face with three to four moist, warm towels, or steam the face with a facial steamer to open the pores.
5. Cover your fingertips with tissue and gently press out blackheads. Do not press so hard as to bruise the skin tissue.

CAUTION

▶ *If it is necessary to cleanse pimples that have come to a head and are open, use rubber or latex gloves. Do not attempt to deal with a skin problem that requires medical attention.*

6. Sponge the face with astringent.
7. Cover the client's eyes with pads moistened with a mild astringent.

8. Apply blue light over the skin for not more than 3 to 5 minutes.
9. Apply massage cream suitable for the skin condition.
10. Give manipulations.
11. Remove cream with a warm, moist towel, cotton pads, or facial sponges.
12. Moisten a cotton pledget with an astringent lotion. Apply it to the face and neck with upward and outward movements to close the pores.
13. Blot the excess moisture with tissues.
14. Apply protective lotion if needed.
15. Complete and clean up, following proper sanitary procedures.

WHITEHEADS (MILIA)

Milia or whiteheads is a common skin disorder, caused by the formation of sebaceous matter within or under the skin. It usually occurs in skin of fine texture. The surface openings of the skin may be so small that the sebum cannot pass out. As a result, it collects under the surface of the skin in small, round, hardened, pearl-like masses that resemble a small grain of sand. This condition may be treated under the supervision of a dermatologist.

FACIAL FOR ACNE

Acne is a disorder of the sebaceous glands; therefore it requires medical direction. If the client is under medical care, the role of the cosmetologist is to work closely with the client's physician to carry out instructions as to the kind and frequency of facial treatments.

Under medical direction, you must limit the cosmetic treatment of acne to the following measures:

1. Reducing the oiliness of the skin by local applications.
2. Removing blackheads, using proper procedures.
3. Cleansing the skin.
4. Using special medicated preparations.

Equipment, Implements, and Materials
Acne cream or lotion
Antiseptic lotion
Cleansing lotion
Astringent lotion for oily skin
Towels
Appropriate mask
High-frequency magnifying lamp

Procedure

Because acne skin contains infectious matter, it is advisable to use rubber or latex gloves and disposable materials such as cotton cleansing pads.

1. Prepare all materials to be used for the facial treatment.
2. Prepare the client.
3. Sanitize your hands.
4. Cleanse the client's face.
5. Place cotton eyepads over the client's eyes; then analyze the skin under the magnifying lamp.
6. Apply warm, wet towels to the face to open the pores for deep cleansing.
7. Extract blackheads and cleanse pimples.
8. Cleanse the face with a wet cotton pad that has been sprinkled with astringent.
9. Apply the acne treatment cream. Leave on the eyepads and turn on the infrared lamp for about 5 to 7 minutes to enable the treatment cream to penetrate the skin. Or, you can apply high-frequency current with direct application (facial electrode) over the affected area for not more than 5 minutes. (See Fig. 19.30) Be guided by your instructor.

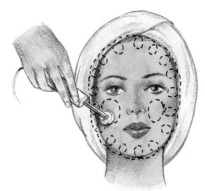

19.30—Applying high-frequency current with facial electrode.

10. Leave the eyepads on and apply a treatment mask that is suitable for the skin condition. Leave it on the face for about 8 to 10 minutes.
11. Remove the mask with moist towels or cotton pads.
12. Apply astringent to the face with a wet cotton pad.
13. Apply protective fluid or special acne lotion.
14. Complete the cleanup procedures.

DIET FOR ACNE

Modern studies show that acne might be due to hereditary and environmental factors. It can be aggravated by emotional stress and faulty diet. Acne is not believed to be caused by any particular food or drink, but foods high in fats, starches, and sugars tend to worsen the condition. The client should consult a physician for a prescribed diet. A well-balanced diet, drinking plenty of water, and following healthful personal hygiene habits are recommended.

Packs and Masks

Masks and packs are somewhat the same, but generally the substances of a heavier consistency such as clay are referred to as packs. Pack facials are recommended for normal and oily skin and are usually applied directly to the skin. Mask facials are recommended for dry skin and are applied to the skin with the aid of gauze layers or masks. Masks are made of many ingredients and combinations such as vegetables, fruits, dairy products, herbs, and oils. Gauze is often used to aid in holding the mask preparation on the face.

CUSTOM-DESIGNED MASKS

You will usually use prepared masks, but there are times when a custom-designed mask prepared from fresh fruits, vegetables, milk, yogurt, or eggs might be preferred. These masks are generally beneficial unless the client is allergic to a particular substance. You should ask the client about allergies before applying a mask. Custom-designed masks are generally left on the face for 10 to 15 minutes during a one-hour treatment. The following is a list of ingredients used in custom-designed masks and their benefits to the skin:

1. *Fresh fruit mask.* Fresh strawberries can be crushed or sliced and applied to the face (usually over or between layers of gauze) for a mildly astringent and stimulating mask. Bananas can be sliced or crushed to make a mask for dry and sensitive skin, since they are rich in vitamins, potassium, calcium, and phosphorus and leave the skin soft and smooth.

2. *Fruits and vegetables that are mildly astringent* and have excellent soothing qualities are: tomatoes, apples, and cucumbers. These fruits or vegetables can be sliced very thin or crushed and applied to the face. Gauze helps to hold the mask in place.

3. *The white of an egg* can be beaten until fluffy and applied to the face as a mask. Egg white has a tightening effect and clears impurities from the skin. It is beneficial to all skin types.

4. *Yogurt and buttermilk* are used for masks on all skin types. Their mildly astringent cleansing action leaves the skin feeling refreshed.

5. *Honey* is used for its toning, tightening, and **hydrating** effect.

6. Some ingredients such as honey and almond meal or oatmeal can be mixed into a paste with milk.

The Use of Gauze for Mask Application

Gauze is a thin, transparent fabric of loosely woven cotton, commonly called *cheesecloth*. Gauze is used to hold certain mask ingredients that do not cling or hold together on the face. Such is the case with sliced or crushed fruits or vegetables, which tend to run. These ingredients can be applied over a layer of gauze. The gauze holds the mask on the face but allows the ingredients to seep through to benefit the skin. In some cases, it is necessary to apply a second layer of gauze over the mask.

Procedure for Applying Gauze

1. Cut a piece of gauze large enough to cover the entire face and neck. (See Fig. 19.31) Cut out spaces for the eyes, nose, and mouth. Although the client is able to breathe through the gauze, the cutout spaces will be more comfortable.

2. Apply the mask ingredients over the gauze. (See Fig. 19.32) Start on the neck and apply upward on the face, ending on the forehead. Apply eyepads for the client's comfort.

3. Allow the mask to remain on the face for the appropriate time; then lift and roll the gauze upward to remove most of the mask. (See Fig. 19.33) Finish cleansing the face with moist cotton pads or facial sponges.

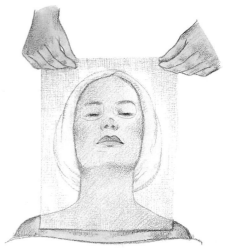

19.31—Cover entire face and neck with gauze.

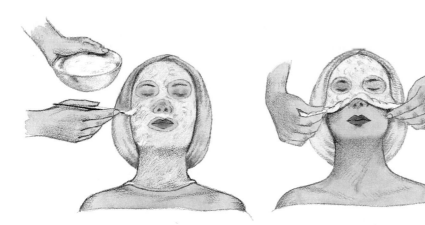

19.32—Apply the mask ingredients over the gauze.

19.33—Lift and roll the gauze upward to remove.

Equipment, Implements, and Materials for Custom-Designed Mask

Assemble all items needed for a plain facial and any special cosmetics or ingredients for the mask. Prepare the gauze.

Procedure for Custom-Designed Mask

1. Give a plain facial, including removal of massage cream after manipulations.
2. Place cotton pads moistened with mild astringent over the eyes.
3. Apply the gauze and the appropriate mask or mask ingredients for the skin condition. Keep the mask from getting into the client's eyes, nostrils, mouth, or on the hairline.
4. Allow the mask to remain on the skin 10 to 15 minutes or until it is dry. Follow the manufacturer's directions if using a prepared mask.
5. Remove the gauze mask carefully and finish cleansing the face with a warm, moist towel or cotton pads.
6. Apply a mild astringent or skin-freshening lotion.
7. Apply moisturizer or protective lotion.
8. Follow the usual completion and cleanup procedures.

HOT OIL MASK FACIAL

A hot oil mask facial is recommended for dry, scaly skin, or skin that is inclined to wrinkle. The mask is applied directly to the skin with the aid of gauze layers. Prepare the gauze in sections large enough to cover the face. Cut openings for the eyes, nose, and mouth.

Equipment, Implements, and Materials

Gather all items needed for a facial plus the following:

Prepared gauze facial mask
Hot oil preparation
Hot oil heater
Infrared lamp

Procedure

1. Give a plain facial, including the removal of massage cream.
2. Cover the eyes with eyepads moistened with mild astringent (skin-freshening lotion).
3. Moisten gauze facial mask with warm oil and place on the face, starting at the throat.
4. Place an infrared lamp about 24″ (60 cm) from the client's face. (See Fig. 19.34)
5. Allow the client to rest for 5 to 10 minutes under the lamp.
6. Remove the gauze facial mask.
7. Apply additional massage or moisturizing cream.
8. Give facial manipulations.
9. Remove cream with a warm, moist towel.
10. Apply an astringent lotion.
11. Apply moisturizer or protective lotion as needed.
12. Complete cleanup procedures.

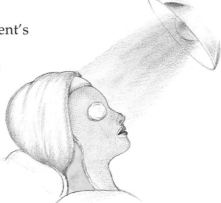

19.34—Infrared lamp.

Reasons a Client Might Find Fault with a Facial Treatment

A client might find fault with a facial treatment if you:

1. Fail to present yourself in a professional manner.
2. Have offensive breath or body odor.
3. Have rough nails that scratch the skin.
4. Have rough, cold hands.
5. Allow cream or other substances to get into the client's eyes, mouth, nostrils, or on the hairline.
6. Use towels that are too hot to be comfortable.
7. Apply substances or towels that are too cold.
8. Fail to follow sanitary procedures at all times.
9. Show no interest in the client's comfort and safety.
10. Fail to allow the client to relax by talking too much.
11. Give rough manipulations or massage muscles in the wrong direction.
12. Are disorganized and need to interrupt the facial to get supplies.
13. Fail to assist the client when necessary.
14. Fail to be courteous at all times.

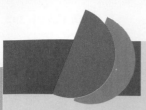

Focus on: Joel Gerson, Esthetician

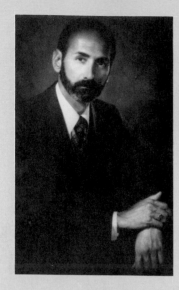

"Some people can't wait for the evening when their jobs are over. I can't wait for the morning so that I can start mine," says Joel Gerson, an internationally known esthetician. "That's because I love my work." Gerson, who has worked in some of the most prestigious salons in the country, says his career in skin care now takes him around the world, presenting seminars and hands-on workshops. "I get paid to travel to places as far away as Monte Carlo and Japan to do the work I love to do," he says.

"I started off as a hairstylist. I was a good hairstylist, but not a terrific one. It was while in cosmetology school that I realized hairstyling came easier to some students than to others." Gerson next tried his hand as a makeup artist, working in a world-famous full-service salon. It was during these years spent as a makeup artist that he became concerned with the importance of skin care. Gerson contends that "the finest makeup in the hands of the most skilled artist does not take the place of naturally beautiful skin glowing with cleanliness and good health." Gerson eventually became a teacher specializing in skin care and facial treatments. After teaching for several years, he wrote the *Standard Textbook for Professional Estheticians*.

Looking back on his journey through the beauty industry, Gerson says that his cosmetology license was the passport that opened the door to several careers over the years. He says, "In order to be successful in the field of skin care and makeup, you must put your creative imagination to work, visualize your goals, work in that direction, love what you do, and ***dare to be different***."

Review Questions

FACIALS

1. What are the benefits of a facial?
2. Why should you analyze a client's skin before giving a facial?
3. Why is it important to use a spatula when removing a product from its container?
4. What causes dry skin?
5. What is another name for blackheads?
6. What causes oily skin or blackheads?
7. What is milia?
8. What is acne and how should it be treated?
9. For what type of skin are masks recommended?
10. For what type of skin are packs recommended?
11. For what type of skin is the hot oil mask recommended?

20

FACIAL MAKEUP

LEARNING OBJECTIVES

After completing this chapter, you should be able to:

1. List the types of cosmetics used for facial makeup and their purposes.
2. Identify the different facial types.
3. Describe correct makeup application procedures.
4. Demonstrate the different procedures for corrective makeup.
5. Describe the technique for properly shaping eyebrows.
6. Demonstrate the application and removal of artificial eyelashes.
7. List the safety precautions to be observed in the application of makeup.

Introduction

The main objective of a makeup application is to emphasize the client's most attractive facial features and to minimize less attractive features. There is no fixed pattern for applying facial makeup. It is important that you analyze each client's face carefully and consider individual needs.

When applying makeup, you must take into consideration the structure of the client's face, the color of the eyes, skin, and hair, how the client wants to look, and the results you can achieve.

Once you know the basic principles, you can use makeup to create optical illusions with shadowing, highlighting, and color. The client's natural beauty can be enhanced by the proper coordination of facial makeup, hairstyle, and clothing colors.

Preparation for Makeup Application

When the client is having hair care services and also wants makeup, the makeup should be applied just before the comb-out (after rollers and clips have been removed) or after the hair has been blown dry and/or curled. Fasten a protective strip of tissue, headband, or turban around the client's head to protect the hair.

The first step in a makeup procedure is to see that your work area is clean and neat and that all the items you use for applying and removing makeup are sanitized. Products must be removed from containers with a sanitized spatula or a clean applicator. Be sure to have disposable items and applicators available. Wash and sanitize your hands before touching the client's face.

EQUIPMENT, IMPLEMENTS, AND MATERIALS

Cleansing creams and lotions

Astringent and skin-freshening lotions

Moisturizer and protective lotion

Cream, liquid, or cake foundation in appropriate colors

Shading and highlighting cosmetics

Liquid, cream, and dry powder cheek colors

Face powder

Lip colors in a variety of colors

Assorted lip liners and brushes

A variety of eye colors (shadows)

Mascara and brushes

Eye makeup applicators (disposable)

Eyeliner pencils and brushes

Tissues

Disposable cotton-tipped applicators

Spatulas

Cotton pads and pledgets

Disposable towels

Draping sheets and towels

Makeup cape

Tissue neckbands

Headband or turban

Eyelash curler

Assorted brushes (eyebrow, powder, etc.)

When selecting and applying makeup, be sure to have a well-lighted makeup mirror and, when possible, check the makeup in natural light.

FOUNDATION FOR MAKEUP

Cosmetics for Facial Makeup

Probably no other item of makeup is as important as *foundation*. Foundation, when properly applied, provides a base for color harmony, evens out the skin color, conceals minor imperfections, and protects the skin from soil, wind, and weather. Skin tones, or pigment, determine the selection of foundation color. Skin tones are generally classified with the following descriptions: very light or white, ivory, cream, pink, florid, sallow, olive, tan, brown, and ebony. Selecting the correct foundation color is of extreme importance to the success of the entire makeup application.

When choosing foundation color for light skin, a shade darker than the natural skin tone is usually best because it adds color. When choosing foundation for dark skin, foundation should be matched to the natural skin tone. For a sallow or pale skin tone, a rosy foundation will give a desirable glow to the skin. For a florid skin tone, a beige foundation will soften the reddish undertones.

For all other skin tones (fair, medium, or dark), select foundation and powder to blend with the lightness or darkness of the natural skin tone. If foundation is too light, it gives an artificial, pasty look to the skin.

When deciding on a foundation, place a small dot or two on the client's jawline and blend it upward on the jawline, then downward on the side of the neck. This will enable you to determine if the foundation color will blend well with the client's natural skin tone. Avoid creating a contrast between the color of the face and the color of the neck. When makeup is correctly matched in color and blended smoothly, no line of demarcation should be seen.

Selecting the Right Foundation

Liquid and cream foundations are the most widely used and give a slight sheen to the skin. Stick, water-base, or cake foundations give a matte (dull) finish.

1. Cream foundation gives the most natural look and is a long-lasting makeup. It is formulated for normal, dry, or oily skin types. Dot a small amount of foundation on the forehead, cheeks, and chin; then blend upward and outward for a smooth finish. A facial sponge can be used to finish the application and remove excess foundation.

2. Liquid (lotion) foundation is color suspended in a semi-liquid, delicate, light oil. For quick and effective blending, apply it on one area of the skin at a time, using long, smooth, upward strokes. A small facial sponge can be used to smooth the foundation and remove any excess.

3. Cake foundation adds color, gives a smooth velvety look, and helps conceal minor skin blemishes and discoloration. Cake foundation is effective for oily skin. If used on normal or dry skin, apply a moisturizer before applying cake makeup. To apply cake makeup, moisten a facial sponge and apply to one area of the face at a time, using upward strokes and smoothing carefully.

4. Stick foundation is particularly useful in concealing minor skin blemishes and discoloration. Because it is of thicker consistency, stick foundation can be patted over a blemish and then blended into the surrounding area for a more natural look. Use a facial sponge to smooth and finish the makeup.

5. Blemish-masking creams and sticks are available in a range of colors to coordinate with, or match, natural skin tones. Blemish-masking creams or sticks can be used to conceal blemishes and discolorations and may be applied before or after foundation. To apply, take a small amount of the product from the container with a spatula; then use your fingertips and a facial sponge to smooth and blend it over the desired area.

FACE POWDERS

Face powders improve the overall attractiveness of the skin by helping to conceal minor blemishes and discolorations and by toning down excessive color, gloss, or sheen. Face powder also enhances the skin's natural color and makes it soft and velvety to the touch.

Face powders come in cake or powdered form, in a variety of tints and shades, and in different weights. Light and medium weights are generally best for dry and normal skin, and a heavier weight is effective on skin that tends to be oily. Face powder should coordinate with or match the natural skin tones and work well with the foundation. Powder may be slightly darker or lighter than the foundation if it achieves the desired effect, but it should never appear caked, spotted, or streaked on the face.

▶ **NOTE:** Translucent powder (colorless) blends with all foundations and will not turn to a color when applied.

Apply face powder (after foundation) using a fresh cotton puff or pledget. Press the powder over the face in the desired areas; then use a powder brush or another puff or pledget to whisk off the excess. Face powder helps to set the makeup.

CHEEK AND LIP COLORS

The purpose of *cheek color* (also called rouge or blush) is to give a soft natural-looking glow of color to the face. It aids in creating more attractive facial contours.

Cheek color should coordinate with, or be the same color as, the lip color. However, when a deeper lip color is worn, generally, a lighter cheek color will appear more natural. Color on the cheeks should be less vivid in daylight than in artificial light. Bright colors call attention to that area of the face and the makeup looks artificial.

There are four types of cheek color: liquid, cream, dry, and brush-on.

1. Liquid cheek color blends well and is suitable for all skin types. Apply over the foundation before powdering the face.
2. Cream cheek color closely resembles pigmented foundation creams and cream makeup. It is generally preferred for dry and normal skin. Apply over the foundation before powdering the face.
3. Dry (compact) cheek color imparts a matte (dull) finish. Apply with a cotton puff or brush.
4. Brush-on powdered (loose) cheek color comes in a variety of shades and tints, and is used to add color and to contour the cheeks. Apply over foundation and powder using a cotton puff or brush.

Lip color (also called lipstick or gloss) adds color to the lips and protects them from becoming dry and chapped. Lip color is also used to enhance or correct the shape of the lips.

Artistry and a keen sense of fashion are essential in selecting the appropriate lip color shade or tint. The prevailing fashion trend might call for a certain look, lighter or darker colors, or style of application. Consider the client's preferences before selecting and applying lip color.

Lip color must not be applied directly from the container unless it belongs to the client. Use a spatula to remove the lip color from the container; then take it from the spatula with a lip brush. Use the tip of the brush to line the lips, beginning at inner peak of the upper lip and working outward to the corner of the mouth.

Do the other side, outline the lower lip, and then apply color on the lips staying within the outline. A lip lining pencil may be used when doing corrective makeup or when a more emphasized lip line is desired.

EYE MAKEUP

Eye makeup is available in a wide range of colors from pastels to deeper shades and tints of blue, gray, green, brown, beige, purple, and in colors with metallic silver and gold added.

When applied to the lids, *eye color* or *shadow* complements the eyes by making them appear brighter and more expressive. Eye colors can match the color of the eyes or be lighter or darker.

Focus on Stan Campbell Place, Makeup Artist

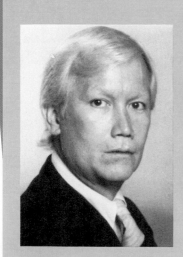

Stan Campbell Place, a master of makeup artistry, likens his craft to art and to magic. "I paint faces," he explains, "but as with a magician, if you can see the trick, it isn't a trick anymore. That's the magic of an invisible art."

To achieve such delicate effects takes years of concrete training, cautions Place. He explains, "The more time you invest in preparing for this career, the longer your career will be and the more you'll get out of it. A makeup artist's clientele demands a rare excellence. Furthermore," he reflects, "you'll work with the cream of society, with people who have so much money that they can pay somebody to paint a picture that will be washed down the drain the same night." Place says he climbed to these artistic and creative heights by starting at the bottom, volunteering to work for free at local community theaters. "I would offer to clean the brushes or carry the makeup case of an artist I wished to learn from," he says.

Absorbed in the profession for more than 20 years, Place says he has explored makeup artistry "in all its possibilities." This veteran artist has worked on Broadway productions as well as for the American Ballet Theater, has served as makeup director for Bergdorf Goodman, and has had his work appear on the cover of every fashion magazine in New York City. Today, he serves as a public spokesperson for Maybelline. "Makeup artistry allows you to be independent, mobile, and employable," he says. "It's a terribly attractive career."

Generally, a darker shade of eye color makes the natural color of the iris appear lighter, and a lighter shade makes the iris appear deeper. However, there are no set rules for selection of eye makeup colors except that they should enhance the client's eyes and be more subtle for daytime wear. Eye makeup colors may match or coordinate with the client's clothing color as desired.

Eye colors and shadows are available in stick, cream, cake, and dry powder form, and usually come with their own applicators. Remove the product from its container and use a fresh applicator. Unless you are doing corrective makeup, apply the eye color close to the lashes on the upper eyelid, sweeping the color slightly upward and outward. Blend to achieve the desired effect. More than one color may be used if a particular effect is desired.

Eyeliners are used to create a line on the eyelid close to the lashes to make the eyes appear larger and the lashes fuller. Eyeliners are manufactured in a variety of colors in pencil, liquid, or cake form. Most clients prefer an eyeliner that is the same color as the lashes or mascara for a more natural look. More dramatic colors may be desired for evening wear. The same rules of sanitation apply to eyeliners as for other makeup application. No applicator may be used on more than one client unless it can be sanitized thoroughly before each use.

Using an eyelining pencil on the lower eyelids is a matter of choice. Some clients prefer lining both the upper and lower eyelids. Be extremely cautious when applying eyeliner. You must have a steady hand and should tell the client to remain still while the makeup is being applied.

Eyebrow pencils are used to modify the natural outline of the eyebrows, usually after tweezing. They can be used to darken the eyebrows, to fill in where the brow is too thin or devoid of hair, and to correct misshapen brows. Eyebrow pencils cannot be sanitized; therefore a fresh pencil must be used for each client. Brush-on brow color comes in powdered form and is applied with a brush. Cream, liquid, and cake brow colors are also applied with a brush. Most brush applicators can be sanitized. Avoid harsh contrasts between hair and eyebrow color; for example, pale blonde or silver hair with black eyebrows.

Mascara is available in liquid, cake, and cream form. Mascara colors are available in a variety of shades and tints. The most popular colors are brown, black, and deep auburn, which enhance natural lashes and make them appear thicker and longer. Mascara is also used to darken eyebrows. Mascara and eyebrow pencils should be the same color or color coordinated so there is no harsh contrast. Usually the lashes should be darker than eyebrows.

PROCEDURE FOR APPLYING A PROFESSIONAL MAKEUP

1. Apply cleansing cream or lotion. Remove a small quantity of cleanser from the container with a spatula and place it in the palm of the left hand, or apply a dab of lotion to an applicator. With the fingertips of the right hand, place dabs of cleanser on the forehead, nose, cheeks, chin, and neck. Spread the cleanser over the face and neck with light upward and outward circular movements. (See Fig. 20.1)

2. Remove the cleanser with tissue mitts or moistened cotton pads, using an upward and outward motion. Be especially gentle around the eyes. If necessary, apply cleanser a second time, to remove heavy makeup or color on the eyes and lips. (See Fig. 20.2)

3. Apply astringent lotion or skin freshener (toner). For oily skin, apply astringent lotion; for dry skin, apply a skin freshener (mild astringent). Moisten a cotton pad with the lotion and pat it lightly over the entire face and under the chin and neck. Blot off excess moisture with tissues or a cotton pad. (See Fig. 20.3)

4. Apply a moisturizing lotion when necessary, usually when the skin is dry and delicate. Dab a small amount of the moisturizer on the forehead, cheeks, and chin. Blend upward over the face. Remove excess with a tissue, cotton pad, or facial sponge.

5. Eyebrows. Eyebrow arching is a complete service in itself. The procedure for arching is given in another section of this chapter. However, you may remove a few straggly hairs before a facial makeup by tweezing the hair in the same direction in which it grows. (See Fig. 20.4)

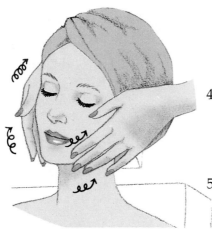

20.1—Apply cleansing cream or lotion.

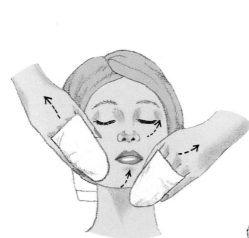

20.2—Remove the cleanser.

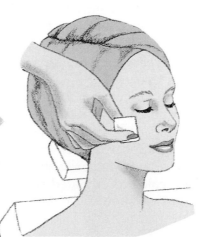

20.3—Apply astringent lotion or skin freshener.

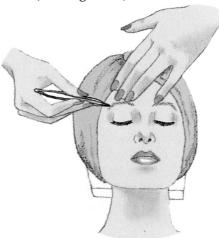

20.4—Eyebrow arching.

6. Apply foundation. Select the appropriate type and color of foundation. Test for color by blending the foundation on the client's jawline. Place a small amount of the foundation in the palm of your hand. With the tips of your fingers, apply sparingly and evenly over the entire face and around the neckline. Use gentle upward and outward motions. Blend near the hairline, and remove excess foundation with a cosmetic sponge or cotton pledget. When a moisturizer is needed, apply it in the same way, but before applying the foundation. (See Fig. 20.5)

7. Apply powder. Following the application of foundation, apply powder with a sanitary puff or cosmetic sponge. Press it over the face and whisk off the excess with a puff or powder brush. A moistened cosmetic sponge may be pressed over the finished makeup to give the face a matte look. (See Fig. 20.6)

8. Apply cheek color. Cheek color is sometimes applied after the application of foundation and before powdering. Select the appropriate type and color. Have the client smile, to raise the cheeks. Apply liquid or cream cheek color with a sanitized applicator, and blend upward and outward toward the temples. (See Fig. 20.7) Powdered cheek color is brushed on following the application of powder. Use the same procedure as with a cream or liquid.

9. Apply corrective makeup, if desired. To minimize a feature, use a darker foundation or contouring makeup. To emphasize a feature, use a lighter foundation or a highlighting product. See corrective techniques in this chapter.

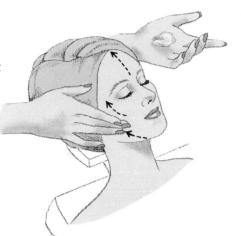

20.5—Apply foundation.

10. Apply eye color. Select the color to match or complement the eyes. Apply color lightly on the upper lid and softly blend outward with the color applicator or your fingertips. Shade a prominent puffy area beneath the brow, or highlight a small space between the eyelid and brow. (See Fig. 20.8)

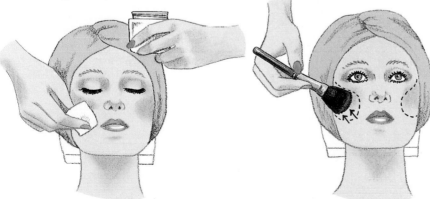

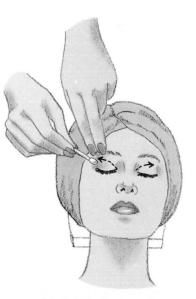

20.6—Apply powder.   20.7—Apply cheek color.   20.8—Apply eye color.

11. Apply eyeliner. Eyeliner is used to make the eyes look larger and lashes appear thicker. Select cake or liquid liner in a color to harmonize with the mascara you will apply. Pull eyelid taut, and gently draw a very fine line along the entire lid, as close to the lashes as possible. If eyeliner pencil is used, the point should be fine and care should be taken to avoid injury or discomfort to the client. (See Fig. 20.9)

12. Apply eyebrow makeup. Brush the brows in place. With light feathery strokes, apply color with a fine pointed pencil. Brush the brows carefully. Excess color can be removed with a cotton-tipped swab. (See Fig. 20.10)

13. Apply mascara to the top and underside of the upper lashes with careful, gentle strokes until the desired effect is achieved. Use a fresh brush or applicator to separate the lashes. Mascara may be applied to lower lashes if desired, but the effect should be subtle. (See Fig. 20.11)

14. Apply lip color (lipstick). Lip color is removed from its container with a sanitized spatula. The lips are first outlined with a sanitized applicator such as a brush or pencil. Rest your ring finger on the client's chin to steady your hand. Ask the client to relax her lips and part them slightly. Brush on the lip color. Ask the client to stretch her lips in a slight smile, to enable you to smooth the lip color in any small crevices. After the lip color application, blot the lips with tissue to remove excess. Blotting will also help to set the lip color. Powdering over the lips is not recommended, because the powder dries the lips and removes the attractive moist look. (See Fig. 20.12)

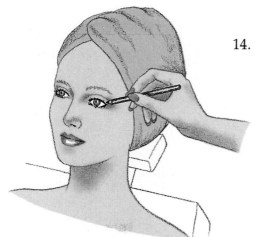

20.9—Apply eyeliner.

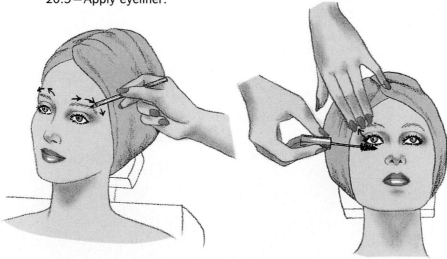

20.10—Apply eyebrow makeup.

20.11—Apply mascara.

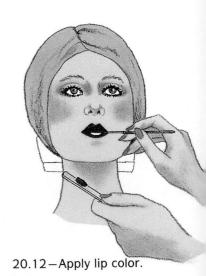

20.12—Apply lip color.

Makeup Techniques for the Black Woman

When applying makeup to any face, many of the same techniques are used. The skin is analyzed and given a facial for its specific condition, and makeup is selected to enhance the client's skin, eyes, and hair color. Most cosmetic manufacturers offer a full range of makeup colors and there are manufacturers who specialize in makeup for black women.

Before applying makeup, thoroughly cleanse the face, use an appropriate astringent, and apply a moisturizer, if needed.

PROCEDURE FOR MAKEUP APPLICATION

1. Choose an appropriate foundation shade and apply evenly. (Figs. 20.13, 20.14)
2. Apply translucent powder. (Fig. 20.15)

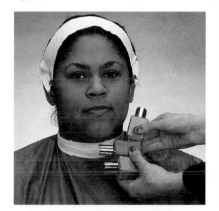
20.13—Select foundation.

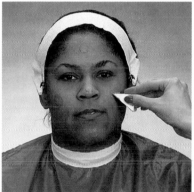
20.14—Apply foundation.

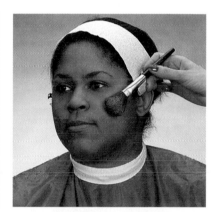
20.15—Apply translucent powder.

3. Apply a contouring (dark) blusher shade below the cheekbone. (Fig. 20.16) Now, using a lighter cheek color, apply blusher high on the cheekbone. (Fig. 20.17)
4. Apply eye shadow to eyelids and brow bone as desired. (Fig. 20.18)

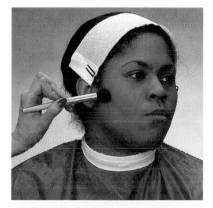
20.16—Contour with blush.

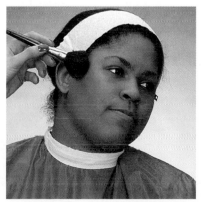
20.17—Apply blusher.

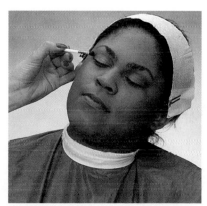
20.18—Apply eye makeup.

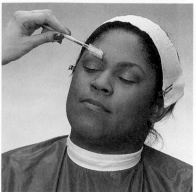

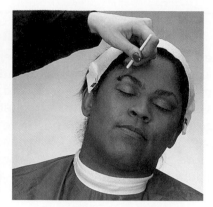

20.19—Brush eyebrow.

20.20—Fill in eyebrows.

5. Using an eyebrow brush, brush eyebrows and fill in sparse areas with an eyebrow pencil or brush. (Figs. 20.19, 20.20)

6. Line the eyes with an eyeliner pencil from the outer corner in toward the nose. (Fig. 20.21)

7. Apply mascara to top lashes, and then to bottom lashes. (Figs. 20.22, 20.23)

8. Line and fill lips with lip color (Figs. 20.24, 20.25)

9. Complement a makeup application with hairstyle, clothing, and accessories. (Fig. 20.26)

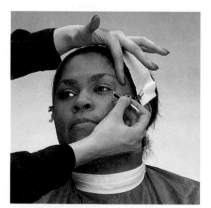

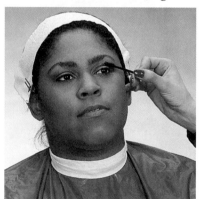

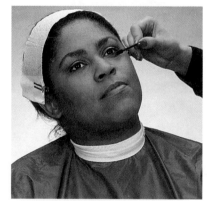

20.21—Line eyes.

20.22—Apply mascara to top lashes.

20.23—Apply mascara to bottom lashes.

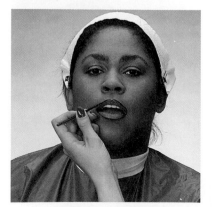

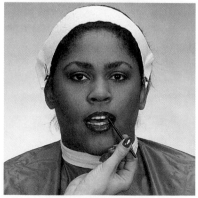

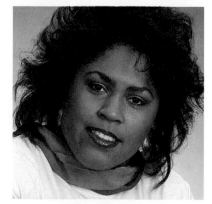

20.24—Line lips.

20.25—Apply lip color.

20.26—Finished look.

Facial Features

Faces are interesting, but few are perfect. When you analyze a client's face, you might see that the nose, cheeks, lips, or jawline are not the same on both sides, or that one eye might be larger than the other, and the eyebrows may not match. However, these subtle imperfections can make the face more interesting. Facial makeup can create the illusion of better balance and proportion when desired.

ANALYZING THE CLIENT'S FACIAL FEATURES AND FACE SHAPE

When applying makeup it is important to emphasize the client's attractive features while minimizing features that are out of proportion or unattractive in relation to the rest of the face. Learning to see the face and its features and to determine the best makeup for the individual takes practice. You might have an unsteady hand at first, especially when working with eye and lip colors. However, diligent practice and experience are the best ways to become proficient. The oval face with well-proportioned features has long been considered to be the ideal shape, but all face shapes are attractive when makeup is applied properly. What counts most is that the client's individuality is enhanced.

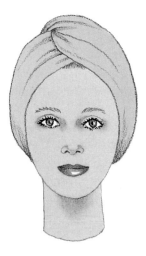

20.27 — The oval face.

CORRECTIVE MAKEUP TECHNIQUES

It is difficult to provide set rules for cheek color application because each person's facial structures are different. In addition, facial features as well as the shape of the face must be taken into consideration.

Oval-Shaped Face

The artistically ideal proportions and features of the oval face are used to form the basis for corrective makeup application. The face is divided into three equal horizontal sections. The first third is measured from the hairline to the point between the eyebrows where they begin. The second third is measured from here to the end of the nose. The last third is measured from the end of the nose to the bottom of the chin.

The ideal oval face is approximately three-fourths as wide as it is long. The distance between the eyes is the width of one eye. (Figs. 20.27, 20.28)

The following suggestions can serve as a guide to face shapes and cheek color application.

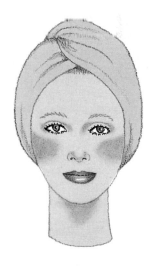

20.28 — Oval face with makeup applied.

Round-Shaped Face

The round face is usually broader in proportion to its length than the oval face. It has a rounding chin and hairline. Corrective makeup can be applied to slenderize and lengthen the face. (Figs. 20.29, 20.30)

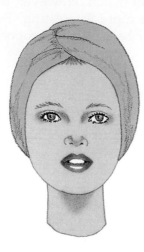

20.29—The round face.

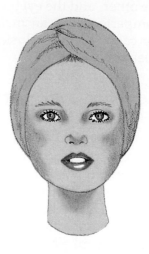

20.30—Round face with corrective makeup.

Square-Shaped Face

The square face is composed of comparatively straight lines with a wide forehead and square jawline. Corrective makeup can be applied to offset the squareness and soften the hard lines around the face. (Figs. 20.31, 20.32)

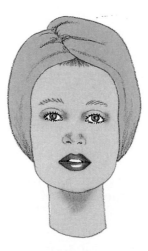

20.31—The square face.

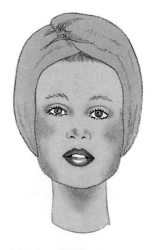

20.32—Square face with corrective makeup.

Pear-Shaped Face

This face is characterized by a jaw that is wider than the forehead. Corrective makeup can be applied to create width at the forehead, to slenderize the jawline, and to add length to the face. (Figs. 20.33, 20.34)

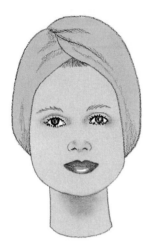 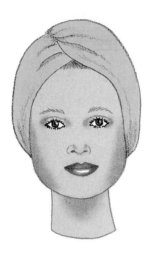

20.33 — The pear-shaped face.

20.34 — Pear-shaped face with corrective makeup.

Heart-Shaped Face

The heart-shaped face has a wide forehead and narrow, pointed chin. Corrective makeup can be applied to minimize the width of the forehead and to increase the width of the jawline. (Figs. 20.35, 20.36)

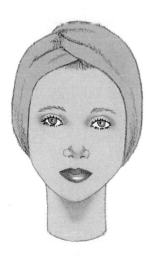 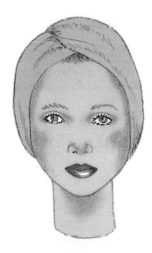

20.35 — The heart-shaped face.

20.36 — Heart-shaped face with corrective makeup.

Diamond-Shaped Face

This face has a narrow forehead. The greatest width is across the cheek bones. Corrective makeup can be applied to reduce the width across the cheekbone line. (Figs. 20.37, 20.38)

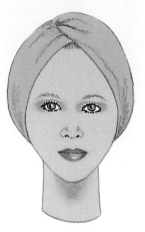

20.37—The diamond-shaped face.

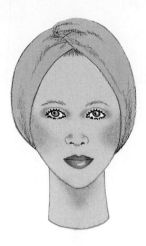

20.38—Diamond-shaped face with corrective makeup.

Oblong-Shaped Face

This face has greater length in proportion to its width than the square or round face. It is long and narrow. Corrective makeup can be applied to create the illusion of width across the cheekbone line, making the face appear shorter. (Figs. 20.39, 20.40)

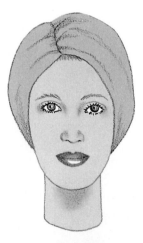

20.39—The oblong-shaped face.

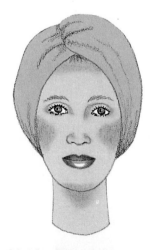

20.40—Oblong-shaped face with corrective makeup.

TIPS FOR APPLYING CHEEK COLOR

Cheek color accents the part of the face where it is applied. The following are general rules for cheek color application:

1. Apply cheek color where natural color would normally appear in the cheeks. Do not apply the color in toward the nose beyond the center of the eye.
2. Keep color above the horizontal line at the tip of the nose.
3. Do not extend color above the outer corner of the eye.
4. Never apply color in a bright, round circle. Blend the color so that it fades softly into the foundation.

BASIC RULES FOR APPLYING CORRECTIVE BASE MAKEUP

The primary objective of corrective makeup is to minimize unattractive features and accent good features. Facial features can be accented with proper highlighting, subdued with correct shadowing or shading, and balanced with the proper hairstyle.

A basic rule for the application of makeup is that highlighting emphasizes a feature, while shadowing minimizes it. A highlight is produced when a shade lighter than the original foundation is used on a particular part of the face. A shadow is formed when the foundation used is darker than the original color. The use of shadows (dark colors and shades) minimizes or subdues prominent features so that they are less noticeable.

When two shades of foundations are used, care must be taken to blend them properly so that there will be no line of demarcation. Color harmony can be achieved when the makeup tones flatter the color of the client's eyes, hair, and skin. To determine what is best for each client, you must:

1. Analyze the color of the client's skin, hair, and eyes.
2. Examine the front and profile views of the facial features.
3. Select and apply those makeup highlights and/or shades that will produce the desired results.

Concealing Wrinkles with Foundation Cream

Age lines and wrinkles due to dry skin can be concealed with foundation cream. It should be used sparingly. Apply foundation cream evenly, in a light outward circular motion over the entire surface of the face. Care should be taken to remove any foundation cream that collects in lines and wrinkles of the face.

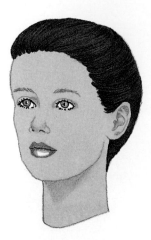

20.41—Protruding forehead.

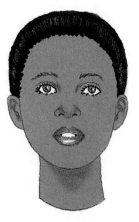

20.42—Short flat nose.

Corrective Makeup for Forehead

For a low forehead, applying a lighter foundation cream gives it a broader appearance between the brows and hairline. For a bulging forehead, applying a darker foundation over the prominent area gives an illusion of fullness to the rest of the face and minimizes the bulging forehead. With a suitable hairstyle, attention can be drawn away from the forehead. (Fig. 20.41)

Corrective Makeup for Nose and Chin

For a *large or protruding nose*, apply a darker foundation on the nose and a lighter foundation on the cheeks at the sides of the nose. This will create fullness in the cheeks and make the nose appear smaller. Avoid placing the cheek color close to the nose.

For a *short and flat nose*, apply a lighter foundation down the center of the nose, stopping at the tip. This will make the nose appear longer and larger. If the nostrils are wide, apply a darker foundation to both sides of the nostrils. (Fig. 20.42)

For a *broad nose*, use a darker foundation on the sides of the nose and nostrils. Avoid carrying this dark tone into the laugh lines because it will accentuate them. The foundation must be carefully blended to avoid visible lines. (Fig. 20.43)

For a *protruding chin and receding nose*, shadow the chin with a darker foundation and highlight the nose with a lighter foundation.

For a *receding (small) chin*, highlight the chin by using a lighter foundation than the one used on the face. (Fig. 20.44)

For a *sagging double chin*, use a darker foundation on the sagging portion, and use a natural skin tone foundation on the face. (Fig. 20.45)

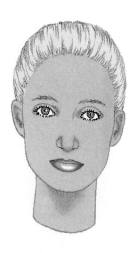

20.43—Broad nose.

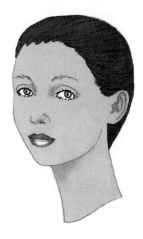

20.44—Receding chin.

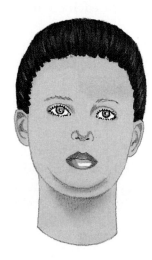

20.45—Double chin.

Corrective Makeup for Jawline and Neck

The neck and jaws are just as important as the eyes, cheeks, and lips. When applying makeup, carry the foundation cream down below the neckline of the client's dress to prevent the appearance of a line of demarcation.

For *broad jaws*, apply a darker shade of foundation over the heavy area of the jaws, starting at the temples. This will minimize the lower part of the face and create an illusion of width in the upper part of the face. (Fig. 20.46)

A *narrow jawline* may be highlighted by using a lighter shade foundation than the one used on the rest of the face.(Fig. 20.47)

For a *round, square, or triangular face*, apply a darker shade of foundation over the prominent area of the jawline. By creating a shadow over this area, the prominent part of the jaw will appear softer and more oval.

For a *small face and a short and thick neck*, use a darker foundation on the neck than the one used on the face. This will make the neck appear thinner.

For a *long, thin neck*, apply a lighter shade foundation on the neck than the one used on the face. This will create fullness and counteract the long, thin appearance of the neck. (Fig. 20.48)

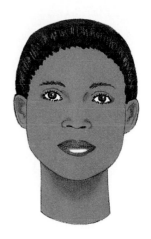

20.46 – Broad jawline.

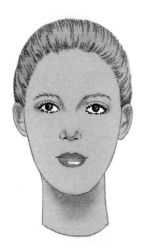

20.47 – Narrow jawline.

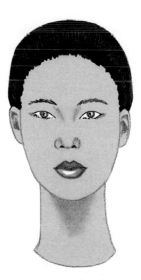

20.48 – Long, thin neck.

Corrective Makeup for Eyes

The eyes are very important features of correct facial balance. Applying eye colors and shadows properly can create the illusion of the eyes being larger or smaller, and enhance the overall attractiveness of the face.

Round eyes can be lengthened by extending the shadow beyond the outer corner of the eyes. (Figs. 20.49, 20.50)

20.49—Round eyes.   20.50—Round eyes with corrective makeup.

Close-set eyes. For eyes that are set too close together, apply shadow lightly up from the outer edge of the eyes. (Figs. 20.51, 20.52)

20.51—Close-set eyes.   20.52—Close-set eyes with corrective makeup.

Bulging eyes can be minimized by blending the shadow carefully over the prominent part of the upper lid, carrying it lightly to the line of the brow. Use dark shadow as in the illustration. (Figs. 20.53, 20.54)

20.53—Bulging eyes.   20.54—Bulging eyes with corrective makeup.

Heavy-lidded eyes. Shadow evenly and lightly across the lid from the edge of the eyelash line to the small crease in the eye socket as in the illustration. (Figs. 20.55, 20.56)

20.55—Heavy-lidded eyes.   20.56—Heavy-lidded eyes with corrective makeup.

Small eyes. To make small eyes appear large, extend the shadow slightly above, beyond, and below the eyes.

Eyes set too far apart. When eyes are set too far apart, use the shadow on the upper inner side of the eyelid.

Deep-sunken eyes. Use very little shadow on the lids nearest the temples and leave untouched the part next to the nose and inner corner of the eyes. (Fig. 20.57)

Dark circles under eyes. Apply a lighter foundation cream over the dark area, blending and smoothing it into the surrounding area. (Fig. 20.58)

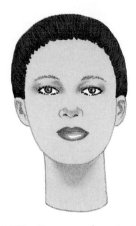

20.57—Deep-sunken eyes.

THE USE OF THE EYEBROW PENCIL

When a client wants to correct misshaped eyebrows, remove all unnecessary hairs and then demonstrate how to use the eyebrow pencil to draw short hair-like lines in the brows until the natural hairs have grown in again. When there are spaces in the brow devoid of hair, they can be filled in with hair-like strokes of an eyebrow pencil. Use an eyebrow brush to soften the pencil marks. (Figs. 20.59–20.62)

When the arch is too high, remove the superfluous hair from the top of the brow and fill in the lower part with eyebrow pencil. When the arch is too low, remove the superfluous hair from the lower part of the brow and build up the shape of the brow using the eyebrow pencil.

In the case of a high forehead, the eyebrow arch may be slightly elevated to detract from a high forehead. Avoid a too thin, too round line. This gives the client a "surprised" look.

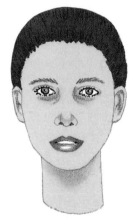

20.58—Dark circles under eyes.

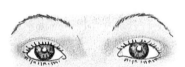

20.59—Thin eyebrows.

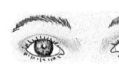

20.60—Corrective technique for thin eyebrows.

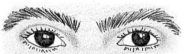

20.61—Thick eyebrows.

20.62—Corrective technique for thick eyebrows.

Corrective Placing and Shaping of the Eyebrows

Low forehead. A low arch gives more height to a very low forehead.

Wide-set eyes. The eyes can be made to appear closer together by extending the eyebrow lines to the inside corners of the eyes. However, care must be taken to avoid giving the client a frowning look.

Close-set eyes. To make the eyes appear farther apart, widen the distance between the eyebrows; also slightly extend the brows outward.

Round face. Arch the brows high to make the face appear narrower. Start on a line directly above the inside corner of the eye and extend to the end of the cheekbone.

Long face. The illusion of a shorter face can be created by making the eyebrows almost straight. Do not extend the eyebrow lines farther than the outside corners of the eyes.

Triangular face. To offset a narrow forehead, arch the eyebrows slightly on the ends only. Start the lines directly above the inside corners of the eyes and continue to the ends of the cheekbones.

Square face. The face will appear more oval if there is a high arch on the ends of the eyebrows. Begin the lines directly above the corners of the eyes and extend them outward.

EYEBROW ARCHING

Correctly shaped eyebrows have a marked effect on the attractiveness of the face. The natural arch of the eyebrow follows the bony structure or the curved line of the **orbit** (eye socket). Most people have a disorderly growth of hairs both above and below the natural line. These hairs should be removed to give a clean and attractive appearance.

Because of the sensitivity of the skin around the eyes, some clients cannot tolerate tweezing. For them, shaving or a wax depilatory may be used. You will find a discussion of wax depilatory in the chapter on removing unwanted hair.

Implements, Supplies, and Materials

Emollient cream	Eyebrow brush	Astringent lotion
Cotton pledgets	Towels	Antiseptic lotion
Cleansing tissue	Tweezers	Eyebrow pencil

Procedure

1. Seat the client in a facial chair in a reclining position, as for a facial massage. Or, if you prefer, seat the client in a half-upright position and work from the side.
2. Discuss with the client the type of eyebrow arch suitable for that person's facial characteristics.

3. Cover the client's eyes with cotton pledgets moistened with witch hazel or a mild astringent.

4. Brush the eyebrows with a small brush to remove any powder or scaliness.

5. Soften brows. Saturate two pledgets of cotton or a towel with hot water and place over the brows. Allow them to remain on the brows long enough to soften and relax the eyebrow tissue. Brows and surrounding skin may be softened by rubbing emollient cream into them.

6. Remove the hairs between the brows. When tweezing, stretch the skin taut with the index finger and thumb (or index and middle finger) of the left hand. Grasp each hair individually with tweezers and pull with a quick motion in the direction in which the hair grows. (Fig. 20.63) Sponge the tweezed area frequently with cotton moistened with an antiseptic lotion to avoid infection. Hairs between the brows and above the brow line are tweezed first, because the area under the brow line is much more sensitive.

7. Remove hairs from above the eyebrow line. Brush the hair downward. Shape the upper section of one eyebrow; then shape the other. Frequently sponge the area with antiseptic. (Fig. 20.64)

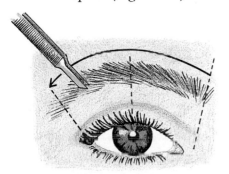

20.63—Remove hair in this direction.

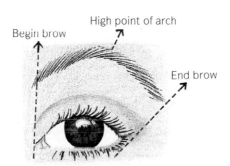

20.64—Correct points for eyebrow arching.

8. Remove hairs from under the eyebrow line. Brush the hairs upward. Shape the lower section of one eyebrow; then shape the other. Sponge the area with antiseptic. (*Optional:* Apply emollient cream and massage brows. Remove cream with tissues.)

9. After the tweezing is completed, sponge the brows and surrounding skin with astringent to contract the skin.

10. Brush the brows, placing the hair in its normal position. Use an eyebrow pencil where necessary. The eyebrows should be treated about once a week.

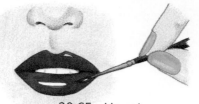
20.65—Lip color application.

CORRECTIVE MAKEUP FOR LIPS

Lips are usually proportioned so that the curves or peaks of the upper lip fall directly in line with the nostrils. (Fig. 20.65) In some cases, one side of the lips may differ from the other. Lips can be very full, very thin, or uneven. The following illustrations show various lip lines and how lip color can be used to create the illusion of better proportions. (Figs. 20.66–20.74)

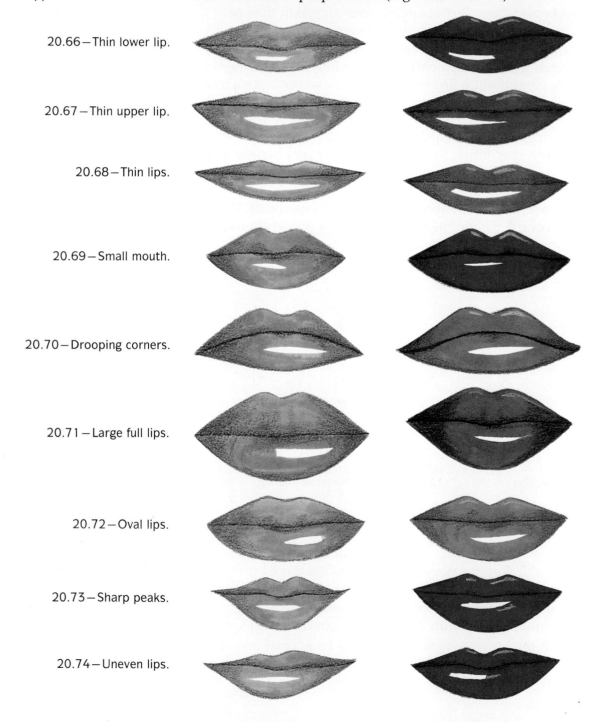

20.66—Thin lower lip.

20.67—Thin upper lip.

20.68—Thin lips.

20.69—Small mouth.

20.70—Drooping corners.

20.71—Large full lips.

20.72—Oval lips.

20.73—Sharp peaks.

20.74—Uneven lips.

An aniline derivative tint should never be used for coloring eye-brows or eyelashes; to do so can cause blindness. Instead a harm-less coloring agent can be used which usually consists of two so-lutions; one that allows the lashes to accept color and the other to deposit color. To temporarily color the lashes, mascara can be used.

Lash and Brow Tint

The choice of color is limited to either brown or black. Although black is favored in most cases, brown is recommended for very light complexions with blonde hair. Follow the specific directions of the manufacturer when applying the coloring agent.

Materials and Implements

Petroleum jelly (Vaseline)	Dish of clear, cool water
Lash and brow tinting solutions (solutions No. 1 and No. 2)	Towels
	Cotton
	Paper eye shields
Stain remover	Applicator sticks and eye pads
Dish of warm, soapy water	

Preparation

1. Follow sanitary measures.
2. Place the client in a partially reclining position in a facial or shampoo chair at approximately a 45° (.785 rad.) angle. Do not permit her to lie in a straight position, because the tinting solution can enter the eyes more easily.

Procedure

1. Wash the lashes and brows with warm, soapy water, using a cotton pledget, and remove all traces of makeup.
2. Apply petroleum jelly below the lower lashes and place paper eye shields as close to the lower lashes as possible. These shields will protect the skin from stains.
3. Adjust the eye shields. Ask the client to look up, adjust the shield, and close the eye gently. Do the same with the other eye.
4. Apply the No. 1 solution to the lashes. Moisten a cotton-tipped applicator. Touch the tip to a towel to remove excess moisture. Apply over and under the lashes close to the skin. Moisten the lashes several times. Break the applicator stick and discard. Use a fresh applicator stick each time the solution is applied.
5. Apply the No. 1 solution to brows, following the natural brow line. Reapply against the natural growth, working the solution in thoroughly. Replace the cap on the No. 1 solution bottle. (If bottle caps are interchanged, oxidation starts and the liquids lose their value.) Moisten a fresh applicator with a stain remover and place it on the edge of the towel for future use. Replace the cap on the stain remover bottle.

6. Apply the No. 2 solution to lashes and brows in the same manner as the No. 1 solution. If stain gets on the skin, use stain remover immediately. Replace the cap on the No. 2 bottle.

7. Remove the eye shields and wash the lashes and brows with cool water, using cotton pledgets.

8. Place moist eye pads over the eyelids. Rewash the brows with soap and water, then remove eye pads. Place a small roll of cotton under the lashes and wash them from above with cool water.

9. Remove any stains with stain remover. Replace the bottle cap.

10. Soothe the skin with lotion or cream. Wash the eyes with a boric acid solution.

11. Clean up in the usual manner.

Artificial Eyelashes

There are a number of reasons a client might want to wear artificial lashes. She might want to wear them for some special occasion because they enhance the eyes, making them appear larger and more expressive, or she might have extremely sparse eyelashes and wants them to appear fuller and more natural. (Figs. 20.75, 20.76)

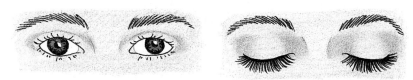

20.75—Sparse eyelashes.   20.76—False eyelashes attached.

Two basic types of artificial (false) eyelashes are in general use:

1. Strip eyelashes
2. Semi-permanent individual eyelashes (eye tabbing)

APPLYING STRIP EYELASHES

Strip eyelashes are available in a variety of types, sizes, and textures. They can be made from human hair or animal hair, such as mink, or synthetic fibers. Synthetic fiber eyelashes are made with a permanent curl and do not react to changes in weather conditions. Artificial eyelashes are available in colors ranging from light to dark brown and black or light to dark auburn to coordinate with the client's hair and brow color. Black and dark brown are the most popular choices.

Equipment, Implements, and Materials

Wet sanitizer for metal implements   Lounge-style makeup chair
Tweezers   Lash adhesive
Cotton swabs   Adhesive tray
Eyelash brushes   Eyelid and eyelash cleanser
Eyelash curler   Eyelash remover
Hand mirror   Cotton pads
Manicure scissors   Eye makeup remover
Adjustable light (gooseneck lamp)   Makeup cape

Procedure

1. Wash and sanitize your hands.
2. Check to see that all required supplies and sanitized implements are on hand.
3. Place the client in the makeup chair with her head at a comfortable working height.
4. The client's face should be well lighted, but avoid shining the light directly into her eyes.
5. If the client has not already done so, remove all eye makeup so that the lash adhesive will adhere properly. Work carefully and gently.
6. If the client wears contact lenses, they must be removed before starting the procedure.
7. Brush the client's eyelashes to make sure they are clean and free of foreign matter such as mascara particles. If the client's lashes are straight, they can be curled with an eyelash curler before you apply the artificial lashes.
8. Discuss with the client the desired length of lashes and the effect she hopes to achieve. Try to create an effect that makes the client's eyelashes fuller, longer, and more attractive without looking unnatural.
9. Work from behind or to the side of the client when applying artificial lashes. Avoid working directly in front of the client whenever possible.
10. Carefully remove the eyelash strip from the package.
11. Follow the manufacturer's directions carefully.
12. Start with the upper lash. If it is too long to fit the curve of the upper eyelid, trim the outside edge. Use your fingers to bend the lash into a horseshoe shape to make it more flexible so it fits the contour of the eyelid. (See Fig. 20.77)
13. Feather the lash by nipping into it with the points of your scissors. This creates a more natural look.
14. Apply a thin strip of lash adhesive to the base of the lash and allow a few seconds for it to set. (See Fig. 20.78)

20.77—Start with the upper lash.

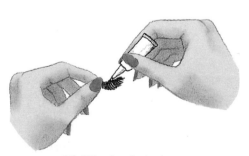

20.78—Apply lash adhesive.

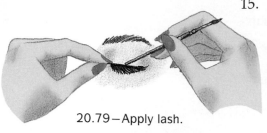

20.79—Apply lash.

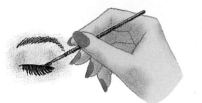

20.80—Retouch the lash.

15. Apply the lash. Start with the shorter part of the lash and place it on the inside of the eye. Position the rest of the artificial lash as close to the client's own lash as possible. Use the rounded end of a lash liner brush to press the lash on. (See Fig. 20.79) Be very careful and gentle when applying the lashes. If eyeliner is to be used the line is usually drawn on the eyelid before the lash is applied and retouched when the artificial lash is in place. (See Fig. 20.80)

16. Apply the lower lash. Trim the lash as necessary and apply adhesive in the same way you did for the upper lash. Place the lash on top of the client's lower lash. Place the shorter lash toward the center of the eye and the longer lash toward the outer part of the lid.

▶ NOTE: Remind the client to be careful with lashes when swimming, bathing, or cleansing the face. Water or cleansing products will loosen the artificial lashes.

REMOVING ARTIFICIAL STRIP EYELASHES

There are commercial preparations, such as pads saturated with specially prepared lotions, to facilitate the removal of false eyelashes. The lash base may also be softened by the application of a face cloth saturated with warm water and a gentle face soap or cleanser. Hold the pad or cloth over the eyes for a few seconds to soften the adhesive. Starting from the outer corner of the lashline, remove lashes carefully to avoid pulling out the client's natural lashes. Cotton tipped swabs may be used to remove makeup and adhesive remaining on the lid.

APPLYING SEMI-PERMANENT INDIVIDUAL EYELASHES (EYE TABBING)

Eye tabbing is the technique of attaching individual, synthetic eyelashes to a client's own eyelashes. Synthetic fibers are used in the manufacture of these false eyelashes because they can be easily curled.

Because synthetic lashes are attached to the client's own and become part of them, they last as long as the natural eyelashes, about 6 to 8 weeks. Hence, they are referred to as "semi-permanent eyelashes." However, due to the fact that natural eyelashes fall out regularly (a few each week), taking the attached false lashes with them, the false lashes should be filled in by periodic visits to the salon.

Equipment, Implements, and Materials

You will need the following for applying individual eyelashes. (Fig. 20.81)

Wet sanitizer to sanitize metal implements

Tweezers

Cotton swabs

Eyelash brush

Hand mirror

Adhesive tray

Eyelash remover

Adhesive container

Eye makeup remover (clear)

Manicure table

Adjustable light (gooseneck lamp)

Makeup or facial chair

Makeup cape

Manicure scissors

Tissues

Trays of eyelashes

Eyelash adhesive

Eyelid and eyelash cleaner

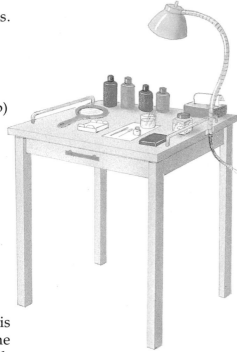

20.81—False eyelash set-up.

Allergy Test

Some clients may be allergic to the adhesive. When in doubt it is advisable to give the client an allergy test before applying the lashes. This test may be accomplished by either one of the following methods:

1. Put a drop of the adhesive behind one ear; or
2. Attach a single eyelash to each eyelid.

In either case, if there is no reaction within 24 hours, it is probably safe to proceed with the application.

Lengths of False Lashes

False lashes usually come in three lengths: short, medium, and long. Some manufacturers have developed a fourth length, extra short. The different lengths are used separately or in combination, in order to achieve certain effects.

1. A natural effect is created by using short lashes intermingled with a few medium size lashes.
2. A luxurious effect can be achieved by using a mixture of short and medium length lashes with a few long ones added for glamour.
3. A very glamorous or high styling effect is achieved by using only long lashes.
4. The extra short lashes are used on lower lashes or in combination with others to achieve special effects.

Procedure for Upper Lashes

1. Wash and sanitize your hands.
2. Check and see that all required supplies and sanitized implements are on hand.
3. Place client in the makeup chair with her head at a comfortable working height.
4. Make sure that the client's face is well lighted, but avoid shining the light directly into the eyes.
5. If the client has not already done so, remove all eye makeup. If the eyelashes are not entirely clean, the adhesive will not adhere properly.
6. Brush the client's lashes to make sure that they are clean and free from foreign matter. Brushing also separates lashes.
7. Discuss with the client the desired length of lashes and the effect she hopes to achieve. Try to create an effect that makes the eyelashes fuller, more attractive, without looking unnatural.
8. Work from behind or to the side of the client when applying lashes. Avoid working in front of the client whenever possible.
9. Place a small amount of adhesive in the adhesive container. This adhesive dries very quickly; therefore, only a small quantity should be used for each lash that is applied. (*Note:* You can make an adhesive container by placing a small piece of aluminum foil over the open end of a bottle cap.)
10. Using the tweezers, remove an eyelash from the tray. Hold the lash as close to the butt (bulb) end as possible. (See Fig. 20.82)
11. When the lash is free from the tray, move the tweezer past the center of the lash.
12. Brush the underside of the individual lash over the adhesive. (See Fig. 20.83)

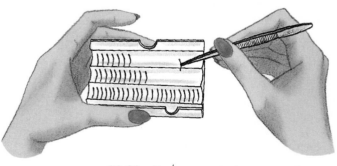

20.82—Remove eyelash from tray.

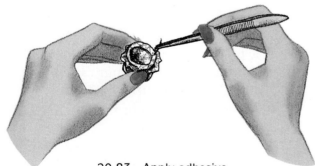

20.83—Apply adhesive.

13. Only a very small amount of adhesive is needed. If too much adhesive is picked up, brush off the excess with your fingertip.

14. If the client wears glasses, place the first lash in the center of the lid. Have the client put her glasses on. If the lash touches the glass, it is too long and a shorter length must be selected. If the lash does not touch, it may be used. (See Fig. 20.84)

15. It is important to remember that the lash is held in the tweezers at exactly the same angle that it will be placed on the natural lash.

16. If you are right-handed you will start applying lashes at the outer corner of the left eye, applying the lashes side by side until you reach the inner corner of the left eye. This method will prove to be the most efficient and time saving. If you are left-handed, follow the same procedure, but start at the outer corner of the right eye and work toward the left. The first two or three lashes applied to the outer corner and the last two or three lashes applied to the inner corner of the eye should be shorter to give a gradual, more natural buildup to the lashes.

17. Start the application procedure by brushing the adhesive from the underside of the individual lash onto the top side of the client's natural lash. Transfer the adhesive to the entire length of the natural lash starting at the base (the part closest to the lid) and brushing out to the tip.

18. The individual lash is placed on top of the natural lash, as close to the eyelid as possible without actually touching the lid. (See Fig. 20.85) For efficient performance, the tweezer must be kept free of adhesive.

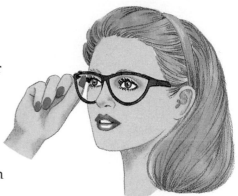

20.84—Be sure eyelashes do not touch glasses.

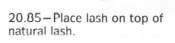

20.85—Place lash on top of natural lash.

19. Start the application of lashes to the other eye by applying the individual lashes to the inside corner of the eye and continue placing the lashes side by side until reaching the outer corner of the eye.

20. For the inside corner of the eye it may be necessary to use the thumb of the free hand to gently extend the eyelid and hold it taut. This exposes the natural inside corner of the eye and permits the placing of the artificial eyelash properly. (See Fig. 20.86)

21. When necessary, the same technique is applied when attaching the outside corner lashes. (See Fig. 20.87)

22. When attaching lashes in the corners of the eyes, the upper and lower lashes must be kept separated for several seconds to permit the adhesive to dry and prevent the eyelids from sticking together.

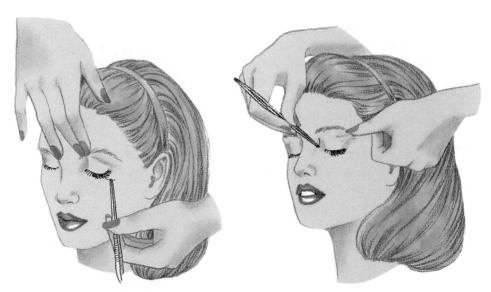

20.86 — Pull eyelid taut to apply.

20.87 — Attach at outside corner.

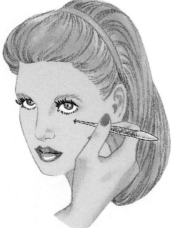

20.88 — Apply lower lashes.

Procedure for Lower Lashes

The application of the lower (bottom) lashes requires a different technique than when applying the upper lashes.

1. Have the client sit facing you. Work from the side rather than directly in front of the client whenever possible.

2. Ask the client to look upward with eyes wide open. (See Fig. 20.88)

3. Use short lashes only.

4. Apply adhesive to the lash the same as for upper lashes. Remove excess adhesive.

5. Ask the client to keep her eyes open for a few extra seconds to permit the adhesive to dry.

6. You might have to use more adhesive when applying lower lashes in order to ensure a more lasting application.

▶ **NOTE:** Advise clients that natural oils from the eyelids tend to dissolve the adhesive. As a result, lower lashes will not stay on as long as upper lashes. Generally, lower lashes begin to fall off about one week after application.

Safety Precautions

1. Wash and sanitize your hands before and after every makeup application or after touching any object unrelated to the procedure.

2. Properly drape the client to protect her clothing and use hairline strip during the makeup procedure.

3. Protect the client's hair and skin from direct contact with the facial chair.

4. Keep your fingernails smooth to avoid scratching the client's skin.

5. Use only sanitized brushes and implements.

6. Use a shaker-type container for loose powder.

7. Pour all lotions from bottle containers.

8. Always use a spatula or cosmetic applicator to remove cosmetics from their containers.

9. Never apply lip color directly from the container to the client's lips. Use a spatula or special applicator to remove the product from the container; then use a brush to apply.

10. Use an antiseptic on tweezed areas of the eyebrow to avoid infection.

11. Place all used items that can be properly sanitized in a container until they can be sanitized.

12. Discard all disposable items, such as sponges, pads, spatulas, and applicators, after use.

13. Discard used pencils or applicators immediately following the makeup application so that they are not used on another client.

14. Place all towels, linens, makeup cape, or other washable items in the proper container until they can be washed and sanitized.

15. Keep your work area clean, neat, and well organized.

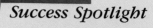

Success Spotlight

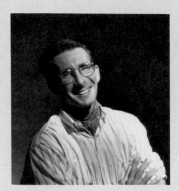

Patrick Poussard is a makeup artist who is much sought after. His editorial work has appeared in French *Vogue, Elle,* and *American Salon,* among many magazines worldwide. Poussard, who spends his time jetting between Paris and New York, says, "Makeup skills translate well beyond the salon, and the career options for the accomplished makeup artist are plentiful. If you think you want to do makeup for magazine editorial shootings, the first thing to realize is that photographic makeup is quite different from salon makeup. It has to be extremely precise and very well blended. Foundations should allow the natural skin tone to show through and never look heavy or caked on.

"You can start by calling photographers and offering to do test shootings with them for free. Working with the photographer's lighting is key, so pay great attention to this as you develop your skills. Once you have a portfolio of your makeup work, find an agent who will help you get bookings."

Poussard has traveled around the world and worked with the top fashion and beauty photographers in every country he's visited. It isn't farfetched to believe that this could be you, if you have persistence and determination, and if you practice, practice, practice.

Review Questions

FACIAL MAKEUP

1. What is the main objective of makeup application?
2. What factors must be taken into consideration when applying makeup?
3. Name the seven facial types.
4. Why is foundation (base) an important part of facial makeup?
5. How is a foundation color selected for a makeup application?
6. Name four types of cheek color.
7. When do you apply lipstick directly from the container?
8. Why do we use mascara?
9. What is the primary objective of applying corrective makeup?
10. Name two basic types of artificial eyelashes.

21

THE SKIN AND ITS DISORDERS

LEARNING OBJECTIVES

After completing this chapter, you should be able to:

1. Describe the structure and composition of the skin (histology).
2. List the functions of the skin.
3. Define important terms relating to skin disorders.
4. Discuss which skin disorders may be handled in the beauty salon and which should be referred to a physician.

Introduction

The skin is the largest and one of the most important organs of the body. The scientific study of the skin and scalp is important to the cosmetologist because it forms the basis for an effective program of skin care, beauty services, and scalp treatments. A cosmetologist who has a thorough understanding of skin, its structure, and functions is in a better position to give clients professional advice on scalp, facial, and hand care. (Fig. 21.1)

A healthy skin is slightly moist, soft, and flexible; possesses a slightly acid reaction; and is free from any disease or disorder. The skin also has immunity responses to organisms that touch or try to enter it. Its *texture* (feel and appearance) ideally is smooth and fine grained. A person with a good complexion has fine skin texture and healthy skin color. Appendages of the skin are hair, nails, and sweat and oil glands.

Skin varies in thickness. It is thinnest on the eyelids and thickest on the palms and soles. Continued pressure on any part of the skin can cause it to thicken and develop into a callous.

The skin of the scalp is constructed similarly to the skin elsewhere on the human body. However, the scalp has larger and deeper hair follicles to accommodate the longer hair of the head. (Fig. 21.2)

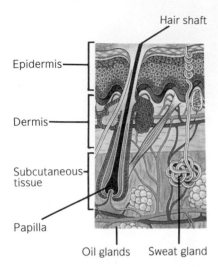

21.1 — Microscopic section of skin.

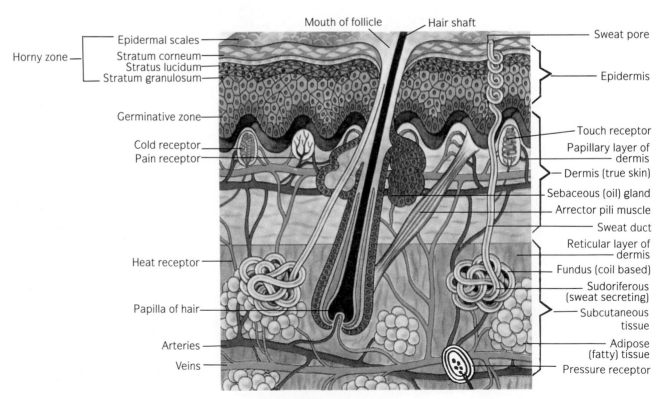

21.2 — Diagram of a section of the scalp.

Histology of the Skin

The skin contains two main divisions: the epidermis and the dermis.

The *epidermis* (ep-i-**DUR**-mis) is the outermost layer of the skin. This layer is commonly called the cuticle (**KYOO**-ti-kel), or *scarf skin*. It is the thinnest layer of skin and forms a protective covering for the body. It contains no blood vessels, but it has many small nerve endings. The epidermis is made up of the following layers:

1. The *stratum corneum* (**STRAT**-um **KOHR**-nee-um), or horny layer, is the outer layer of the skin. Its scale like cells are continually being shed and replaced by underneath cells coming to the surface. These cells contain the protein keratin, and combined with a thin covering layer of oil help make the stratum corneum almost waterproof.

2. The *stratum lucidum* (**LOO**-si-dum), or clear layer, consists of small, transparent cells through which light can pass.

3. The *stratum granulosum* (gran-yoo-**LOH**-sum), or granular layer, consists of cells that look like distinct granules. These cells are almost dead and are pushed to the surface to replace cells that are shed from the stratum corneum.

4. The *stratum germinativum* (jur-mi-nah-**TIV**-um), formerly known as the *stratum mucosum* (myoo-**KOH**-sum) and also referred to as the basal or Malpighian layer, is composed of several layers of different-shaped cells. The deepest layer is responsible for the growth of the epidermis. It also contains a dark skin pigment, called melanin, which protects the sensitive cells below from the destructive effects of excessive ultra violet rays of the sun or of an ultra violet lamp. These special cells are called *melanocytes* (**MEL**-uh-no-sights). They produce melanin, which determines skin color.

The *dermis* (**DUR**-mis) is the underlying, or inner, layer of the skin. It is also called the *derma*, *corium* (**KOH**-ree-um), *cutis* (**KYOO**-tis), or *true skin*. It is about 25 times thicker than the epidermis. It is a highly sensitive and vascular layer of connective tissue. Within its structure there are numerous blood vessels, lymph vessels, nerves, sweat glands, oil glands, hair follicles, arrector pili muscles, and papillae. The dermis is made up of two layers: the papillary, or superficial layer, and the reticular, or deeper layer.

1. The *papillary layer* (pa-**PIL**-ah-ry) lies directly beneath the epidermis. It contains small cone-shaped projections of elastic tissue that point upward into the epidermis. These projections are called *papillae* (pah-**PIL**-e). Some of these

papillae contain looped *capillaries* (**KAP**-i-ler-ees); others contain nerve fiber endings, called *tactile corpuscles* (**TAK**-til **KOR**-pus-ls), which are nerve endings for the sense of touch. This layer also contains some of the melanin skin pigment.

2. The *reticular layer* (re-**TIK**-u-lar) contains the following structures within its network:

Fat cells	Sweat glands
Blood vessels	Hair follicles
Lymph vessels	Arrector pili muscles
Oil glands	

This layer also supplies the skin with oxygen and nutrients.

Subcutaneous tissue (sub-kyoo-**TAY**-nee-us) is a fatty layer found below the dermis. Some histologists consider this tissue as a continuation of the dermis. This tissue is also called *adipose* (**AD**-i-pohs), or *subcutis* (sub-**KYOO**-tis) tissue and varies in thickness according to the age, sex, and general health of the individual. It gives smoothness and contour to the body, contains fats for use as energy, and also acts as a protective cushion for the outer skin. Circulation is maintained by a network of *arteries* and *lymphatics*.

HOW THE SKIN IS NOURISHED

Blood and lymph supply nourishment to the skin. As they circulate through the skin, the blood and lymph contribute essential materials for growth, nourishment, and repair of the skin, hair, and nails. In the subcutaneous tissue are found networks of arteries and lymphatics that send their smaller branches to hair papillae, hair follicles, and skin glands.

NERVES OF THE SKIN

The skin contains the surface endings of many nerve fibers. They are:

1. *Motor nerve fibers,* which are distributed to the arrector pili muscles attached to the hair follicles. This muscle can cause gooseflesh when you are frightened or cold.
2. *Sensory nerve fibers,* which react to heat, cold, touch, pressure, and pain. These sensory receptors send messages to the brain. (Fig. 21.3)
3. *Secretory nerve fibers,* which are distributed to the sweat and oil glands of the skin. These nerves regulate the excretion of perspiration from the sweat glands and control the flow of sebum to the surface of the skin.

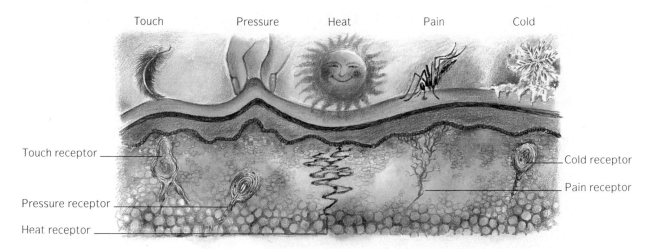

Touch   Pressure   Heat   Pain   Cold

Touch receptor

Cold receptor

Pain receptor

Pressure receptor

Heat receptor

21.3—Sensory nerves of the skin.

Sense of Touch

The papillary layer of the dermis houses the nerve endings that provide the body with the sense of touch. These nerve endings register basic sensations; touch, pain, heat, cold, pressure, or deep touch. Nerve endings are most abundant in the fingertips. Complex sensations, such as vibrations, seem to depend on the sensitivity of a combination of these nerve endings.

SKIN ELASTICITY

The pliability of the skin depends on the elasticity of the dermis. For example, healthy skin regains its former shape almost immediately after being expanded.

Aging Skin

The aging process of the skin is a subject of vital importance to everyone. Perhaps the most outstanding characteristic of the aged skin is its loss of elasticity. One factor that contributes to the loss of elasticity is that as we age subcutaneous tissue shrinks and is not as effective a support system in preventing the skin from wrinkling.

SKIN COLOR

The color of the skin, whether fair, medium, or dark, depends, in part, on the blood supply to the skin and primarily on melanin, the coloring matter that is deposited in the stratum germinativum and the papillary layers of the dermis. The color of pigment varies from person to person. The distinctive color of the skin is a hereditary trait and varies among races and nationalities. Melanin protects sensitive cells from sunburn and tanning beds with ultra violet rays. A sun protection factor (SPF) should be used to help the melanin in the skin protect it from burning.

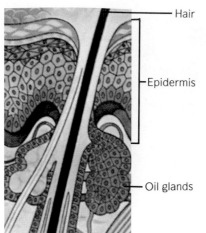

21.4—Body hair and follicle.

GLANDS OF THE SKIN

The skin contains two types of duct glands that extract materials from the blood to form new substances: the *sudoriferous* (soo-dohr-**IF**-er-us), or *sweat glands*, and the *sebaceous* (si-**BAY**-shus), or *oil glands*. (Figs. 21.4–21.6)

Sweat Glands

The sweat glands (tubular type), which excrete sweat, consist of a coiled base, or *fundus* (**FUN**-dus), and a tubelike duct that terminates at the skin surface to form the sweat pore. Practically all parts of the body are supplied with sweat glands, which are more numerous on the palms, soles, forehead, and in the armpits.

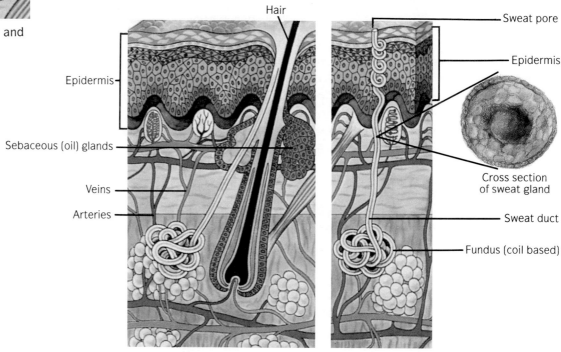

21.5—Scalp hair, follicle and oil glands.

21.6—Sweat gland.

The sweat glands regulate body temperature and help to eliminate waste products from the body. Their activity is greatly increased by heat, exercise, emotions, and certain drugs.

The excretion of sweat is controlled by the nervous system. Normally, 1 to 2 pints of liquids containing salts are eliminated daily through sweat pores in the skin.

Oil Glands

The oil glands (saccular type) consist of little sacs whose ducts open into the hair follicles. They secrete sebum, which lubricates the skin and preserves the softness of the hair. With the exception of the palms and soles, these glands are found in all parts of the body, particularly in the face and scalp where they are larger.

Sebum is an oily substance produced by the oil glands. Ordinarily, it flows through the oil ducts leading to the mouths of the hair follicles. However, when the sebum becomes hardened and the duct becomes clogged, a blackhead is formed.

FUNCTIONS OF THE SKIN

The principal functions of the skin are protection, sensation, heat regulation, excretion, secretion, and absorption.

1. *Protection.* The skin protects the body from injury and bacterial invasion. The outermost layer of the epidermis is covered with a thin layer of sebum, thus rendering it waterproof. It is resistant to wide variations in temperature, minor injuries, chemically active substances, and many forms of bacteria.

2. *Sensation.* By stimulating sensory nerve endings, the skin responds to heat, cold, touch, pressure, and pain. When the nerve endings are stimulated, a message is sent to the brain. You respond by saying "ouch" if you feel pain, by scratching an itch, or pulling away when you touch something hot. Sensory nerve endings, responsive to touch and pressure, are located near hair follicles.

3. *Heat regulation* means that the skin protects the body from the environment. A healthy body maintains a constant internal temperature of about 98.6° Fahrenheit (37° Celsius). As changes occur in the outside temperature, the blood and sweat glands of the skin make necessary adjustments and the body is cooled by the evaporation of sweat.

4. *Excretion.* Perspiration from the sweat glands is excreted through the skin. Water lost through perspiration takes salt and other chemicals with it.

5. *Secretion.* Sebum, or oil, is secreted by the sebaceous glands. This oil lubricates the skin, keeping it soft and pliable. Oil also keeps hair soft. Emotional stress can increase the flow of sebum.

6. *Absorption* is limited, but it does occur. Female hormones, when an ingredient of a face cream, can enter the body through the skin and influence it to a minor degree. Fatty materials, such as lanolin creams, are absorbed largely through hair follicles and sebaceous gland openings. Research is being conducted with mink oil, turtle oil, and caviar as catalysts for absorption.

Disorders of the Skin

In your work as a cosmetologist in a salon you will come in contact with skin and scalp disorders. You must be prepared to recognize certain common skin conditions and must know what you can and can not do with them. Some skin and scalp disorders can be treated in cooperation with, and under the supervision of, a physician. Medicinal preparations, available only by prescription, must be applied in accordance with the physician's directions. If a client has a skin condition that the cosmetologist does not recognize as a simple disorder, the person should be referred to a physician.

Most important is that a client who has an inflamed skin disorder, infectious or not, should not be served in the beauty salon. The cosmetologist should be able to recognize these conditions and suggest that proper measures be taken to prevent more serious consequences. Thus, the health of the cosmetologist as well as the health of the public is safeguarded.

DEFINITIONS PERTAINING TO SKIN DISORDERS

Listed below are a number of important terms that should be familiar to the cosmetologist for an understanding of the subject of skin, scalp, and hair disorders.

Dermatology (dur-mah-**TOL**-o-jee)—The study of the skin, its nature, structure, functions, diseases, and treatment.

Dermatologist (dur-mah-**TOL**-o-jist)—A medical skin specialist.

Pathology (pa-**THOL**-o-jee)—The study of disease.

Trichology (treye-**KOL**-o-jee)—The study of the hair and its diseases.

Etiology (ee-ti-**OL**-o-jee)—The study of the causes of disease.

Diagnosis (deye-ag-**NOH**-sis)—The recognition of a disease by its symptoms.

Prognosis (prog-**NOH**-sis)—The foretelling of the probable course of a disease.

LESIONS OF THE SKIN

A lesion is a structural change in the tissues caused by injury or disease. There are three types: primary, secondary, and tertiary. The cosmetologist is concerned with primary and secondary lesions only. If you are familiar with the principal skin lesions you will be able to distinguish between conditions that may or may not be treated in a beauty salon. (Fig. 21.7)

The symptoms or signs of diseases of the skin are divided into two groups:

1. *Subjective symptoms* are those that can be felt, such as itching, burning, or pain.
2. *Objective symptoms* are those that are visible, such as pimples, pustules, or inflammation.

DEFINITIONS PERTAINING TO PRIMARY LESIONS

The following is a list of important terms and definitions that should be familiar to the cosmetologist.

Macule (**MAK**-ul)—A small, discolored spot or patch on the surface of the skin, such as freckles. These are neither raised nor sunken.

Papule (**PAP**-yool)—A small, elevated pimple on the skin, containing no fluid, but which might develop pus.

Wheal (**HWEEL**)—An itchy, swollen lesion that lasts only a few hours. Examples include hives, or the bite of an insect, such as a mosquito.

Tubercle (**TOO**-ber-kel)—A solid lump larger than a papule. It projects above the surface or lies within or under the skin. It varies in size from a pea to a hickory nut.

Tumor (**TOO**-mohr)—An abnormal cell mass, varying in size, shape, and color. *Nodules* are also referred to as tumors, but they are smaller.

Vesicle (**VES**-i-kell)—A blister with clear fluid in it. Vesicles lie within or just beneath the epidermis; for example, poison ivy produces small vesicles.

Bulla (**BYOO**-lah)—A blister containing a watery fluid, similar to a vesicle, but larger.

Pustule (**PUS**-chool)—An elevation of the skin having an inflamed base, containing pus.

Cyst (**SIST**)—A semisolid or fluid lump above and below the skin.

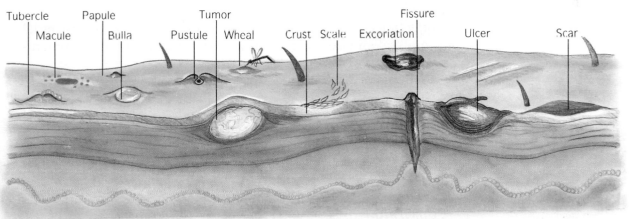

21.7—Primary and Secondary skin lesions.

DEFINITIONS PERTAINING TO SECONDARY LESIONS

Secondary skin lesions are those that develop in the later stages of disease. These are:

Scale—An accumulation of epidermal flakes, dry or greasy. (Example: abnormal or excessive dandruff)

Crust (scab)—An accumulation of serum and pus, mixed perhaps with epidermal material. (Example: the scab on a sore)

Excoriation (ek-skohr-i-**AY**-shun)—A skin sore or abrasion produced by scratching or scraping. (Example: a raw surface due to the loss of the superficial skin after an injury)

Fissure (**FISH**-ur)—A crack in the skin penetrating into the dermis, as in the case of chapped hands or lips.

Ulcer (**UL**-ser)—An open lesion on the skin or mucous membrane of the body, accompanied by pus and loss of skin depth.

Scar (cicatrix) (**SIK**-a-triks)—Likely to form after the healing of an injury or skin condition that has penetrated the dermal layer.

Stain—An abnormal discoloration remaining after the disappearance of moles, freckles, or liver spots, sometimes apparent after certain diseases.

DEFINITIONS PERTAINING TO DISEASE

Before describing the diseases of the skin and scalp so that they will be recognizable to the cosmetologist, it is necessary to understand what is meant by disease.

Disease is any departure from a normal state of health.

Skin disease—Any infection of the skin characterized by an objective lesion (one that can be seen), which may consist of scales, pimples, or pustules.

Acute disease—One with symptoms of a more or less violent character such as fever and usually of short duration.

Chronic disease—One of long duration, usually mild but recurring.

Infectious (in-**FEK**-shus) *disease*—One due to germs (bacterial or viral) taken into the body as a result of contact with a contaminated object or lesion.

Contagious disease—One that is communicable by contact.

▶ NOTE: The terms "infectious disease," "communicable disease," and "contagious disease" are often used interchangeably.

Congenital disease—One that is present in the infant at birth.

Seasonal disease—One that is influenced by the weather, as prickly heat in the summer, and forms of eczema, which is more prevalent in cold weather.

Occupational disease (such as dermatitis)—One that is due to certain kinds of employment, such as coming in contact with cosmetics, chemicals, or tints.

Parasitic disease—One that is caused by vegetable or animal parasites, such as pediculosis and ringworm.

Pathogenic disease—One produced by disease-causing bacteria, such as staphylococcus and streptococcus (pus-forming bacteria), or viruses.

Systemic disease—Due to under- or over-functioning of the internal glands. It can be caused by faulty diet.

Venereal disease—A contagious disease commonly acquired by contact with an infected person during sexual intercourse.

Epidemic—The appearance of a disease that simultaneously attacks a large number of persons living in a particular locality. Infantile paralysis, influenza, or smallpox are examples of epidemic-causing diseases.

Allergy—A sensitivity that some people develop to normally harmless substances. Skin allergies are quite common. Contact with certain types of cosmetics, medicines, and tints or eating certain foods all can cause an itching eruption, accompanied by redness, swelling, blisters, oozing, and scaling.

Inflammation—A skin disorder characterized by redness, pain, swelling, and heat.

DISORDERS OF THE SEBACEOUS (OIL) GLANDS

There are several common disorders of the sebaceous (oil) glands that the cosmetologist should be able to identify and understand.

Comedones (**KOM**-e-donz), or blackheads, are wormlike masses of hardened sebum, appearing most frequently on the face, especially the forehead and nose.

Blackheads accompanied by pimples often occur in youths between the ages of 13 and 20. During this adolescent period, the activity of the sebaceous glands is stimulated, thereby contributing to the formation of blackheads and pimples. (Fig. 21.8)

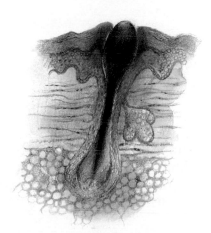

21.8—Blackhead (plug of sebaceous matter and dirt) forming around mouth of hair follicle.

When the hair follicle is filled with an excess of oil from the sebaceous gland, a blackhead forms and creates a blockage at the mouth of the follicle. Should this condition become severe, medical attention is necessary.

To treat blackheads, the skin's oiliness must be reduced by local applications of cleansers and the blackheads removed under sterile conditions. Thorough skin cleansing each night is a very important factor. Cleansing creams and lotions often achieve better results than common soap and water.

Milia (**MIL**-ee-uh), or whiteheads, is a disorder of the sebaceous (oil) glands caused by the accumulation of sebaceous matter beneath the skin. This can occur on any part of the face, neck, and, occasionally, on the chest and shoulders. Whiteheads are associated with fine-textured, dry types of skin.

Acne (**AK**-nee) is a chronic inflammatory disorder of the sebaceous glands, occurring most frequently on the face, back, and chest. The cause of acne is generally believed to be microbic, but predisposing factors are adolescence and perhaps certain foods in the diet. Acne, or common pimples, is also known as *acne simplex* or *acne vulgaris*. (Fig. 21.9)

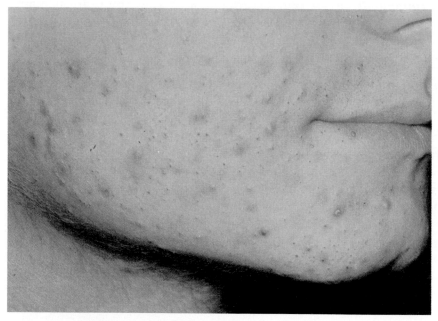

21.9 — Acne.

Acne appears in a variety of different types, ranging from the simple (noncontiguous) pimple, to serious, deep-seated skin conditions. It is always advisable to have the condition examined and diagnosed by a physician before any service is given in a beauty salon.

Seborrhea (seb-o-**REE**-ah) is a skin condition caused by an excessive secretion of the sebaceous glands. An oily or shiny condition of the nose, forehead, or scalp indicates the presence of seborrhea. On the scalp, it is readily detected by an unusual amount of oil on the hair.

Asteatosis (as-tee-ah-**TOH**-sis) is a condition of dry, scaly skin, characterized by absolute or partial deficiency of sebum, due to senile changes (old age) or some bodily disorders. It can be caused by alkalis, such as those found in soaps and washing powders.

Rosacea (ro-**ZA**-se-a), formerly called acne rosacea, is a chronic inflammatory congestion of the cheeks and nose. It is characterized by redness, dilation of the blood vessels, and the formation of papules and pustules. The cause of rosacea is unknown. Certain things are known to aggravate rosacea in some individuals. These include consumption of hot liquids, spicy foods or alcohol, being exposed to extremes of heat and cold, exposure to sunlight, and stress. (Fig. 21.10)

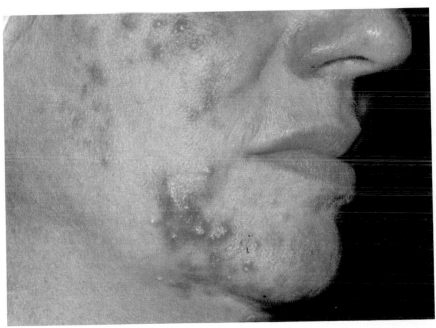

21.10—Rosacea.

Steatoma (stee-ah-**TOH**-mah), or sebaceous cyst, is a subcutaneous tumor of the sebaceous gland. It is filled with sebum and ranges in size from a pea to an orange. It usually appears on the scalp, neck, and back. A steatoma is sometimes called a wen. (Fig. 21.11)

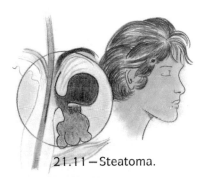

21.11—Steatoma.

DEFINITIONS PERTAINING TO DISORDERS OF THE SUDORIFEROUS (SWEAT) GLANDS

Bromidrosis (broh-mi-**DROH**-sis), or *osmidrosis* (ah-smi-**DROH**-sis)—Foul-smelling perspiration, usually noticeable in the armpits or on the feet.

Anhidrosis (an-i-**DROH**-sis), or lack of perspiration—Often a result of fever or certain skin diseases. It requires medical treatment.

Hyperhidrosis (heye-per-heye-**DROH**-sis), or excessive perspiration—Caused by excessive heat or general body weakness. The most commonly affected parts are the armpits, joints, and feet. Medical treatment is required.

Miliaria rubra (mil-ee-**AY**-ree-ah **ROOB**-rah), or *prickly heat*—An acute inflammatory disorder of the sweat glands, characterized by an eruption of small red vesicles and accompanied by burning and itching of the skin. It is caused by exposure to excessive heat.

DEFINITIONS PERTAINING TO INFLAMMATIONS

Dermatitis (dur-mah-**TEYE**-tis)—A term used to indicate an inflammatory condition of the skin. The lesions come in various forms, such as vesicles or papules.

Eczema (**EK**-se-mah)—An inflammation of the skin, of acute or chronic nature, presenting many forms of dry or moist lesions. It is frequently accompanied by itching or a burning sensation. All cases of eczema should be referred to a physician for treatment. Its cause is unknown.

Psoriasis (so-**REYE**-a-sis)—A common, chronic, inflammatory skin disease whose cause is unknown. It is usually found on the scalp, elbows, knees, chest, and lower back, rarely on the face. The lesions are round, dry patches covered with coarse, silvery scales. If irritated, bleeding points occur. It is not contagious.

Herpes simplex (**HUR**-peez **SIM**-pleks)—A recurring virus infection, commonly called fever blisters. It is characterized by the eruption of a single vesicle or group of vesicles on a red swollen base. The blisters usually appear on the lips, nostrils, or other part of the face, and rarely last more than a week. It is contagious. (Fig. 21.12)

Occupational Disorders in Cosmetology

Abnormal conditions resulting from contact with chemicals or tints can occur in the course of performing services in the beauty salon. Some individuals may develop allergies to ingredients in cosmetics, antiseptics, cold waving lotions, and aniline derivative tints. These can cause eruptive skin infections known as *dermatitis venenata* (**VEN**-e-na-tah). It is important that cosmetologists employ protective measures, such as the use of rubber gloves or protective creams whenever possible.

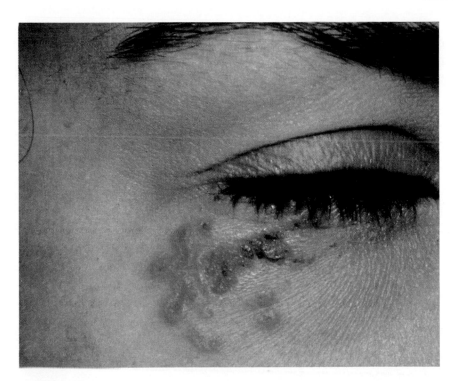

21.12—Herpes simplex, or fever blisters.

DEFINITIONS PERTAINING TO PIGMENTATIONS OF THE SKIN

In abnormal conditions, *pigment* can be affected from inside or outside the body. Abnormal colors accompany every skin disorder and many systemic disorders. A change in pigmentation is observed when certain drugs are being taken internally.

Tan—Caused by excessive exposure to the sun.

Lentigines (len-ti-**JEE**-neez) (singular, lentigo), or freckles—Small yellow-to-brown-colored spots on parts exposed to sunlight and air.

Stains—Abnormal brown skin patches, having a circular and irregular shape. Their permanent color is due to the presence of darker pigment. They occur during aging, after certain diseases, and after the disappearance of moles, freckles, and liver spots. The cause of these stains is unknown.

Chloasma (kloh-**AZ**-mah)—Characterized by increased deposits of pigment in the skin. It is found mainly on the forehead, nose, and cheeks. Chloasma is also called *moth patches* or *liver spots*.

Naevus (**NEE**-vus)—Commonly known as birthmark. It is a small or large malformation of the skin due to abnormal pigmentation or dilated capillaries.

Leucoderma (loo-ko-**DUR**-mah)—Abnormal white patches in the skin, due to congenital defective pigmentation. It is classified as:

Vitiligo (vit-i-**LEYE**-goh)—An acquired condition of leuco-derma, affecting the skin or the hair. The only treatment is a matching cosmetic color, making it less conspicuous. Must be protected from over-exposure to the sun.

Albinism (**AL**-bi-niz-em)—Congenital absence of melanin pigment of the body, including the skin, hair, and eyes. The silky hair is white. The skin is pinkish white and will not tan. Eyes are pink. Skin ages early.

Business Tips

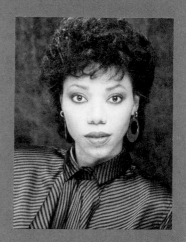

Nina Curtis, a senior instructor at the International Dermal Institute in Marina del Ray, California, says there is no better time than now to get involved in esthetics because the prestige of estheticians has grown tremendously in the United States in the past few years, particularly with medical professionals. According to Curtis, the Dermal Institute receives frequent requests from dermatologists and plastic surgeons for recent graduates to work with them in their offices.

Says Curtis, "Plastic surgeons in particular see the value of pre- and postoperative skin care services and are convinced that these services help the skin heal faster."

Curtis recommends that estheticians who are looking toward the future focus on the benefits of makeup applications for face-lift patients, because makeup enhances the results of the operation. "Many women who go out in public after a recent face-lift need proper makeup instruction," she says.

According to Curtis, there are two ways to work with a medical doctor: on staff or through a referral system. Working with dermatologists requires additional expertise in paramedical techniques, such as extraction, so estheticians who are more interested in the scientific side of esthetics will find this path exciting and rewarding. Once a relationship is established, the medical professional refers clients to you, and you to him or her.

Adds Curtis, "Just remember that when working with a medical professional, you should establish a good rapport and a relationship of equality. Estheticians should be as proud of their profession as doctors are and realize that they are every bit as much of a professional. Estheticians see the same client more than a doctor does, so they are doubly responsible for spotting a potentially dangerous skin disease before it becomes serious. When you do see a suspicious mole on a client, encourage him or her to seek a medical consultation immediately."

Curtis herself has received much praise and respect from medical professionals for doing just that.

DEFINITIONS PERTAINING TO HYPERTROPHIES (NEW GROWTHS) OF THE SKIN

Keratoma (ker-a-**TOH**-ma), or callous—An acquired, superficial, round, thickened patch of epidermis, due to pressure or friction on the hands and feet. If the thickening grows inward, it is called a corn.

Mole—A small, brownish spot, or blemish, on the skin. Moles are believed to be inherited. They range in color from pale tan to brown or bluish black. Some moles are small and flat, resembling freckles; others are more raised and darker in color. Large, dark hairs often occur in moles. Any change in a mole requires medical attention.

Melanotic sarcoma—Fatal skin cancer that starts with a mole.

CAUTION

▶ *Do not treat or remove hair from moles.*

Verruca (ve-**ROO**-kah)—Technical term for *wart*. It is caused by a virus and is infectious. It can spread from one location to another, particularly along a scratch in the skin.

DEFINITIONS PERTAINING TO PLASTIC SURGERY

Estheticians are being added to the staff of many dermatologists and plastic surgeons. Estheticians are people who specialize in skin care. More specifically, they help clients preserve the youthful look of the face and neck. To be effective assisting in a medical office, you should be familiar with the following terms and procedures.

Rhytidectomy (rit-i-**DECK**-tuh-mee)—A face-lift is an operation designed to diminish the changes of aging in the face and neck. It involves lifting and removing the excess skin of the face, neck, and temple.

Blepharoplasty (**BLEF**-uh-ro-plas-tee)—Eyelid surgery is the procedure often combined with a forehead or eyebrow lift to improve the overall appearance of the upper face. It involves incisions in the natural skin fold of the eyelids to remove skin and protruding fatty tissue.

Chemical peeling—A technique for improving the appearance when wrinkles of the skin are present. In this procedure, a specially formulated chemical solution is applied to the areas to be treated. The chemical causes a mild, controlled burn of the skin.

Rhinoplasty (**RYE**-no-plas-tee)—Plastic surgery of the nose. The procedure is sometimes performed in conjunction with a face-lift to adjust the aging nose's tendency to droop and lose definition. Incisions are hidden just inside the rim of the nostrils and sometimes across the skin between the nostrils. The cartilage and bone of the nose are then reshaped to give the nose a more pleasing appearance.

Mentoplasty (**MEN**-to-plas-tee)—Chin surgery involves a small incision made either inside the mouth or just underneath and behind the most prominent part of the chin to change a person's profile by building up a small chin. It is often performed at the same time as plastic surgery of the nose.

Dermabrasion (dur-muh-**BRAY**-zhun)—A technique to smooth scarred skin by "sanding" irregularities so that scars blend better with the surrounding skin. This procedure is usually performed with a rotary abrasive instrument that actually thins the skin, making the sharp edges of facial scars less prominent.

Injectable fillers—When there are deep scars, severe acne scarring, or deep aging lines around the mouth or forehead, tiny injections of collagen may be used to raise depressions closer to the normal skin level. Collagen, a natural product derived from cowhide, blends well with skin tissue.

Retina (**RET**-i-nuh) *A*—*Retinoic* (ret-i-**NO**-ick) *acid*, *Tretinoin* (tre-**TIN**-o-in), *Vitamin A acid* are all names for Retina A, which is a prescription cream used in the treatment of acne. Recently the general public has begun to use it as a sloughing off (shedding) agent to bring new cells to the epidermis more quickly. The purpose is to control and slow down the formation of wrinkles.

Review Questions

THE SKIN AND ITS DISORDERS

1. What is skin?
2. Briefly describe healthy skin.
3. Name the two main divisions of the skin.
4. How is the skin nourished?
5. What determines the color of the skin?
6. What are the glands contained within the skin?
7. What are the six important functions of the skin?
8. Define dermatology.
9. What is a lesion of the skin?
10. Define acne.
11. Define herpes simplex. What is it commonly called?
12. Define albinism.
13. What is a mole?

22

REMOVING UNWANTED HAIR

LEARNING OBJECTIVES

After completing this chapter, you should be able to:

1. List the two general classifications of unwanted hair removal.

2. Identify acceptable techniques involved in the three methods of permanent hair removal.

3. Demonstrate the methods of temporary hair removal.

Introduction

Hirsuties (hur-**SUE**-shee-eez) or *hypertrichosis* (hi-per-**TRIK**-osis) means hairiness, or superfluous hair. It is recognized by the growth of hair in unusual amounts or locations, as on the faces of women. Unwanted hair is not a new problem. It has plagued individuals throughout the ages. Unwanted hair is a problem that concerns many men as well as women.

One of the earliest methods of hair removal was the use of an abrasive, such as pumice stone to wear away the hair. Excavations of early Egyptian tombs revealed that abrasives were used for this purpose. Ancient Greek and Roman women were known to remove most of their body hair by abrasion. Native Americans used sharpened stones and seashells to rub off and pluck out hair.

History also records chemical means of removing excess hair. For example, the ancient Turks used *rusma*, a combination of yellow sulfide of arsenic, quicklime, and rose water, as a crude *depilatory*. Most depilatories today also have an alkaline pH to assist in the decomposition of the hair.

Today, there are two types of hair removal: permanent and temporary. Several means of temporary hair removal are covered later in this chapter. This section covers the permanent hair removal method called *electrology*.

Permanent Methods of Hair Removal

The first effective technique of permanent hair removal invented was electrolysis. This technique was devised by ophthalmologist Charles E. Michel of St. Louis, Missouri, in 1875 as he was trying to solve the problem of ingrown eyelashes. Michel attached a very fine conductor wire to a dry-cell battery. He then attached the wire to a surgical needle and inserted it into the follicle of the eyelash. In most cases after the treatment, the hair did not grow back. History was made.

The electrolysis treatment devised by Michel used a *galvanic* or direct current of electricity. The galvanic current chemically decomposed the *dermal papilla*, the lower hair root and source of nourishment of the hair follicle. The galvanic process was very time-consuming and tedious. In 1916 Professor Paul Kree developed a multiple galvanic machine or *epilator*. This allowed the electrologist to insert up to ten needles in time sequence instead of spending several minutes on each hair.

In 1924, Dr. H. Brodier of Paris developed *thermolysis* (thur-**MOL**-e-sis), a method of hair removal using high-frequency or alternating current. This method created heat to destroy the papilla. It soon became popular because it was a much faster technique than the galvanic process.

In 1945, Henri St. Pierre and Arthur Hinkel successfully blended galvanic current with low intensity high-frequency short-wave current running simultaneously through a single needle. Known as the blend method, the purpose was to destroy hair growth more quickly using galvanic current with the aid of the heat from high-frequency current.

GENERAL INFORMATION

The importance of training. The electrologist is dealing with the skin, and an inefficient or unskilled operator could cause irreparable damage. Therefore, every electrologist must be thoroughly trained, both in the theory and in the practice of electrology. This means that she or he must use live models to practice on, under the direct supervision of an instructor, until proper skill, certificate (if required), and confidence are achieved.

Machines. Some shortwave machines have many safety factors. They are automatically timed and F.C.C. (Federal Communications Commission) approved. Pain is kept to a minimum by the rapid shut-off of current.

Areas that may be treated. Upper lips, chin, cheeks, arms, legs, eyebrows, hairline, and underarms may receive electrology treatments.

Areas that may not be treated. Do not treat the lower eyelids, inside the ears, or nostrils. Obtain permission from a physician before treating clients who have conditions such as diabetes or pregnancy, and those who have pacemakers or who are receiving hormone treatments.

Causes of unwanted hair. The growth of hair is due to hormonal imbalance in the body. No one knows the exact cause, although authorities agree that heredity often plays a large role in excessive hair growth. Certain drugs, pregnancy, and weight problems are also known to influence hair growth.

SHORTWAVE OR THERMOLYSIS METHOD

The shortwave method, also known as the thermolysis method, is the quickest of permanent hair removal methods and the one most generally used. (Fig. 22.1) In fact, because it is the overwhelming choice of electrologists today, we will describe it in detail. We will not discuss the other permanent removal methods.

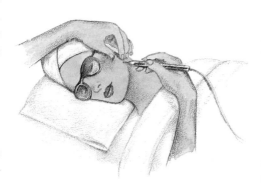

22.1—Inserting needle in shortwave method.

Equipment, Implements, and Materials

You will need the following equipment and accessories to perform thermolysis treatment:

Shortwave epilator and stand (Fig. 22.2)
Needles
Patient chair or table
Electrologist's stool
Antiseptic solution
Sterilizer
Sterile cotton
Facial tissue
Protective eye shields
Magnification mirror and regular mirror
Magnification treatment lens lamp or glasses
Tweezers
Apron for client
After-treatment lotion
Small blunt-end scissors
Small treatment pillow
Covered waste container

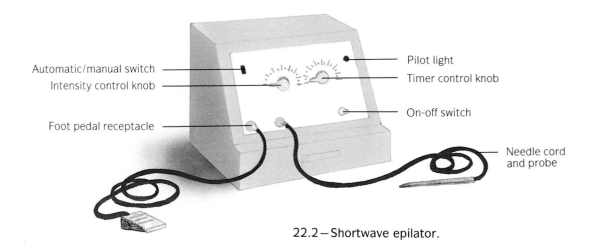

22.2 — Shortwave epilator.

Thermolysis Controls

Thermolysis epilators are also known as shortwave epilators. They use radio frequency and operate on alternating current (AC). All thermolysis epilators have the same control systems:

1. Plug to power source
2. On/off switch
3. Indicator light—indicates machine is on or off
4. Timer or manual switch
5. Intensity control—regulates current flow (rheostat)
6. Needle holder jack (negative electrode)
7. Foot pedal—on/off current flow
8. Intensity light—comes on when pedal is depressed
9. Timer light—stays on as long as pedal is depressed

Beyond the basic controls, manufacturers may add their own innovations. Some, for example, have incorporated two *negative jacks* to allow needle holders for different sized needles. Others may have radio frequency (RF) meters. Because machines may vary slightly, it is wise to follow the instruction manual provided by each manufacturer.

Client Comfort
The care and comfort of the client should always be of utmost importance to the electrologist. The comfort of the electrologist is also important. The treatment given will be of better quality if the electrologist is comfortable.

Procedure for Thermolysis
1. Position aproned client on chair.
2. Wash your hands.
3. Apply an astringent to the treatment area.
4. Sterilize tweezers.
5. Determine the size of needle required and sterilize it.
6. Turn on the epilator and wait 1 minute.
7. Set the timer on low.
8. Set the intensity on low.
9. Make the first insertion until slight resistance is felt.
10. Depress the foot switch.
11. Test the hair with tweezer for easy release.
12. Raise the intensity and timer controls accordingly, until hair is easily released.

Inserting the Needle into the Hair Follicle
Insertion is the most critical technique in electrology treatment. The size of the needle corresponds to the diameter of the hair being treated. Hold the needle holder as you would a pen or pencil, but not as firmly. The index finger and thumb must not touch. The needle holder may lean gently on the middle finger, which serves as a guide.

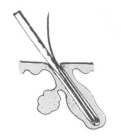

22.3 – Needle inserted correctly.

The angle at which the needle is inserted depends on the angle at which the hair is growing. For example, a hair that grows straight up requires that the needle be inserted straight down into the follicle. If a hair is growing at an angle, the needle should be inserted at an angle. (Figs. 22.3–22.6) When there is an excessive amount of hair and the hairs are long, it is difficult to see the hair follicle and the angle of growth. Simply cut the hair to a length where the follicle and angle of growth can be observed easily.

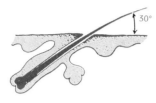

22.4 – Hair growing at a 30° (.523 rad.) angle on the neck.

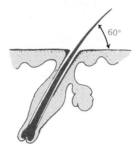

22.5 – Hair growing at a 60° (1.05 rad.) angle on the front of the chin.

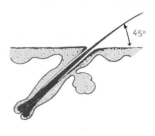

22.6 – Hair growing at a 45° (.785 rad.) angle on the face.

Tweezer Manipulation

It is necessary to use a tweezer to gently remove the hair. Once the current is turned off, remove the wire from the follicle and use your tweezer to remove the hair. You should not have to use any pressure. The needle holder and the tweezer should not be held tightly. You must practice a light touch and practice maneuvering the needle holder and tweezer in one hand while the fingers of the other hand hold the treatment area firmly but without causing discomfort to the client.

Developing an expert skill of insertion, tweezer manipulation, and correct intensity and timer judgments increase treatment efficiency.

After treatment is completed, turn the machine off. Saturate a pad of sterile cotton with a strong after-treatment lotion and press it gently on the area treated. This cools and soothes the skin and aids in the healing process.

Temporary Methods of Hair Removal

SHAVING

Shaving is usually recommended when the unwanted hairs cover a large area, such as under arms and on the legs. A shaving cream is applied before shaving.

An electric clipper may also be used. The application of a pre-shaving lotion helps to reduce any irritation. An electric clipper is most often used to remove unwanted hair at the nape.

Shaving does not cause the hair to grow thicker or stronger, it only seems that way because the razor blunts the hair ends and makes them feel stiff.

TWEEZING

Tweezing is commonly used for shaping the eyebrows. Tweezing can also be used for removing undesirable hairs from around the mouth and chin. (The procedure for tweezing the eyebrows will be found in the chapter on facial makeup.)

ELECTRONIC TWEEZER METHOD OF HAIR REMOVAL

Another method for the removal of superfluous hair that is used in salons is the electrically charged tweezer. This method transmits radio frequency energy down the hair shaft into the follicle area. It is claimed that the papilla is thus dehydrated and eventually destroyed.

The tweezer is used to grasp a single strand of hair. The energy is then applied, first at a low level to pre-warm and then at a higher level for up to 2 minutes to remove the hair. Most manufacturers suggest that the area be steamed first in order to increase efficiency.

The electronic tweezer is not a method of permanent hair removal. Further, the process of clearing any area of hair by this method is slow.

DEPILATORIES

Depilatories also belong to the group of temporary methods for the removal of superfluous hair. There are *physical* (wax) and *chemical* types of depilatories.

HOT WAX

The hot wax depilatory is applied either heated or cold as recommended by the manufacturer. It may be applied over such parts of the body as the cheeks, chin, upper lip, nape area, arms, and legs. Do not remove lanugo hair; doing so may cause the skin to lose its softness. (Fig. 22.7)

Waxing and tweezing may cause the hair to grow stronger because it stimulates the circulation and increases the blood supply to the hair follicle.

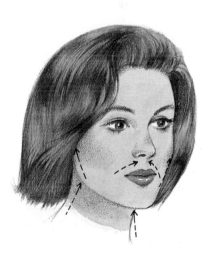

22.7—Superfluous hair.

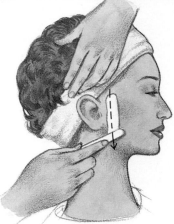

22.8—Spread wax downward.

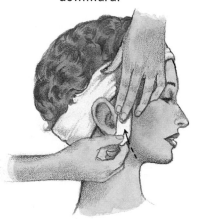

22.9—Pull wax off upward.

Procedure for Hot Waxing

1. Melt wax in a double boiler on a stove or in a heater.
2. Remove clothing from the area to be treated and seat the client comfortably.
3. Wash the skin area with a mild soap and water. Rinse thoroughly and dry.
4. Spread talcum powder over the skin surface.
5. Test temperature and consistency of heated wax by applying a little of it on your arm.
6. Using a spatula or brush, spread warm wax evenly over the skin surface in the same direction as the hair growth. Apply a sanitized cloth strip in the same direction as the hair growth. (Figs. 22.8, 22.10)
7. Allow the wax to cool and harden.
8. Quickly pull off the adhering wax against the direction of hair growth. (Figs. 22.9, 22.11)
9. Gently massage treated area.
10. Dust off remaining powder from the skin.
11. Apply an emollient cream or antiseptic lotion to the treated area.

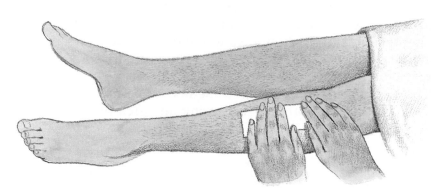

22.10—Applying wax to skin.

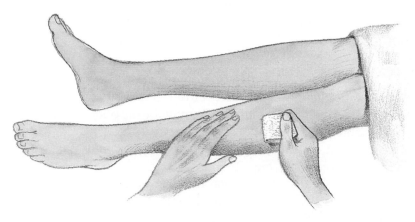

22.11—Removing wax from skin.

Safety Precautions

1. To prevent burns, test the temperature of the heated wax before applying it to the client's skin.
2. Use caution so the wax does not contact the eyes.
3. Do not use a wax depilatory under the arms, if the client's skin is sensitive, over warts, on moles, abrasions, irritated or inflamed skin.

COLD WAX

For those clients who cannot tolerate heated wax, a cold wax method of hair removal also is available. This technique has all the advantages of hot wax in a ready-to-use form. It removes the hair in the same manner as warm wax, but needs no heating or special equipment.

Procedure for Cold Waxing

1. Apply wax at room temperature.
2. Using a spatula, spread a thin coat of wax in the direction of the hair growth.
3. Apply a strip of cellophane or cotton cloth and press down firmly so that the wax adheres correctly.
4. Holding the skin taut with one hand, use the other hand to grasp the wax strip, and with one fast movement, pull off the strip against the direction of the hair growth.

CHEMICAL DEPILATORIES

Chemical depilatories are available as a cream, paste, or powder mixed with water into a paste. These depilatories are generally used to remove hair from the legs.

A *skin test* is advisable to determine whether the individual is sensitive to the action of this type of depilatory.

To give such a test, select a hairless part of the arm, apply a portion of the depilatory according to the manufacturer's directions, and leave it on the skin from 7 to 10 minutes. If at the end of this time there are no signs of redness or swelling, the depilatory can probably be used with safety over a large area of the skin.

Procedure

1. The cream type is applied directly from the container, while the powder type is mixed to form a smooth paste according to the manufacturer's directions.
2. After the skin has been cleansed and dried, a thick layer of the depilatory is applied over the area where the hair is to be removed.
3. The surrounding skin is protected with petroleum jelly or cream.

4. The depilatory is kept on the hair for 5 to 10 minutes depending on the thickness of the hair. The thicker the hair, the longer the depilatory is kept on.
5. Wash off the depilatory and hair with warm water.
6. Pat the skin dry and apply cold cream.

Business Tips

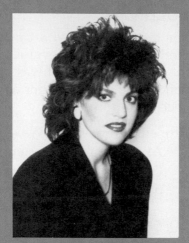

Waxing is one of the fastest growing salon services, and one you shouldn't miss out on because it is relatively quick and lucrative. But how do you build up a clientele for this business as a beginner? Through promotion, professionalism, and personality, according to Rhonda Lyon, national sales manager and educator for GiGi Laboratories.

"Nine out of ten clients won't know waxing exists unless you tell them," says Lyon, who is also a licensed esthetician. "Promote the service by posting signs throughout the salon and by making certain that waxing is added to the salon's service menu. Work out joint promotions with other staff members, such as a free eyebrow arch or lip wax with every makeup application."

To keep new clients on your permanent list, professionalism and personality are essential. "Clients are usually in some state of undress during waxing," says Lyon. "Making them feel comfortable is important. Don't be afraid to touch the client and help her overcome her possible fear that she'll feel pain or discomfort during waxing.

"Always call the client a day or two after the service to ask her how she likes the results, to find out if she has had any irritation, and to tell her that you look forward to seeing her again.

"Most important, have a clean, sanitary room. The key area of concern to most clients is the treatment table. I prefer the paper table covers like those used in doctors' offices because the client knows that she is the only one who will be using that surface."

Review Questions

REMOVING UNWANTED HAIR

1. Define hirsuties.
2. What are two types of hair removal?
3. What was the first effective technique of permanent hair removal and who invented this method?
4. What is thermolysis?
5. What technique did Henri St. Pierre and Arthur Hinkel successfully develop in 1945?
6. Name three temporary methods of hair removal.
7. Name three areas that may not be treated by the electrologist.
8. What is the quickest method of permanent hair removal?
9. Name three safety precautions when waxing.

23

CELLS, ANATOMY, AND PHYSIOLOGY

LEARNING OBJECTIVES

After completing this chapter, you should be able to:

1. Define the functions of human cells.

2. Describe the structures and functions of the human body.

3. Discuss why a basic understanding of the various organs and systems and how they function will help to improve the professional skill of the cosmetologist.

4. Describe the many tissues, organs, and systems of the human body and how they function.

5. Discuss how the malfunction of a body system or organ can affect cosmetology services.

6. Discuss the effect of the various organs and systems on the general health of the client.

Introduction

In the first part of this chapter we discuss the cell, the basic structure from which all other body structures are made. In the second part of the chapter we discuss the body structures themselves, the anatomy and physiology of the human body, and its relationship to the cosmetology profession.

The human organism is made of a vast variety of parts that vary in complexity. These include organ systems, organs, tissues, cells. These cellular parts are composed of molecules, which are made of atoms or groups of atoms. And, as you will see in the chemistry chapter, atoms are made up of even smaller, submicroscopic particles called protons, neutrons, and electrons.

Cells

Cells are the basic units of all living things, including bacteria, plants, and animals. The human body is composed entirely of cells, fluids, and cellular products. As the basic functional units, the cells carry on all life processes. Cells also have the ability to reproduce, providing new ones for growth and replacement of worn and injured tissues. (Fig. 23.1)

Cells are made up of *protoplasm* (**PROH**-toh-plaz-em), a colorless, jellylike substance in which food elements such as protein, fats, carbohydrates, mineral salts, and water are present. The principal parts of a cell are the *cytoplasm* (**SEYE**-toh-plaz-em), *centrosome* (**SEN**-tro-sohm), *nucleus* (**NOO**-klee-us), and *cell membrane* (**MEM**-brayn). The thin cell membrane or cell wall permits soluble (dissolvable) substances to enter and leave the protoplasm. The nucleus, near the center of the cell, is contained in a nuclear membrane. Outside of the nucleus are the cytoplasm and a centrosome. The nucleus and the cytoplasm are made of protoplasm. The centrosome and the nucleus control cell reproduction.

The protoplasm of the cells contains the following important structures:

Nucleus (dense protoplasm), found in the center, which plays an important part in the reproduction of the cell.

Cytoplasm (less dense protoplasm), which is found outside of the nucleus and contains food materials necessary for the growth, reproduction, and self-repair of the cell.

Centrosome, a small, round body in the cytoplasm, which also affects the reproduction of the cell.

Cell membrane encloses the protoplasm. It permits soluble substances to enter and leave the cell.

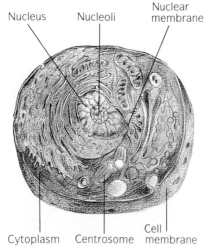

Nucleus Nucleoli Nuclear membrane

Cytoplasm Centrosome Cell membrane

23.1 — Cells consist of protoplasm and contain essential elements.

CELL GROWTH

As long as the cell receives an adequate supply of food, oxygen, and water, eliminates waste products, and is favored with proper temperature, it will continue to grow and thrive. However, if these conditions do not exist and there is the presence of toxins (poisons) or pressure, then the growth and the health of the cells are impaired. Most body cells are capable of growth and self-repair during their life cycle. (Fig. 23.2)

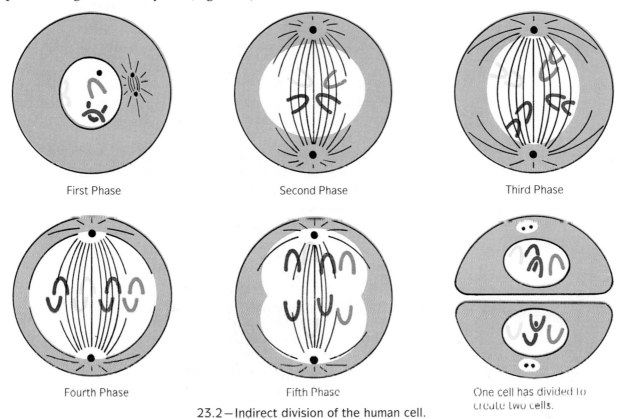

First Phase	Second Phase	Third Phase

Fourth Phase	Fifth Phase	One cell has divided to create two cells.

23.2—Indirect division of the human cell.

CELL METABOLISM

Metabolism (meh-**TAB**-o-lis-em) is a complex chemical process whereby the body cells are nourished and supplied with the energy needed to carry on their many activities.

There are two phases of metabolism:

1. *Anabolism* (ah-**NAB**-o-lizm) is the process of building up larger molecules from smaller ones. During this process the body stores water, food, and oxygen for the time when these substances are needed for cell growth and repair.

2. *Catabolism* (kah-**TAB**-o-liz-em) is the breaking down of larger substances or molecules into smaller ones. This process releases energy that can be stored by special molecules to be used for muscle contraction, secretion, or heat production.

Anabolism and catabolism are carried out simultaneously and continuously in the cells. Their activities are closely regulated so that the breaking down, energy-releasing reactions are balanced with the building up, energy-consuming reactions. Therefore, *homeostasis* (the maintenance of normal, internal stability in the organism) is maintained. However, if we use less energy than we manufacture, we may notice a weight gain. If molecules of energy are not used, they turn to fat. To get rid of the built-up fat, more energy must be used (exercise) or less energy (food) taken in.

Tissues

Tissues are composed of groups of cells of the same kind. Each tissue has a specific function and can be recognized by its characteristic appearance. Body tissues are classified as follows:

1. *Connective tissue* serves to support, protect, and bind together other tissues of the body. Bone, cartilage, ligament, tendon, fascia (separates muscles), and fat tissue are examples of connective tissue.
2. *Muscular tissue* contracts and moves various parts of the body.
3. *Nerve tissue* carries messages to and from the brain, and controls and coordinates all body functions.
4. *Epithelial* (ep-i-**THE**-le-al) *tissue* is a protective covering on body surfaces, such as the skin, mucous membranes, linings of the heart, digestive and respiratory organs, and glands.
5. *Liquid tissue* carries food, waste products, and hormones by means of the blood and lymph.

Organs

Organs are structures designed to accomplish a specific function. The most important organs of the body are the brain, which controls the body; the heart, which circulates the blood; the lungs, which supply oxygen to the blood; the liver, which removes toxic products of digestion; the kidneys, which excrete water and other waste products; and the stomach and intestines, which digest food.

Systems

Systems are groups of organs that cooperate for a common purpose, namely the welfare of the entire body. The human body is composed of the following important systems. (These systems are discussed in detail later in the chapter.)

Integumentary (in-**TEG**-yu-men-ta-ree) *system*—skin.

Skeletal (**SKEL**-e-tahl) *system*—bones.

Muscular (**MUS**-kyoo-lahr) *system*—muscles.

Nervous (**NUR**-vus) *system*—nerves.

Circulatory (**SUR**-kyoo-lahr-tohr-ee) *system*—blood supply.

Endocrine (**EN**-doh-krin) *system*—ductless glands.

Excretory (**EK**-skre-tohr-ee) *system*—organs of elimination.

Respiratory (**RES**-pi-rah-tohr-ee) *system*—lungs.

Digestive (deye-**GES**-tiv) *system*—stomach and intestines.

Reproductive (ree-proh-**DUK**-tiv) *system*—organs for reproducing.

The *integumentary system* is made up of the skin and its various accessory organs such as the oil and sweat glands, sensory receptors, hair, and nails and is composed of two distinct layers, the dermis and epidermis. It functions as a protective covering, contains sensory receptors, and plays a major role in the body's heat regulation.

The *skeletal system* is the physical foundation or framework of the body. The function of the skeletal system is to serve as a means of protection, support, and locomotion (movement).

The *muscular system* covers, shapes, and supports the skeleton. Its function is to produce all the movements of the body.

Introduction to Anatomy and Physiology

Although you may have groaned when you saw a chapter on anatomy and physiology, these are important subjects in the practice of cosmetology. A basic understanding of the structure and functions of the human body forms the scientific basis for the proper application of cosmetic services. The cosmetologist should know which cosmetic service is best for a client's condition, and how to adjust and control the service for the best results.

Very generally, *anatomy* (ah-**NAHT**-o-mee) is the study of the structure of the body and what it is made of, for example, bones, muscles, and skin. *Physiology* (fiz-i-**OL**-o-jee) is the study of the functions or activities performed by those structures. The cosmetologist is concerned with *histology* (hi-**STOL**-o-jee), the study of the minute structural parts of the body, such as hair, nails, sweat glands, and oil glands.

Although the names of bones, muscles, arteries, veins, and nerves are seldom used in the beauty salon, an understanding of body structures will help make you more proficient in performing many of the salon services such as facials and hand and arm massage.

The Skeletal System

The *skeletal system* is the physical foundation of the body. It is composed of different shaped bones that are connected by movable and immovable joints.

Bone, except for the tissue that forms the major part of the tooth, is the hardest tissue of the body. It is composed of connective tissues consisting of about one-third animal matter, such as cells and blood, and two-thirds mineral matter, mainly calcium carbonate and calcium phosphate. The scientific study of bones, their structure, and functions is called *osteology* (os-tee-**OL**-oh-jee). *Os* is the technical term for bone.

The following are the primary functions of the bones:

1. Give shape and support to the body.
2. Protect various internal structures and organs.
3. Serve as attachments for muscles and act as levers to produce body movement.
4. Produce various blood cells in the red bone marrow.
5. Store various minerals such as calcium, phosphorus, magnesium, and sodium.

BONES OF THE SKULL

The *skull* is the skeleton of the head and is divided into two parts: the *cranium*, an oval, bony case that shapes the top of the head and protects the brain, and the skeleton of the face, which is made up of fourteen facial bones. (Fig. 23.3)

Bones of the Cranium

Occipital (ok-**SIP**-i-tal) *bone* forms the lower back part of the cranium.

Two *parietal* (pa-**REYE**-e-tal) *lones* form the sides and top (crown) of the cranium.

Frontal (**FRUNT**-al) *bone* forms the forehead.

Two *temporal* (**TEM**-po-rahl) *bones* form the sides of the head in the ear region (below the parietal bones).

The *ethmoid* (**ETH**-moid) *bone* is a light spongy bone between the eye sockets and forms part of the nasal cavities.

Sphenoid (**SFEEN**-oid) *bone* joins together all the bones of the cranium. *(The ethmoid and sphenoid bones are not affected by massage.)*

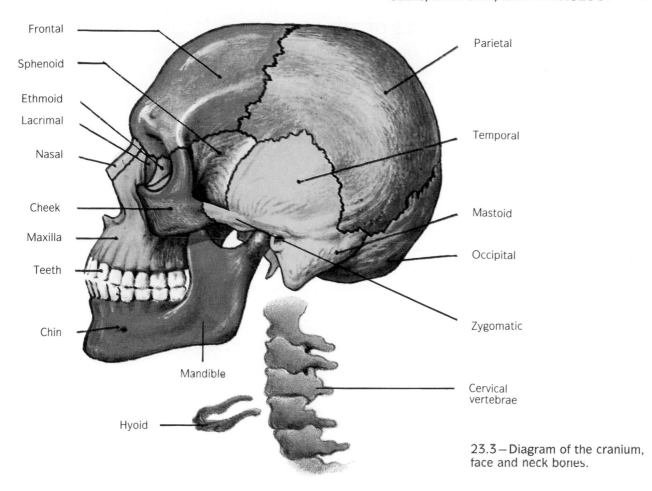

Frontal
Sphenoid
Ethmoid
Lacrimal
Nasal
Cheek
Maxilla
Teeth
Chin
Mandible
Hyoid
Parietal
Temporal
Mastoid
Occipital
Zygomatic
Cervical vertebrae

23.3 — Diagram of the cranium, face and neck bones.

Bones of the Face

Two *nasal* (**NAY**-zal) *bones* form the bridge of the nose.

Two *lacrimal* (**LAK** ri mahl) *bones* are small fragile bones located at the front part of the inner wall of the eye sockets.

Two *zygomatic* (zcye-goh-**MAT**-ik), or *malar bones* form the prominence of the cheeks.

Two *maxillae* (mak-**SIL**-ee) are the upper jawbones which join to form the whole upper jaw.

Mandible (**MAN**-di-bel) is the lower jawbone and is the largest and strongest bone of the face. It forms the lower jaw.

Facial bones that do not appear in Fig. 23.3 are two *turbinal* (**TUR**-bi-nahl) *bones*, which are thin layers of spongy bone on either of the outer walls of the nasal depression; *vomer* (**VOH**-mer), which is a single bone that forms part of the dividing wall of the nose; two *palatine* (**PAL**-i-teyen) *bones*, which form the floor and outer wall of the nose, roof of the mouth, and floor of the orbits.

BONES OF THE NECK
(See Fig. 23.3)

Hyoid (**HEYE**-oid) *bone*, a U-shaped bone, is located in the front part of the throat, and is referred to as the "Adam's apple."

Cervical vertebrae (**SUR**-vi-kal **VER**-te-bray) form the top part of the spinal column located in the neck region.

BONES OF THE CHEST (THORAX)

The *thorax* (**THO**-racks), or chest, is an elastic bony cage that serves as a protective framework for the heart, lungs, and other delicate internal organs. This framework is constructed of twelve *thoracic vertebrae*, twelve ribs on each side, the *sternum* (**STUR**-num) (breastbone), and the cartilage that connects the ribs to the sternum.

BONES OF THE SHOULDER, ARM, AND HAND
(See Figs. 23.4, 23.5)

The *shoulder girdle*, each side of which is made up of one clavicle and one scapula.

Humerus (**HYOO**-mo-rus) is the uppermost and largest bone of the arm.

Ulna (**UL**-nah) is the large bone on the little finger side of the forearm.

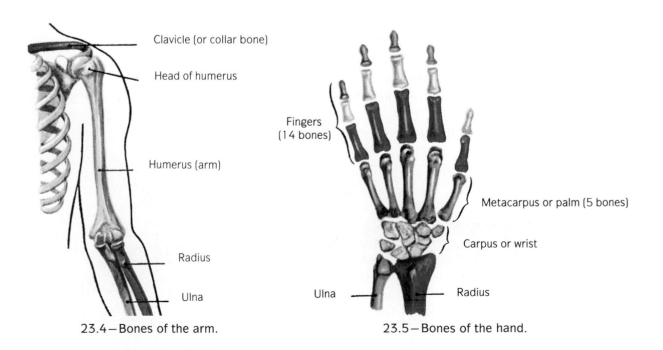

23.4 — Bones of the arm.

23.5 — Bones of the hand.

Radius (**RAY**-dee-us) is the small bone on the thumb side of the forearm.

The *wrist*, or *carpus* (**KAHR**-pus), is a flexible joint composed of eight small, irregular bones, held together by ligaments.

The *palm*, or *metacarpus* (met-a-**KAHR**-pus), consists of five long, slender bones, called metacarpal bones.

The *fingers*, or *digits* (**DIJ**-its), consist of three *phalanges* (fa-**LAN**-jeez) in each finger, and two in the thumb, totaling fourteen bones.

The Muscular System

The *muscular* (**MUS**-kyoo-lahr) *system* covers, shapes, and supports the skeleton. Its function is to produce all movements of the body. *Myology* (meye-**OL**-oh-jee) is the study of the structure, functions, and diseases of the muscles.

The muscular system consists of over 500 muscles, large and small, comprising 40 to 50% of the weight of the human body.

Muscles are fibrous tissues that have the ability to stretch and contract according to our movements. Different types of movements, for example, stretching and bending, depend on muscles to perform in specific ways.

There are three kinds of muscular tissue:

1. *Striated* (striped) or voluntary, which is controlled by will. Facial, arm, and leg muscles are voluntary muscles. (Fig. 23.6)
2. *Non-striated* (smooth) or involuntary muscles such as those of the stomach and intestines. They function automatically. (Fig. 23.7)
3. *Cardiac* (heart muscle) which is the heart itself, and is not found anywhere else in the body. (Fig. 23.8)

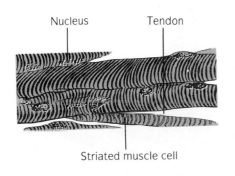

23.6—Striated muscle cells.

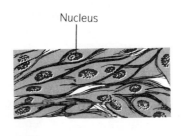

23.7—Non-striated muscle cells.

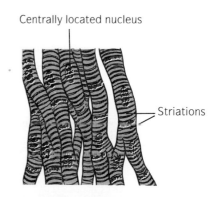

23.8—Cardiac muscle cells.

MUSCLES

There are three parts to a muscle: the origin, the insertion, and the belly. The *origin* is the part that does not move. It is attached to the skeleton, and is usually part of a skeletal muscle. The *insertion* is the part that moves, and the *belly* is the middle part.

Stimulation of Muscles

Muscular tissue can be stimulated by any of the following:

Massage (hand massage and electric vibrator)
Electric current (high-frequency and faradic current)
Light rays (infrared rays and ultra violet rays)
Heat rays (heating lamps and heating caps)
Moist heat (steamers or moderately warm steam towels)
Nerve impulses (through the nervous system)
Chemicals (certain acids and salts)

Muscles Affected by Massage

The cosmetologist is concerned with the voluntary muscles of the head, face, neck, arms, and hands. It is essential to know where these muscles are located, and what they control. Pressure in massage is usually directed from the insertion to the origin. (Fig. 23.9)

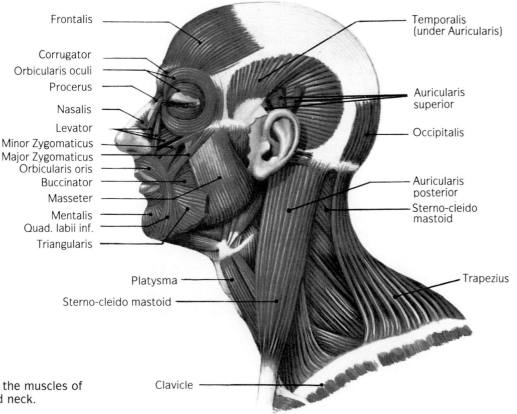

23.9—Diagram of the muscles of the head, face and neck.

Muscles of the Scalp

Epicranius (ep-i-**KRAY**-ne-us), or *occipito-frontalis* (ok-**SIP**-i-toh-fron-**TAY**-lis), is a broad muscle that covers the top of the skull. It consists of two parts: the *occipitalis* (ok-**SIP**-i-ta-lis), or back part, and the *frontalis* (fron-**TAY**-lis), or front part. Both are connected by a tendon *aponeurosis* (ap-o-noo-**ROH**-sis). The frontalis raises the eyebrows, draws the scalp forward, and causes wrinkles across the forehead. (Fig. 23.10)

Muscles of the Eyebrow

Orbicularis oculi (or-bik-yoo-**LAY**-ris **OK**-yoo-leye) completely surrounds the margin of the eye socket and enables you to close your eyes.

Corrugator (**KOR**-oo-gay-tohr) muscle is beneath the frontalis and orbicularis oculi, and draws the eyebrow down and in. It produces vertical lines, and is the muscle used for frowning. (Fig. 23.11)

Muscles of the Nose

The *procerus* (proh-**SEE**-rus) covers the bridge of the nose, depresses the eyebrow, and causes wrinkles across the bridge of the nose. (Fig. 23.12)

(The other nasal muscles are small muscles around the nasal openings which contract and expand the openings of the nostrils.)

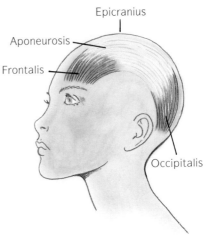

23.10 — Muscles of the scalp.

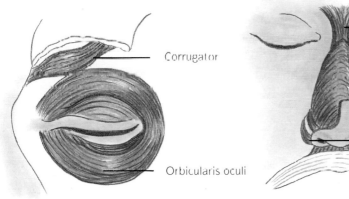

23.11 — Muscles of the eyebrow.

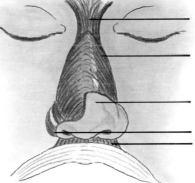

23.12 — Muscles of the nose.

Muscles of the Mouth

Quadratus labii superioris (kwah-**DRAY**-tus **LAY**-bee-eye suu-**PEER**-ee-or-ihs) consists of three parts. It surrounds the upper part of the lip, raises and draws back the upper lip, and elevates the nostrils, as in expressing distaste.

Quadratus labii inferioris (in-**FEER**-ee-or-ihs) surrounds the lower part of the lip. It depresses the lower lip and draws it a little to one side, as in the expression of sarcasm.

Buccinator (**BUK**-si-nay-tor) is the muscle between the upper and lower jaws. It compresses the cheeks and expels air between the lips, as in blowing. (Fig. 23.13)

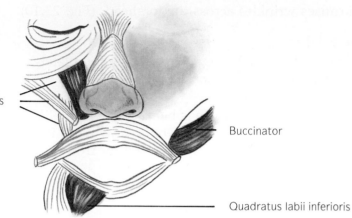

Quadratus labii superioris

Buccinator

Quadratus labii inferioris

23.13—Muscles of the upper and lower lips, and jaw.

Caninus (kay-**NIGH**-nus) lies under the quadratus labii superioris. It raises the angle of the mouth, as in snarling.

Mentalis (men-**TAL**-is) is situated at the tip of the chin. It raises the lower lip, causing wrinkling of the chin, as in doubt or displeasure. (Fig. 23.14)

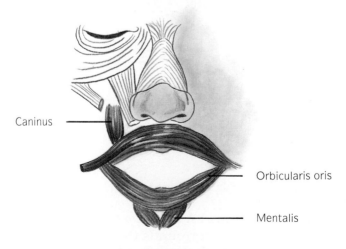

Caninus

Orbicularis oris

Mentalis

23.14—Muscles of the mouth and chin.

Orbicularis oris (or-bik-yoo-**LAY**-ris **OH**-ris) forms a flat band around the upper and lower lips. It compresses, contracts, puckers, and wrinkles the lips, as in kissing or whistling.

Risorius (ri-**ZOHR**-ee-us) extends from the masseter muscle to the angle of the mouth. It draws the corner of the mouth out and back, as in grinning.

Zygomaticus (zeye-goh-**MAT**-i-kus) extends from the zygomatic bone to the angle of the mouth. It elevates the lip, as in laughing.

Triangularis (treye-an-gyoo-**LAY**-ris) extends along the side of the chin. It draws down the corner of the mouth. (Fig. 23.15)

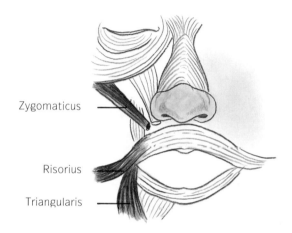

Zygomaticus

Risorius

Triangularis

23.15—Muscles of the jaw.

Muscles of the Ear

Three muscles of the ear are practically functionless:

Auricularis (aw-rik-yoo-**LAHR**-is) *superior* is above the ear.
Auricularis posterior is behind the ear.
Auricularis anterior is in front of the ear. (Fig. 23.16)

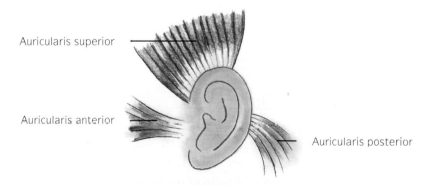

Auricularis superior

Auricularis anterior

Auricularis posterior

23.16—Muscles of the ear.

Muscles of Mastication

Masseter (ma-**SEE**-tur) and *temporalis* (tem-po-**RAY**-lis) are muscles that coordinate in opening and closing the mouth, and are referred to as chewing muscles. (Fig. 23.17)

Muscles of the Neck

Platysma (pla-**TIZ**-mah) is a broad muscle that extends from the chest and shoulder muscles to the side of the chin. It depresses the lower jaw and lip, as in the expression of sadness. (Fig. 23.18)

Sterno-cleido-mastoid (**STUR**-noh-**KLE**-i-doh-**MAS**-toid) extends from the collar and chest bones to the temporal bone in back of the ear. It rotates and bends the head, as in nodding. (Fig. 23.19)

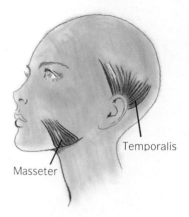

23.17—Muscles of mastication.

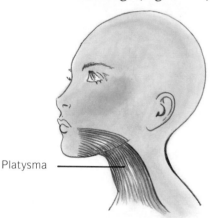

23.18—Muscles of the jaw and neck.

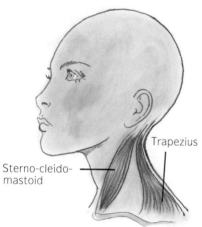

23.19—Muscles of the neck.

Muscles that Attach the Arms to the Body

The principal muscles that attach the arms to the body and permit movements of the shoulders and arms are:

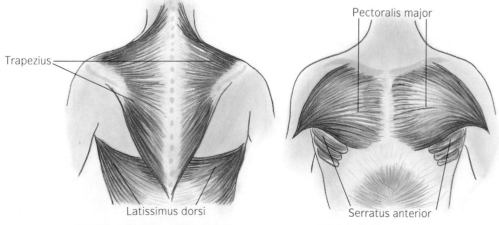

23.20—Muscles of the back and neck.

23.21—Muscles of the chest.

Trapezius (tra-**PEE**-zee-us) and *latissimus dorsi* (la-**TIS**-i-mus **DOR**-see) cover the back of the neck and upper and middle region of the back. They rotate the shoulder blade and control the swinging movements of the arm. (Fig. 23.20)

Pectoralis (pek-tohr-**AL**-is) *major* and *pectoralis minor* cover the front of the chest. They also assist in swinging movements of the arm.

Serratus anterior (ser-**RAT**-us an-**TEER**-ee-or) assists in breathing and in raising the arm. (Fig. 23.21)

Muscles of the Shoulder, Arm, and Hand

The principal muscles of the shoulder and upper arm are given below. (Fig. 23.22)

Deltoid (**DEL**-toid) is the large, thick triangular-shaped muscle that covers the shoulder and lifts and turns the arm.

Biceps (**BEYE**-seps) is the two-headed and principal muscle in the front of the upper arm. It lifts the forearm, flexes the elbow, and turns the palm outward.

Triceps (**TREYE**-seps) is the three-headed muscle of the arm that covers the entire back of the upper arm and extends the forearm.

The forearm is made up of a series of muscles and strong tendons. The cosmetologist is concerned with the following:

Pronators (pro-**NAY**-tors) are found in the forearm and turn the hand inward, so that the palm faces downward.

Supinators (**SUE**-pi-nay-tors) turn the hand outward and the palm upward.

Flexors (**FLEKS**-ors) bend the wrist, draw the hand up, and close the fingers toward the forearm.

Extensors (eck-**STEN**-surs) straighten the wrist, hand, and fingers to form a straight line.

The hand has many small muscles that overlap from joint to joint, giving flexibility and strength. When the hands are properly cared for, these muscles will remain supple and graceful. They close and open the hands and fingers.

Abductor (ab-**DUK**-tohr) and *adductor* (a **DUK**-tohr) muscles are located at the base of each digit. The abductor muscles separate the fingers and the adductor muscles draw them together. (Fig. 23.23)

Opponent muscles are located in the palm of the hand and act to bring the thumb toward the fingers, allowing the grasping action of the hands.

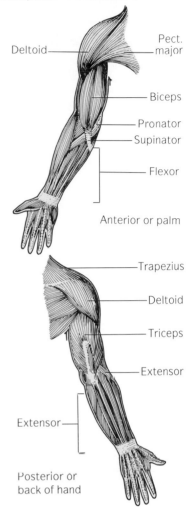

Deltoid — Pect. major

— Biceps

— Pronator
— Supinator

— Flexor

Anterior or palm

— Trapezius

— Deltoid

— Triceps

— Extensor

Extensor —

Posterior or back of hand

23.22—Muscles of the shoulders, arms, and hands.

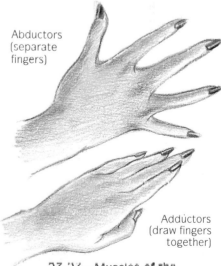

Abductors (separate fingers)

Adductors (draw fingers together)

23.23—Muscles of the hand.

The Nervous System

Neurology (nuu-**ROL**-o-jee) is the branch of anatomy that deals with the nervous system and its disorders.

The *nervous* (**NUR**-vus) *system* is one of the most important systems of the body. It controls and coordinates the functions of all the other systems and makes them work harmoniously and efficiently. Every square inch of the human body is supplied with fine fibers, which we know as *nerves.*

The main purpose in studying the nervous system are to understand:

1. How the cosmetologist administers scalp and facial services for the client's benefit.
2. What effects these treatments have on the nerves in the skin and scalp, and on the body as a whole.

DIVISIONS OF THE NERVOUS SYSTEM

The principal parts that compose the nervous system are the brain and spinal cord and their nerves. Generally, the nervous system is composed of three main divisions:

1. The *cerebro-spinal* (ser-**EE**-broh **SPEYE**-nahl), or *central,* nervous system (CNS).
2. The *peripheral* (pe-**RIF**-er-al) nervous system.
3. The *autonomic* (aw-toh-**NAHM**-ik) nervous system (ANS), which includes the sympathetic (sim-pah-**THET**-ik) and parasympathetic (**PA**-rah-sim-pah-**THET**-ik) systems.

The *central nervous system* consists of the brain and spinal cord. The following are its functions:

1. Controls consciousness and all mental activities.
2. Controls voluntary functions of the five senses: seeing, smelling, tasting, feeling, and hearing.
3. Controls voluntary muscle actions, such as all body movements and facial expressions.

The *peripheral nervous system* is made up of the sensory and motor nerve fibers that extend from the brain and spinal cord and are distributed to all parts of the body. Its function is to carry messages to and from the central nervous system.

The *autonomic nervous system* is the portion of the nervous system that functions without conscious effort and regulates the activities of the smooth muscles, glands, blood vessels, and heart. This system has two divisions: the *sympathetic and parasympathetic systems*, which act in direct opposition to each other to regulate such things as heart rate, blood pressure, breathing rate, and body temperature to aid the body in the maintenance of homeostasis (balance). The sympathetic division is primarily activated during stressful, energy-demanding, or emergency situations; the parasympathetic division is most active in ordinary restful situations.

THE BRAIN AND SPINAL CORD

The brain is the largest mass of nerve tissue in the body and is contained in the cranium. The weight of the average brain is 44 to 48 ounces (1232 to 1344 g). It is considered to be the central power station of the body, sending and receiving telegraphic messages. Twelve pairs of cranial nerves originate in the brain and reach various parts of the head, face, and neck.

The spinal cord is composed of masses of nerve cells, with fibers running upward and downward. It originates in the brain, extends the length of the trunk, and is enclosed and protected by the spinal column. Thirty-one pairs of spinal nerves, extending from the spinal cord, are distributed to the muscles and skin of the trunk and limbs. Some of the spinal nerves supply the internal organs controlled by the sympathetic nervous system. (Fig. 23.24)

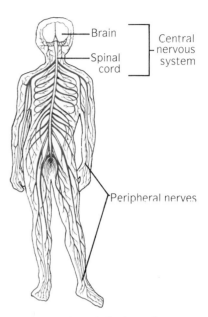

23.24—Spinal cord.

NERVE CELLS AND NERVES

A *neuron* (**NOOR**-on), or *nerve cell*, is the primary structural unit of the nervous system. (Fig. 23.25) It is composed of a cell body, *dendrites* (**DEN**-dreyets), which receive messages from other neurons, and an *axon* (**AK**-son) and *axon terminal*, which send messages to other neurons, glands, or muscles.

Nerves are long, white cords made up of fibers that carry messages to and from various parts of the body. Nerves have their origin in the brain and spinal cord, and distribute branches to all parts of the body.

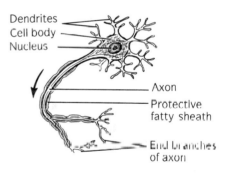

23.25—A neuron or nerve cell.

Types of Nerves

Sensory nerves, called *afferent* (**AF**-fer-ent) *nerves*, carry impulses or messages from sense organs to the brain, where sensations of touch, cold, heat, sight, hearing, taste, smell, pain, and pressure are experienced.

Motor nerves, called *efferent* (**EF**-e-rent) *nerves*, carry impulses from the brain to the muscles. The transmitted impulses produce movement.

Mixed nerves contain both sensory and motor fibers and have the ability to both send and receive messages.

Sensory nerve endings called receptors are located near the surface of the skin. As impulses pass from the sensory nerves to the brain and back over the motor nerves to the muscles, a complete circuit is established and movement of the muscles results.

A *reflex* is an automatic response to a stimulus that involves the movement of an impulse from a sensory receptor along an *afferent* nerve to the spinal cord, and a responsive impulse along an *efferent* neuron to a muscle causing a reaction. (Example: the quick removal of the hand from a hot object.) A reflex act does not have to be learned.

Nerves of the Head, Face, and Neck

The *fifth cranial, trifacial,* or *trigeminal nerve* is the largest of the cranial nerves. It is the chief sensory nerve of the face, and the motor nerve of the muscles that control chewing. It consists of three branches: *ophthalmic, mandibular,* and *maxillary.*

The following are the important branches of the fifth cranial nerve that are affected by massage. (Fig. 23.26)

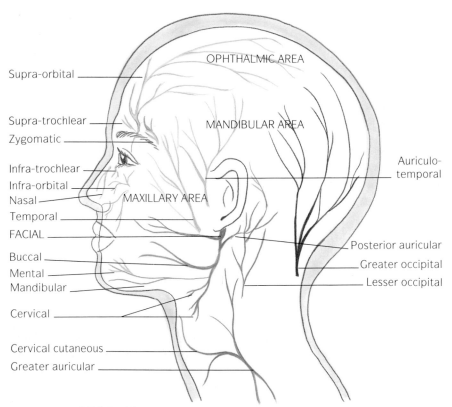

23.26—Diagram of the nerves of the head, face, and neck.

1. *Supra-orbital* (soo-prah-**OHR**-bi-tahl) *nerve* affects the skin of the forehead, scalp, eyebrow, and upper eyelid.
2. *Supra-trochlear* (soo-prah-**TROK**-lee-ahr) *nerve* affects the skin between the eyes and upper side of the nose.
3. *Infra-trochlear* (in-frah-**TROK**-lee-ar) *nerve* affects the membrane and skin of the nose.

4. *Nasal* (**NAY**-zal) *nerve* affects the point and lower side of the nose.
5. *Zygomatic* (zeye-goh-**MAT**-ik) *nerve* affects the skin of the temple, side of the forehead, and upper part of the cheek.
6. *Infra-orbital* (in-frah-**OR**-bi-tal) *nerve* affects the skin of the lower eyelid, side of the nose, upper lip, and mouth.
7. *Auriculo-temporal* (o-**RIK**-yoo-loh **TEM**-po-rahl) *nerve* affects the external ear and skin above the temple, up to the top of the skull.
8. *Mental* (**MEN**-tahl) *nerve* affects the skin of the lower lip and chin.

The *seventh (facial) cranial nerve* is the chief motor nerve of the face. It emerges near the lower part of the ear; its divisions and their branches supply and control all the muscles of facial expression, and extend to the muscles of the neck.

The following are the most important branches of the facial nerve:

1. *Posterior auricular* (po-**STEER**-i-ohr aw-**RIK**-yoo-lahr) *nerve* affects the muscles behind the ear at the base of the skull.
2. *Temporal* (**TEM**-po-rahl) *nerve* affects the muscles of the temple, side of forehead, eyebrow, eyelid, and upper part of the cheek.
3. *Zygomatic* (zeye-goh-**MAT**-ik) *nerve (upper and lower)* affects the muscles of the upper part of the cheek.
4. *Buccal* (**BUK**-ahl) *nerve* affects the muscles of the mouth.
5. *Mandibular* (man-**DIB**-yoo-lahr) *nerve* affects the muscles of the chin and lower lip.
6. *Cervical* (**SUR**-vi-kal) *nerve* (branch of the facial nerve) affects the side of the neck and the platysma muscle.

The *eleventh* (accessory) *cranial nerve* (spinal branch) affects the muscles of the neck and back.

Cervical nerves originate at the spinal cord, and their branches supply the muscles and scalp at the back of the head and neck, as follows:

1. *Greater occipital* (ok-**SIP**-i-tal) *nerve*, located in the back of the head, affects the scalp as far up as the top of the head.
2. *Smaller (lesser) occipital nerve*, located at the base of the skull, affects the scalp and muscles of this region.
3. *Greater auricular* (aw-**RIK**-yoo-lahr) *nerve*, located at the side of the neck, affects the external ear, and the area in front and back of the ear.

4. *Cervical cutaneous* (kyoo-**TAY**-nee-us), or *cutaneous colli* (**CO**-li) *nerve*, located at the side of the neck, affects the front and side of the neck as far down as the breastbone.

Nerves of the Arm and Hand

The principal nerves supplying the superficial parts of the arm and hand are as follows. (Fig. 23.27)

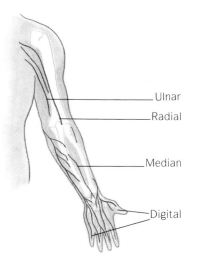

1. The *ulnar* (**UL**-nar) *nerve* (sensory-motor) with its branches, supplies the little finger side of the arm and the palm of the hand.
2. The *radial* (**RAY**-dee-al) *nerve* (sensory-motor) with its branches, supplies the thumb side of the arm and the back of the hand.
3. The *median* (**MEE**-di-an) *nerve* (sensory-motor), a smaller nerve than the ulnar and radial nerves. With its branches, supplies the arm and hand.
4. The *digital* (**DIJ**-it-tal) *nerve* (sensory-motor) with its branches, supplies all fingers of the hand.

23.27—Nerves of the arm and hand.

The Circulatory System

The *circulatory* (**SUR**-kyoo-lah-tohr-ee), or *vascular* (**VAS**-kyoo-lahr), *system* is vitally related to the maintenance of good health. The vascular system controls the steady circulation of the blood through the body by means of the *heart* and the blood vessels (the *arteries* [**AHR**-te-rees], *veins*, and *capillaries* [**KAP**-i-lar-ees]).

The vascular system is made up of two divisions:

1. The *blood-vascular* (**BLUD VAS**-kyoo-lahr) *system* consists of the heart and blood vessels (arteries, capillaries, and veins) for the circulation of the blood.
2. The *lymph-vascular* (**LIMF VAS**-kyoo-lahr), or *lymphatic* (lim-**FAT**-ik) *system* consists of lymph glands and vessels through which the lymph circulates.

These two systems are intimately linked with each other. Lymph is derived from the blood and is gradually shifted back into the bloodstream.

THE HEART

The heart is a muscular, conical-shaped organ, about the size of a closed fist. It is located in the chest cavity, and is enclosed in a membrane, the *pericardium* (per-i-**KAHR**-dee-um). It is an efficient pump that keeps the blood moving within the circulatory system. (Fig. 23.28) At the normal resting rate, the heart beats about 72 to 80 times a minute. The *vagus* (tenth cranial nerve) and nerves from the *autonomic nervous system* regulate the heartbeat.

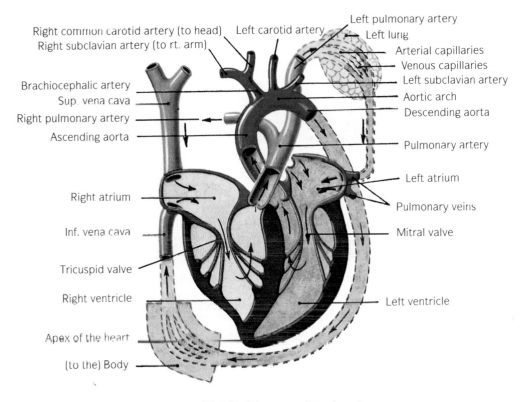

Right common carotid artery (to head)
Right subclavian artery (to rt. arm)
Brachiocephalic artery
Sup. vena cava
Right pulmonary artery
Ascending aorta
Right atrium
Inf. vena cava
Tricuspid valve
Right ventricle
Apex of the heart
(to the) Body

Left carotid artery
Left pulmonary artery
Left lung
Arterial capillaries
Venous capillaries
Left subclavian artery
Aortic arch
Descending aorta
Pulmonary artery
Left atrium
Pulmonary veins
Mitral valve
Left ventricle

23.28—Diagram of the heart.

The interior of the heart contains four chambers and four valves. The upper thin-walled chambers are the *right atrium* (**AY**-tree-um) and *left atrium*. The lower thick-walled chambers are the *right ventricle* (**VEN**-tri-kel) and *left ventricle*. *Valves* allow the blood to flow in only one direction. With each contraction and relaxation of the heart, the blood flows in, travels from the *atria* (**AY**-tri-a) to the ventricles, and is then driven out, to be distributed all over the body. The atrium is also called the *auricle* (**OR**-ik-kel).

BLOOD VESSELS

The arteries, capillaries, and veins are tube-like in construction. They transport blood to and from the heart and to various tissues of the body.

Arteries are thick-walled muscular and elastic tubes that carry pure blood from the heart to the capillaries.

Capillaries are minute, thin-walled blood vessels that connect the smaller arteries to the veins. Through their walls, the tissues receive nourishment and eliminate waste products.

Veins are thin-walled blood vessels that are less elastic than arteries. They contain cup-like valves to prevent back flow, and carry impure blood from the various capillaries back to the heart. Veins are located closer to the outer surface of the body than arteries. (Fig. 23.29)

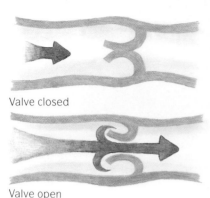

Valve closed

Valve open

23.29—Cross sections of veins.

THE BLOOD

Blood is the nutritive fluid circulating through the circulatory system. It is a sticky, salty fluid with a normal temperature of 98.6° Fahrenheit (37° Celsius), and it makes up about one-twentieth of the weight of the body. Approximately 8 to 10 pints (3.76 to 4.7 l) of blood fill the blood vessels of an adult. Blood is bright red in color in the arteries (except in the pulmonary artery) and dark red in the veins (except in the pulmonary vein). This change in color is due to the exchange of carbon dioxide for oxygen as the blood passes through the lungs and the exchange of oxygen for carbon dioxide as the blood circulates throughout the body.

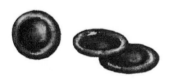

23.30—Red corpuscles.

Circulation of the Blood

The blood is in constant circulation from the moment it leaves until it returns to the heart. There are two systems that take care of this circulation:

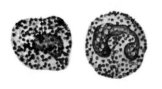

23.31—White corpuscles.

1. *Pulmonary* (**PUUL**-mo-ner-ee) *circulation* is the blood circulation that goes from the heart to the lungs to be purified.
2. *Systemic* or *general circulation* is the blood circulation from the heart throughout the body and back again to the heart.

Composition of the Blood

The blood is composed of red and white corpuscles, platelets, plasma. (Figs. 23.30–23.32)

The function of *red corpuscles* (red blood cells) is to carry oxygen to the cells. *White corpuscles* (white blood cells), or *leucocytes* (**LOO**-ko-seyets), perform the function of destroying disease-causing germs.

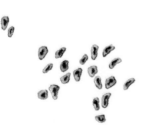

23.32—Platelets.

Blood platelets are much smaller than the red blood cells. They play an important part in the clotting of the blood.

Plasma is the fluid part of the blood in which the red and white blood cells and blood platelets flow. It is straw-like in color. About nine-tenths of plasma is water. It carries food and secretions to the cells and carbon dioxide from the cells.

Chief Functions of the Blood

The following are the primary functions of the blood:

1. Carries water, oxygen, food, and secretions to all cells of the body.
2. Carries away carbon dioxide and waste products to be eliminated through the lungs, skin, kidneys, and large intestine.
3. Helps to equalize the body temperature, thus protecting the body from extreme heat and cold.
4. Aids in protecting the body from harmful bacteria and infections, through the action of the white blood cells.
5. Clots the blood, thereby closing injured minute blood vessels and preventing the loss of blood.

THE LYMPH-VASCULAR SYSTEM

The *lymph-vascular* (**LIMF-VAS**-kyoo-lahr) *system*, also called *lymphatic system*, acts as an aid to the blood system, and consists of lymph spaces, lymph vessels, lymph glands, and *lacteals* (**LAK**-teels).

Lymph is a colorless, watery fluid that is derived from the plasma of the blood, mainly by filtration through the capillary walls into the tissue spaces. By bathing all cells, the tissue fluid acts as a medium of exchange, trading its nutritive materials to the cells in return for the waste products of metabolism. This fluid is absorbed into the lymphatics or lymph capillaries to become lymph and is then filtered and detoxified as it passes through the lymph nodes and is eventually reintroduced into the blood circulation.

The following are the primary functions of lymph:

1. Reaches the parts of the body not reached by blood and carries on an interchange with the blood.
2. Carries nourishment from the blood to the body cells.
3. Acts as a bodily defense against invading bacteria and toxins.
4. Removes waste material from the body cells to the blood.
5. Provides a suitable fluid environment for the cells.

ARTERIES OF THE HEAD, FACE, AND NECK

The *common carotid* (kah-**ROT**-id) *arteries* are the main sources of blood supply to the head, face, and neck. They are located on either side of the neck and divide into internal and external carotid arteries. The *internal division* of the common carotid artery supplies the brain, eye sockets, eyelids, and forehead, while the *external division* supplies the superficial parts of the head, face, and neck. (Fig. 23.33)

The external carotid artery subdivides into a number of branches, which supply blood to various regions of the head, face, and neck. Of particular interest to the cosmetologist are the following arteries:

Facial artery (external maxillary) (**MAK**-si-ler-ee) supplies blood to the lower region of the face, mouth, and nose. Some of its branches are:

1. *Submental* (sub-**MEN**-tahl) *artery* supplies the chin and lower lip.
2. *Inferior labial* (**LAY**-bi-al) *artery* supplies the lower lip.
3. *Angular* (**ANG**-gew-lur) *artery* supplies the side of the nose.
4. *Superior labial artery* supplies the upper lip, septum, and wing of the nose.

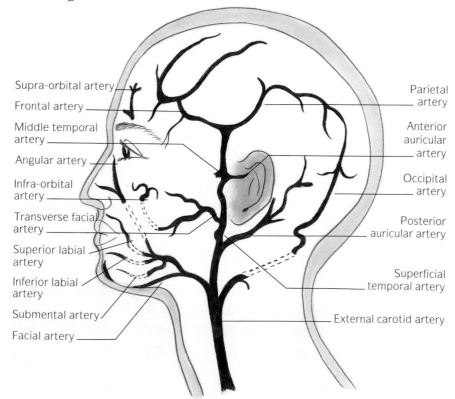

Supra-orbital artery
Frontal artery
Middle temporal artery
Angular artery
Infra-orbital artery
Transverse facial artery
Superior labial artery
Inferior labial artery
Submental artery
Facial artery

Parietal artery
Anterior auricular artery
Occipital artery
Posterior auricular artery
Superficial temporal artery
External carotid artery

23.33—Diagram of the arteries of the head, face, and neck.

Superficial temporal (**TEM**-po-rahl) *artery* is a continuation of the external carotid artery, which supplies muscles, skin, and scalp to the front, side, and top of the head. Some of its important branches are:

1. *Frontal* (**FRUNT**-al) *artery* supplies the forehead.
2. *Parietal* (pa-**REYE**-e-tal) *artery* supplies the crown and side of the head.
3. *Transverse* (trans-**VURS**) *facial artery* supplies the masseter.
4. *Middle temporal* (**TEM**-po-rahl) *artery* supplies the temples.
5. *Anterior auricular* (aw-**RIK**-yoo-lahr) *artery* supplies the anterior part of the ear.

The *supra-orbital* (soo-prah-**OHR**-bi-tal) *artery*, a branch of the internal carotid artery, supplies part of the forehead, the eye socket, eyelid, and upper muscles of the eye.

Infra-orbital (in-frah-**OR**-bi-tal) *artery* originates from the internal maxillary artery, and it supplies the muscles of the eye.

Occipital (ok-**SIP**-i-tal) *artery* supplies the back of the head, up to the crown.

Posterior auricular (aw-**RIK**-yoo-lahr) *artery* supplies the scalp, the area back and above the ear, and the skin behind the ear.

VEINS OF THE HEAD, FACE, AND NECK

The blood returning to the heart from the head, face, and neck flows on each side of the neck in two principal veins: the *internal jugular* and *external jugular*. The most important veins of the face and neck are parallel to the arteries and take the same names as the arteries.

BLOOD SUPPLY FOR THE ARM AND HAND

The *ulnar* and *radial* arteries are the main blood supply for the arm and hand. (Fig. 23.34)

The ulnar artery and its numerous branches supply the little finger side of the arm and the palm of the hand.

The radial artery and its branches supply the thumb side of the arm and the back of the hand.

The important veins are located almost parallel with the arteries and take the same names as the arteries. While the arteries are found deep in the tissues, the veins lie nearer to the surface of the arms and hands.

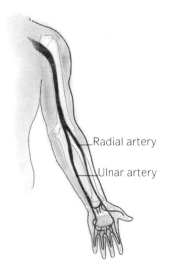

Radial artery

Ulnar artery

23.34—Arteries of the hand and arm.

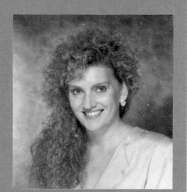

Camouflage makeup or clinical cosmetology is an exciting new field opening up to cosmetologists. Incorporating medicine with cosmetology, this field proves to be intellectually stimulating as well as personally and financially rewarding.

Nancy Dugan is director of esthetics for the Plastic Surgery Center of Montclair, New Jersey, and camouflage makeup instructor for the Esthetic Research Group. She says that many dermatologists and plastic surgeons are working with cosmetologists on a referral system and even hiring esthetic personnel for their offices.

Services and benefits to patients are numerous, including pre-operative skin care treatments and home care programs. These are designed to clarify and soften dry, dehydrated, flaking, and impure skin. Post-operative treatments benefit the healing process, reduce swelling, bruising, and some post-operative discomfort.

To become a clinical cosmetologist, you need a license to practice cosmetology, followed up with private or seminar instruction in skin care and illusionary makeup techniques. These classes may be titled Stage Makeup or Camouflage Makeup and are held at either advanced schools or through manufacturers. You will learn the relationship of light to shadow, color matching, the effect of light on color, and other illusionary techniques that you can practice on your everyday clients to conceal undereye circles, puffiness, small scars, shadows, and over- or under-pigmented areas on the skin.

Your success will depend on how much research you do, how often you practice, and how well you keep up on developments in plastic surgery, patient psychology, and related product and treatment developments.

In addition to treating elective plastic surgery patients, you will help those with vitiligo (loss of pigment), burn victims, and patients undergoing reconstructive surgery following accidents or cancer treatments.

According to Dugan, it's a great way for beauty professionals to use their skills on the people who need them the most.

Endocrine System

Glands are specialized organs that vary in size and function. The blood and nerves are intimately connected with the glands. The nervous system controls the functional activities of the glands. The glands have the ability to take certain elements from the blood and convert them into new compounds.

There are two main sets of glands:

1. One group is called the *exocrine*, or *duct glands*, with canals that lead from the gland to a particular part of the body. Sweat and oil glands of the skin and intestinal glands belong to this group.

2. The other group, known as *endocrine*, or *ductless glands*, have secretions called hormones delivered directly into the bloodstream, which in turn influences the welfare of the entire body.

The Excretory System

The *excretory* (**EK**-skre-tohr-ee) *system*, including the kidneys, liver, skin, intestines, and lungs, purifies the body by eliminating waste matter.

Each of the following plays a part in the excretory system:

1. The *kidneys* excrete urine.
2. The *liver* discharges bile.
3. The *skin* eliminates perspiration.
4. The *large intestine* evacuates decomposed and undigested food.
5. The *lungs* exhale carbon dioxide.

Metabolism of the cells of the body forms various toxic substances which, if retained, might poison the body.

The Respiratory System

The *respiratory* (**RES**-pi-rah-tohr-ee) *system* is situated within the chest cavity, which is protected on both sides by the ribs. The *diaphragm* (**DI**-a-fram), a muscular partition that controls breathing, separates the chest from the *abdominal* (ab-**DOM**-i-nal) region.

The *lungs* are spongy tissues composed of microscopic cells which take in air. These tiny air cells are enclosed in a skin-like tissue. Behind this, the fine capillaries of the vascular system are found.

With each respiratory, or breathing cycle, an exchange of gases takes place. During *inhalation* (in-ha-**LAY**-shon), oxygen is absorbed into the blood, while carbon dioxide is expelled during *exhalation* (eks-ha-**LAY**-shun). Oxygen is more essential than either food or water. Although a man or woman may live more than 60 days without food, and a few days without water, if they are deprived of oxygen, they will die in a few minutes.

Nose breathing is healthier than mouth breathing because the air is warmed by the surface capillaries, and the bacteria in the air are caught by the hairs that line the mucous (**MYOO**-kus) membranes of the nasal passages.

The rate of breathing depends on the activity of the individual. Muscular activities and energy expenditures increase the body's demands for oxygen. As a result, the rate of breathing is increased. A person requires about three times more oxygen when walking than when standing.

The Digestive System

Digestion (di-**JES**-chun) is the process of converting food into a form that can be assimilated by the body. The *digestive* (deye-**GES**-tiv) *system* changes food into *soluble* (**SOL**-yu-bel) form, suitable for use by the cells of the body. Digestion begins in the mouth and is completed in the small intestine. From the mouth, the food passes down the *pharynx* (**FAR**-ingks) and the *esophagus* (i-**SOF**-a-gus), or food pipe, and into the stomach. The food is completely digested in the stomach and small intestine and is assimilated or absorbed into the bloodstream. The large intestine (colon) stores the refuse for elimination through the rectum. The complete digestive process of food takes about nine hours.

Responsible for the chemical changes in food are the *enzymes* (**EN**-zeyems) present in the digestive secretions. *Digestive enzymes* are chemicals that change certain kinds of food into a form capable of being used by the body. Intense emotions, excitement, and fatigue seriously disturb digestion. On the other hand, happiness and relaxation promote good digestion.

Review Questions

CELLS, ANATOMY, AND PHYSIOLOGY

1. What are the functions of human cells?
2. How do cells grow?
3. What is metabolism?
4. What are the functions of organs?
5. What are systems?
6. What is anatomy?
7. What is physiology?
8. What is histology?
9. What are the primary functions of the bones?
10. What is the structure of the muscular system and what is its function?
11. Give two reasons why the cosmetologist should study the nervous system.
12. What is the function of the heart?
13. What is the composition of blood?
14. What is lymph?
15. What are the two types of glands in the endocrine system?
16. Name the five important organs of the excretory system.
17. Describe a respiratory cycle.
18. What is the function of the digestive system?

24

ELECTRICITY AND LIGHT THERAPY

LEARNING OBJECTIVES

After completing this chapter, you should be able to:

1. Define the nature of electricity and name two forms of electricity.

2. Demonstrate the proper use of the different types of electricity.

3. Define the four types of current and explain the benefits derived from the various currents.

4. List and describe electrical appliances available for use in the salon.

5. Explain the safety precautions that must be followed when using electricity.

6. Explain light therapy.

7. Demonstrate the proper uses of light therapy.

Electricity

The beneficial effects of electricity have long been recognized to be valuable to the cosmetology profession. When used intelligently and safely, electricity can be a valuable tool. It supplies light and heat, operates appliances, and is essential to the operation of a modern salon.

Electricity is a form of energy that produces *magnetic, chemical,* and *heat* effects. There are some basic terms that you should learn and some that you may already be familiar with. An *electric current* is the movement of electricity along a conductor.

A *conductor* is a substance that permits electric current to pass through it easily. Metals like copper, silver, and aluminum are good conductors of electricity as are carbon, wet cotton, the human body, and water solutions of acids and salts. A *nonconductor* or *insulator* is a substance that resists the passage of an electric current, such as rubber, silk, dry wood, glass, cement, or asbestos. An *electric wire* is composed of twisted fine metal threads (conductor) covered with rubber or silk (insulator or nonconductor).

Using Electricity

There are two types of electricity:

1. *Direct current* (DC) is a constant, even-flowing current, traveling in one direction. This current produces a chemical reaction. A battery-operated instrument such as a portable radio or a flashlight uses direct current.
2. *Alternating current* (AC) is a rapid and interrupted current, flowing first in one direction and then in the opposite direction. This current produces a mechanical action. When you plug an appliance, such as a hair dryer, into a wall socket you are using an alternating current.

If necessary, one type of current can be changed to the other type by means of a converter or rectifier. A *converter* is used to change direct current into alternating current. A *rectifier* is used to change alternating current to direct current.

A *complete circuit of electricity* is the path traveled by the current from its generating source through the conductors (wire, electrode, or body) and back to its original source.

ELECTRICAL MEASUREMENTS

Electrical measurements are expressed in terms of the following units:

A *volt* (V) is a unit for measuring the pressure that forces the electric current forward. A higher voltage increases the strength of the current. If the voltage is lower, the current is weaker.

An *amp* (A), short for *ampere* (**AM**-peer), is the unit of measurement for the amount of current running through a wire. A cord must be heavy duty enough to handle the amps put out by the appliance. For example, an appliance that puts out 40 amps of current requires a cord that is thicker than the one for an appliance that puts out 20 amps of current. If the current—or number of amps—is too strong, your appliances can overheat or the wires can even burn out. If the current is not strong enough, your appliance will not operate at full strength or might not operate at all.

A *milliampere* (mil-i-**AM**-peer), is 1/1000th part of an ampere. The current for facial and scalp treatments is measured in milliamperes by a milliamperemeter (mil-i-**AM**-peer-**MEE**-ter); an ampere current would be much too strong.

An *ohm* (O) is a unit for measuring the resistance of an electric current. Unless the force (volts) is stronger than the resistance (ohms), current will not flow through the wire.

A *watt* (W) is a measurement of how much electric energy is being used in one second. A 40-watt bulb uses 40 watts of energy per second.

A *kilowatt* (K) equals 1000 watts. The electricity in your house is measured in kilowatt hours (kwh).

SAFETY DEVICES

A *fuse* is a safety device that prevents the overheating of electric wires. It blows out or melts when the wire becomes too hot from overloading the circuit with too much current from too many appliances or if faulty equipment is used. To reestablish the circuit, you must disconnect the appliance and insert a new fuse.

The *circuit breaker* has largely replaced the fuse in modern electric wiring. This device has all the safety features offered by the fuse and does not require replacement every time it shuts off. It is a switch device that automatically shuts down at the first indication of overheating or circuit trouble. When the problem is corrected the switch is simply reset and all the safety factors are restored.

CAUTION

▶ *If, after resetting the circuit breaker, it continues to shut down, call in a licensed electrician to check for further problems.*

Safety of Electrical Equipment

The protection and safety of the client is the primary concern of the cosmetologist. All electrical equipment should be inspected regularly to determine whether or not it is in safe working condition. If you are careless when making electrical connections or if you do not check that you use the right amount of current, a shock or a burn can result. Observing safety precautions helps to eliminate accidents and ensure greater satisfaction to the client. (Figs. 24.1–24.4) Here is a list of useful hints about using electricity:

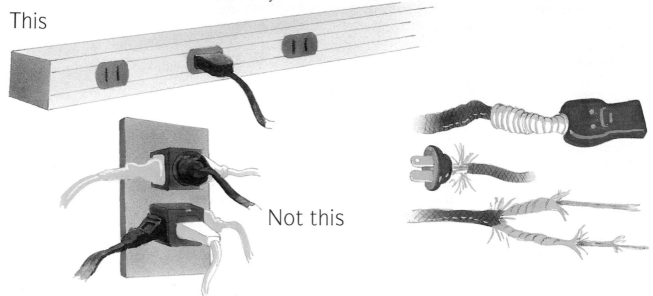

This

Not this

24.1 – Use only one plug to each outlet. Overloading, as in illustration on the right, may cause fuse to blow out.

24.2 – Examine cords regularly.

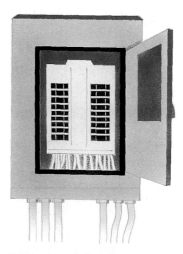

24.3 – Carefully replace blown-out fuses.

24.4 – Circuit breakers automatically disconnect any current of a defective appliance.

1. Study the instructions before using any electrical equipment.
2. Disconnect appliances when you have finished using them.
3. Keep all wires, plugs, and equipment in good repair.
4. Inspect all electrical equipment frequently.
5. Avoid wetting electrical cords.
6. When using electrical equipment, protect the client at all times.
7. Do not touch any metal while using an electrical appliance.
8. Do not handle electrical equipment with wet hands.
9. Do not allow the client to touch any metal surfaces while being treated with electrical equipment.
10. Do not leave the room when your client is connected to an electrical device.
11. Do not attempt to clean around an electric outlet while equipment is plugged in.
12. Do not touch two metallic objects at the same time if either is connected to an electric current.
13. Do not step on or set objects on electrical cords.
14. Do not allow electrical cords to become twisted or bent; the fine wires inside the cord will break and the insulation will wear away from the wires.
15. Disconnect the appliance by pulling on the plug, not the cord.
16. Do not repair electrical appliances unless you are qualified to do so.

Electrotherapy

A *wall plate* (facial stimulator) is an instrument that, when plugged into an ordinary socket, can produce particular currents used for electronic facial treatments. An electronic facial treatment is called *electrotherapy*. These currents are referred to as *modalities*. Each produces a different effect on the skin. There are many types of modalities, but cosmetologists are concerned with only the *galvanic* (gal-**VAN**-ik), *sinusoidal* (si-nu-**SOID**-al), *faradic* (fa-**RAD**-ik), and the *Tesla high-frequency* (**TES**-lah hi-**FREE**-kwen-see). Some wall plates have all four currents and some have only the galvanic current.

An *electrode* is an apparatus that conducts the electric current from the machine to the client's skin. It is usually made of carbon, glass, or metal. Each of the modalities requires two electrodes (one negative and one positive) to conduct the flow of electricity through the body, except the Tesla high-frequency.

MODALITIES

Polarity

Before discussing the various modalities, it will be useful to discuss the test for polarity. *Polarity* is the negative or positive state of electric current. Electrotherapy equipment has a negatively charged pole and a positively charged pole. If the electrodes are not marked with negative or positive indicators, a simple test will tell you which is which.

1. Separate the tips of two conducting cords from each other and immerse them into a glass of saltwater. Turn the selector switch of the appliance to galvanic current, and then turn up the intensity. As the water is decomposed, more active bubbles will accumulate at the negative pole than at the positive pole.

2. Place the tips of two conducting cords on two separate pieces of blue moistened litmus paper. The paper under the positive pole will turn red, while the paper under the negative pole will stay blue. If you use red litmus instead of blue, the positive pole will keep the red litmus the same and the negative pole will turn the red litmus blue.

CAUTION

▶ *Do not let the tips of the cords touch or you will cause a short circuit.*

Galvanic Current

The most commonly used modality is the *galvanic* current. It is a constant and direct current (DC), reduced to a safe, low-voltage level. Chemical changes are produced when this current is used. Galvanic current produces two different chemical reactions depending on the polarity (negative or positive) used on the area treated. A positive electrode is called an *anode,* is red, and is marked with a "P" or a plus (+) sign. A negative electrode is called a *cathode,* is black, and is marked with an "N" or a minus (−) sign.

The positive pole:

Produces acidic reactions
Closes the pores
Soothes nerves
Decreases blood supply
Contracts blood vessels
Hardens (firms) tissues
Forces alkaline solutions into the skin

The negative pole:

Produces alkaline reactions

Opens the pores

Stimulates (irritates) the nerves

Increases the blood supply to the skin

Expands the blood vessels

Softens tissues

Softens and liquifies grease deposits in the hair follicles and
   pores

Note that the effects to the body of the positive pole are just
the opposite of those produced by the negative pole.

CAUTION

▶ *Do not use the negative galvanic current on skin with broken
capillaries, pustular acne conditions, or on a client with high
blood pressure or metal implants.*

The effects of the galvanic current are experienced by your
client as the current passes through the body from one electrode
to the other and completes a circuit. Both the active and inactive
(positive and negative) poles must be functioning to complete the
circuit. Both the active and inactive carbon (ball and cylinder) electrodes must be lightly wrapped with a moistened cotton pledget.

The ***active electrode*** is the electrode used on the area to be
treated. For instance, if negative reactions (e.g., opened pores,
softened tissue) are desired on the face, the negative pole is the
active electrode. Apply the carbon ball or carbon roller to the
active electrode.

The ***inactive electrode*** is the opposite pole from the active electrode. Either your client can hold the carbon stick (inactive electrode) wrapped in a moistened cotton pledget or you can place
the wet pad somewhere on the client's body.

Procedure to Close Pores

1. Wrap the carbon ball electrode (active) in cotton
    moisturized with astringent.
2. Wrap the cylinder electrode (inactive) in cotton moisturized
    with water.
3. Have the client hold the inactive electrode or place the wet
    pad on a comfortable spot on the client's body.
4. After a good contact is established with the two electrodes,
    slowly turn up the current to the desired strength.
5. When the treatment is completed, slowly turn down the
    current before breaking contact with the client.

Phoresis

The process by which chemical solutions are forced into the unbroken skin using a galvanic current is called *phoresis* (foh-**REE**-sis). *Cataphoresis* (KAT-ah-fo-**REE**-sis) is the use of the positive pole to pull a positively charged substance (an acid pH astringent solution) into the skin. *Anaphoresis* (**AN**-o-foh-**REE**-sis) is the use of the negative pole to force, or push, a negatively charged substance (an alkaline pH solution) into the skin. *Disincrustation* is a process used to soften and liquify grease deposits (oil) in the hair follicles and pores. This process is used frequently to treat acne, milia, and comedones.

Faradic Current

The *faradic* current is an alternating and interrupted current that produces a mechanical reaction without a chemical effect. The faradic current is used during scalp and facial manipulations to cause muscular contractions that tone the facial muscles. In some states it is illegal to cause visible muscle contractions with the faradic or sinusoidal currents.

Benefits derived from the use of the faradic current include:

1. Improves muscle tone.
2. Promotes removal of waste products.
3. Increases circulation of the blood.
4. Relieves congested blood.
5. Increases glandular activity.
6. Stimulates hair growth.
7. Increases metabolism.

Sinusoidal Current

The *sinusoidal* current is similar to the faradic current and is used also during scalp and facial manipulations. It is an alternating current that produces mechanical contractions that tone the muscles. The manner of application is the same as that for the faradic current.

The sinusoidal current has the following advantages:

1. It supplies greater stimulation, deeper penetration, and is less irritating than the faradic current.
2. It soothes the nerves and penetrates into the deeper muscle tissue.
3. It is best suited for the nervous client.

Caution When Using Faradic and Sinusoidal Currents

Do not use the faradic current if it causes pain or discomfort, if the face is very florid, or if your client has any of the following: many gold-filled teeth, high blood pressure, broken capillaries, or pustular conditions of the skin. The faradic and sinusoidal currents are never used longer than 15 to 20 minutes.

Application of Faradic and Sinusoidal Current

Two electrodes (one negative and one positive) are required to complete the faradic or sinusoidal circuit.

Indirect method. In the indirect method, you wear a wrist electrode covered with a moistened pad while your client holds the carbon stick electrode wrapped in damp absorbent cotton, or you can place the wet pad on the client's body. Before turning on the current, establish contact with the client's forehead. During treatment, use your fingertips to perform the massage movements. When you have completed the treatment, slowly turn down the current before breaking contact with your client.

Direct method. In the direct method of applying the faradic and sinusoidal currents, two felt-tipped electrodes are used. The cosmetologist should move the two electrodes around the face in circular movements without allowing them to touch. The circuit is completed between the two felt disks.

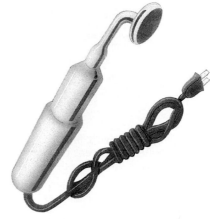

24.5—Facial electrode using Tesla current.

High-Frequency Current

The *high-frequency (Tesla)* current is characterized by a high rate of oscillation, or vibration. It is commonly called the *violet ray*, and is used for both scalp and facial treatments. The Tesla current may be used to treat thinning hair, itchy scalp, and excessively oily or dry skin and scalp. The primary action of this current is thermal or heat producing. Because of its rapid vibration, there are no muscular contractions. The physiological effects are either stimulating or soothing, depending on the method of application.

The electrodes for high-frequency current are made of glass or metal, and you only need one electrode to perform a service. The facial electrode is flat, and the scalp electrode is rake shaped. As the current passes through the glass electrode, tiny violet sparks are emitted. Some units use a neon gas in the tube, which produces an orange glow. Both units produce the same effects. All treatments given with high-frequency current should start with a mild current and gradually increase to the required strength. The length of the treatment depends on the condition to be treated. Allow about 5 minutes for a general facial or scalp treatment. (Figs. 24.5–24.7)

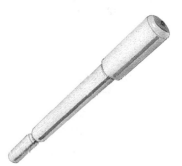

24.6—Metal electrode attachment for Tesla current.

▶ **NOTE:** For proper use, follow the instructions provided by the manufacturer of Tesla equipment.

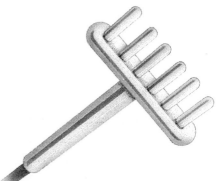

24.7—Scalp electrode attachment for Tesla current.

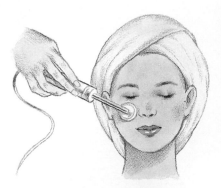

24.8—Applying high-frequency current to face using facial electrode.

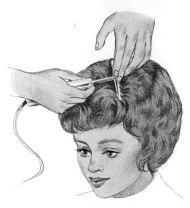

24.9—Applying high-frequency current to scalp using rake electrode.

Application of High-Frequency Current

There are three methods for using the Tesla current:

1. ***Direct surface application.*** Apply a nonalcohol, noncombustible facial cream to the client's face. The cosmetologist holds the electrode and applies it directly to the client's skin. To obtain a stimulating effect, lift the electrode slightly from the area to be treated and apply the current through gauze or a towel. The direct method is more drying to the skin and is recommended for acne-prone and oily skin. When you apply and remove the electrode from the skin, you must hold your finger on the electrode to prevent shock. Remove your finger once the electrode has been placed on the skin. (Figs. 24.8, 24.9)

2. ***Indirect application.*** The client holds the electrode while you use your fingers to massage the surface being treated. At no time do you hold the electrode. To prevent shock, turn on the current after the client has firmly grasped the electrode. Turn the current off before you remove the electrode from the client's hand.

CAUTION

▶ *The client should avoid any contact with metal, such as chair arms and stools. A burn may occur if such contact is made.*

3. ***General electrification.*** Place the electrode in the client's hand and turn on the unit. The client's body will be charged with a small amount of electricity.

Benefits derived from the use of Tesla high-frequency current are as follows:

1. Stimulates circulation of the blood.
2. Increases glandular activity.
3. Aids in elimination and absorption.
4. Increases metabolism.
5. Germicidal action occurs during use.
6. Relieves congestion.

CAUTION

▶ *High-frequency current should not be used with clients who are pregnant, epileptic, asthmatic, who have high blood pressure, excessive fillings in the teeth, sinus blockage, a pacemaker, or metal implants.*

Other Electrical Equipment

The *vibrator* is an electrical appliance used in massage to produce a mechanical succession of manipulations. It has a stimulating effect on the muscular tissues, increases the blood supply to the areas treated, is soothing to the nerves, and increases glandular activities.

By attaching the vibrator to the back of the hand the vibrations are transmitted through the hand or fingers to the areas being treated. The vibrator is used over heavy muscular tissue, such as the scalp, shoulders, and upper back. It is never used on a woman's face, but can be used on a man's face.

CAUTION

▶ *The vibrator should never be used when there is heart disease or when fever, abscesses, or inflammation are present.*

The *steamer*, or *vaporizer*, is applied over the head or face to produce a moist, uniform heat. The steamer may be used instead of hot towels to cleanse and steam the face. The steam warms the skin, inducing the flow of both oil and sweat. It thus helps to cleanse the skin, clean out the pores, and soften any scaliness on the surface of the skin.

The steamer also may be used for scalp and hair conditioning treatments. When fitted over the scalp, it produces controlled moist heat. Its action is to soften the scalp, increase perspiration, and promote the effectiveness of applied scalp cosmetics. Another use for the steamer is to speed up the action of a lightener.

Electrically heated curling irons come in various types and sizes. They have built-in heating elements and operate from electric outlets. One type has perforations. Oil is injected into the barrel of the curling irons where it is vaporized. The vapor is released through small perforations in the irons and conditions the hair as it curls.

Heating caps are electrical devices, which, when placed on the head, provide a uniform source of heat. Their main use is as part of corrective treatments for the hair and scalp. They recondition dry, brittle, and damaged hair, and also serve to activate a sluggish scalp.

The *processing machine*, or *accelerating machine*, has been designed as an aid to the professional hair colorist. Its function is to reduce the processing time for lightening and tinting the hair. The machine accelerates the molecular movement of the chemicals in the color so that they work much faster.

Accelerating machines may be used efficiently and successfully for various hair coloring treatments, such as hair lightening, tinting, frosting, tipping, streaking, and stripping. Accelerating machines must not be used with powdered lighteners.

The *electric chair hair dryer* delivers hot, medium, or cold air for the proper drying of the hair. It consists of an adjustable hood, or helmet, with deflectors that distribute the air evenly, and is capable of drying heavy hair in a relatively short time. The *hand dryer* also delivers hot, medium, and cold air.

The *small electric oil heater* is used to heat oil and to keep the oil warm when giving an oil manicure.

Light Therapy

Light therapy refers to skin treatment using light rays. The sun is the basic source of light rays. In salon work we are concerned with the white rays of the visible spectrum which make up 12% of natural sunlight and the invisible infrared and ultra violet rays, which respectively make up 80% and 8% of natural sunlight. The infrared rays produce heat, and the ultra violet rays produce chemical and germicidal reactions. When the white light of the visible spectrum is passed through a prism, it produces the colors of the rainbow: red, orange, yellow, green, blue, indigo, and violet. These colors are referred to as the visible spectrum. (Fig. 24.10) We are concerned with the white, blue, and red lights. Each of these produces a different effect on the skin.

HOW LIGHT RAYS ARE REPRODUCED

Artificial light rays are produced by using an electrical apparatus called a *therapeutic* (ther-a-**PYOO**-tik) *lamp*. These lamps or bulbs are capable of producing the same rays that are originated by the sun. The lamp used to reproduce these light rays is usually a dome-shaped reflector mounted on a pedestal with a flexible neck. The dome usually has a highly polished metal lining capable of reflecting the rays from the different types of light.

PROTECTING THE EYES

The client's eyes always should be protected during any light ray treatment. Use cotton pads saturated with boric acid solution, witch hazel, or distilled water. The eyepads protect the eyes from the glare of the reflecting rays.

CAUTION

▶ *The cosmetologist and the client always should wear safety goggles when using ultra violet rays to avoid damage to the eyes.*

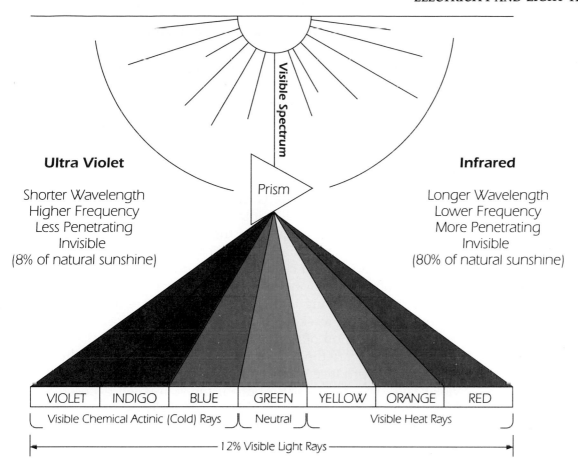

| VIOLET | INDIGO | BLUE | GREEN | YELLOW | ORANGE | RED |

Ultra Violet

Shorter Wavelength
Higher Frequency
Less Penetrating
Invisible
(8% of natural sunshine)

Visible Spectrum

Prism

Infrared

Longer Wavelength
Lower Frequency
More Penetrating
Invisible
(80% of natural sunshine)

Visible Chemical Actinic (Cold) Rays   Neutral   Visible Heat Rays

— 12% Visible Light Rays —

INFRARED RAYS

Infrared rays are located beyond the visible red rays of the spectrum. Infrared rays are long, have the greatest (deepest) penetration, and can produce the most heat. The infrared lamp is red and produces a reddish glow when turned on. Infrared lamps can also be white.

The lamp should be operated at an average distance of 30″ (76.2 cm). Check the comfort of your client frequently.

CAUTION

▶ *NEVER leave your client unattended during the exposure time. The exposure time should be about 5 minutes.*

Use and Effects of Infrared Ray Treatment

1. Heats and relaxes the skin without increasing the temperature of the body as a whole.
2. Dilates blood vessels in the skin, thereby increasing the blood circulation.
3. Increases metabolism and chemical changes within the skin tissues.

4.   Increases the production of perspiration and oil on the skin.

5.   Relieves pain in sore muscles because of the ray's deep penetration.

6.   Is soothing to the nerves.

ULTRA VIOLET RAYS

Ultra violet rays are located beyond the visible spectrum. They are the shortest and least penetrating of the light rays. The ultra violet ray is also referred to as the *cold ray* or *actinic ray*. Ultra violet (UV) rays are divided into three categories: UVA, UVB, and UVC. The farther away from the visible light spectrum, the shorter and less penetrating the ultra violet rays. UVC rays are the most germicidal and chemical of the ultra violet rays, as well as being the farthest away from the visible spectrum. These rays cause the most burning to the skin. UVC rays are destructive to bacteria as well as to skin tissue if the skin is exposed to them for too long a period of time.

The UVB rays are the therapeutic rays in the middle of the UV range, which produce some effects from both ends of the ultra violet rays. This ray will also burn if the skin is left exposed too long. The UVA ray is the tonic UV ray. It is closest to the visible spectrum, is the deepest penetrating, and is the longest of all the UV rays. The UVA ray is used in tanning booths. This ray does not burn the skin but penetrates deeply into the skin tissue, and can destroy the elasticity of the skin, causing premature aging and wrinkling.

It was once thought that the slightest obstruction would keep the ultra violet rays from reaching the skin. Recent studies have proved that ultra violet rays can penetrate up to 3 feet (91.4 cm) below the water and that approximately 50% of the ultra violet rays can penetrate to the skin through a wet T-shirt. It you want to receive full benefit from ultra violet rays, the area treated should be bare and no cream or lotion should be applied so that you can receive the full benefits of the rays.

Application of Ultra Violet Rays

Ultra violet rays are applied with a lamp at a distance of 30″ to 36″ (76.2 to 91.4 cm) from the skin. If the shorter rays are needed, the lamp can be held as close as 12″ (30.4 cm) from the skin. Extra precautions must be used when the lamp is held at such a close range to avoid damage to skin tissue. (Fig. 24.11)

Time Limit

The average exposure can produce redness of the skin and overdoses will cause blistering. It is well to start with a short exposure of 2 to 3 minutes and gradually increase the exposure over a period of days to 7 to 8 minutes.

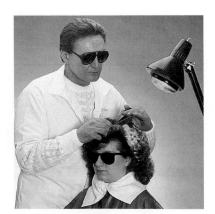
24.11 – Applying ultra violet rays to scalp.

People Skills

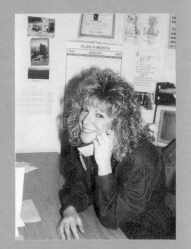

Correct handling of dissatisfied clients can't be stressed enough. Karen Bilbo, a full-time customer service specialist for the Hair Cuttery salon chain, spends her entire day listening to clients face-to-face and over the phone. Here are her quick tips to keep in mind when things go astray:

There is potential conflict when the client is distraught, angry, embarrassed, or has received conflicting information. Also, be on the alert if none of the staff is being straightforward in accepting responsibility for the situation, or if the client was shown indifference or given a smart reply.

If you see potential conflict, be positive, listen, express full interest, offer to be of service, maintain your poise, apologize if necessary, use the client's name, take action quickly, and most important, keep your promises.

Do not interrupt the client, get sidetracked, raise your voice, be defensive, mumble, or fill in pauses with "you know's" or "uh's."

Says Bilbo, "Remember, that clients are the most important people in the world; we depend on them, not the other way around. They are not an interruption of our work; they are our reason for doing what we do. In truth, the client is doing you a favor by giving you the opportunity to serve her."

While this might be tough news to swallow, think about all the other places your client could go for services, and you'll realize that it's really good news because it conveys exactly the attitude you must take to win clients from other salons and ensure your future.

Benefits of Ultra Violet Rays

Ultra violet rays increase resistance to disease by increasing iron and vitamin D content and the number of red and white cells in the blood. They also increase elimination of waste products, restore nutrition where needed and stimulate the circulation by improving the flow of blood and lymph. The rays also have a tendency to increase the fixation of calcium in the blood. Ultra violet rays are used to treat acne, tinea, seborrhea, and to combat dandruff. They also promote healing and can stimulate the growth of hair as well as produce a tan by increasing skin pigment if the skin is exposed in short doses over a long period of time.

Disadvantages of Ultra Violet Rays

Ultra violet rays destroy hair pigment. Continued exposure to the sun's rays causes premature aging of the skin, painful sunburn, and a higher risk of skin cancer, especially for fair- or light-skinned individuals.

VISIBLE LIGHT RAYS OR VISIBLE SPECTRUM

The visible lights are the primary source of lights used for facial and scalp treatments. The bulbs used for the visible light therapy are available in white, red, or blue.

White Light

White light is referred to as a combination light because it is a combination of all the visible rays of the spectrum. White light also has the benefits of all the rays of the visible spectrum. Used for normal skin, the benefits of the white light include: it relieves pain, especially in congested areas, and more particularly, around the nerve centers, such as in the back of the neck and across the shoulders; has some chemical and germicidal actions; and is slightly relaxing to the muscles.

Blue Light

Blue light is used on oily skin that is bare. The blue light contains few heat rays, is soothing to the nerves, produces good skin tone, has some germicidal and chemical effects, and is used for mild cases of skin eruptions. Blue light does not penetrate.

Red Light

Red light is used on dry skin in combination with oils and creams. The red light is the deepest penetrating of the visible spectrum, is good for dry, scaly wrinkled skin, and relaxes tissues.

Review Questions

ELECTRICITY AND LIGHT THERAPY

1. What is electricity?
2. What is a conductor?
3. What is a nonconductor or insulator? Give six examples.
4. What is a direct current (DC)?
5. What is an alternating current (AC)?
6. Describe galvanic current.
7. Give the chemical action of the positive pole; the negative pole.
8. Name three effects of the positive pole on the body.
9. Name three effects of the negative pole on the body.
10. In what cases should faradic current never be used?

25

CHEMISTRY

LEARNING OBJECTIVES

After completing this chapter, you should be able to:

1. Define organic and inorganic chemistry and know the differences between them.

2. Discuss the types of matter.

3. Describe the composition of elements, compounds, and mixtures.

4. Describe the properties of matter, elements, compounds, and mixtures.

5. Define acids and alkalies and know the differences between them.

6. Describe the chemistry of water.

7. Discuss the basic chemistry, types, and action of professional products.

Introduction

Professional cosmetologists are more than just practicing technicians. You will be working with chemicals and performing services that change the hair both chemically and physically. For your client's protection as well as your own, you must understand the safety and health standards of the chemicals you will be working with.

A basic knowledge of modern chemistry is an essential requirement for an intelligent understanding of the multitude of products and cosmetics currently used in the salon. In addition, the science of chemistry brings us a constant flow of new and advanced products. It is important for you, as a professional, to understand these products and learn to use them in a way that is beneficial to your clients.

The Science of Chemistry

Chemistry (**KEM**-i-stree) is the science that deals with the composition, structure, and properties of matter and how matter changes under different chemical conditions. The broad subject of chemistry is divided into two areas: organic chemistry and inorganic chemistry.

Organic (or-**GAN**-ik) *chemistry* is the branch of chemistry that deals with all substances in which carbon is present. Carbon can be found in all plants, animals, petroleum, soft coal, natural gas, and in many artificially prepared substances.

Most organic substances will burn. They are not soluble (not able to be liquefied) in water, but they do dissolve in organic solvents such as alcohol and benzene.

Examples of organic substances are grass, trees, gasoline, oil, soaps, detergents, plastics, and antibiotics.

Inorganic (in-or-**GAN**-ik) *chemistry* is the branch of chemistry that deals with all substances that do not contain carbon. Inorganic substances will not burn and are usually soluble in water. Examples of inorganic substances are water, air, iron, lead, minerals, and iodine.

Matter

Since chemistry is the science that deals with matter, it is essential that we develop an understanding of what matter really is. *Matter* is defined as anything that occupies space, has physical and chemical properties, and exists in one of the following three forms: solids, liquids, or gases.

Solids. Look around your classroom and note what you see: hair, students, teachers, desks, chairs, walls. These are all matter in a solid state.

Liquids. In the clinic area of your school you see water, shampoos, lotions, and hydrogen peroxide. These are matter in a liquid state.

Gases. Take a deep breath. The air you have just brought into your lungs also is matter. It is in a *gaseous state*.

It is not the purpose of this text to train you to be a scientist. But it will help you learn enough about matter so that you are comfortable talking about it in relation to your profession. Therefore, we will briefly examine the nature and structure of matter.

FORMS OF MATTER

Matter exists in the form of elements, compounds, and mixtures.

Elements. An *element* is the basic unit of all matter. An element, being composed of a single part or unit, cannot be reduced to a more simple substance. There are more than 109 known elements.

Each element is identified by a letter symbol, which is generally made up of the principal letter or letters of either the English or Latin name of the element. For example, the letter symbol that identifies sulfur is S; oxygen, O; carbon, C; iron, Fe; lead, Pb; and silver, Ag. The symbols for each element can be obtained by referring to the Periodic Table of Elements found in almost any chemistry textbook.

Atoms

An *atom* (**AT**-om) is the smallest particle of an element that is capable of showing the properties of that element. If you took a piece of gold (an element) and divided it into smaller and smaller pieces, you would eventually come to a particle so small that it no longer showed the properties of the element.

Molecules

A *molecule* is two or more atoms that are joined together chemically.

When two of the *same* atoms are joined, the result is an element. When two *different* atoms are joined, the result is a compound.

Compounds. A *compound* is any substance made up of two or more different elements chemically joined together in definite proportions by weight. When joined, each element loses its characteristic properties and a new set of properties called a compound is created. For example, the combining of nitrogen (N) and hydrogen (H) at a ratio of 1 nitrogen molecule for every 3 hydrogen molecules (NH_3) creates ammonia. A compound can be altered only by chemical means, not by mechanical methods. Compounds can be divided into four classes.

1. *Oxides* are compounds of any element combined with oxygen. For example, a combination of elements you will work with as a cosmetologist is 2 parts hydrogen and 2 parts oxygen, which create the compound known as hydrogen peroxide.

2. *Acids* are compounds of hydrogen, a non-metal, and sometimes oxygen that release hydrogen in a solution. For example, nitrogen + hydrogen + oxygen = nitric acid (NHO), which is used in making dyes. You can test for acidity with litmus paper. Acids turn blue litmus paper red. Acids also have a sour taste, for example, vinegar and lemons.

3. *Alkalies*, also known as *bases*, are compounds of hydrogen, a metal, and oxygen. For example, sodium + oxygen + hydrogen = sodium hydroxide (NaOH), which is used in making soap and hair relaxers. Alkalies neutralize acids and turn red litmus paper blue.

4. *Salts* are substances formed when the hydrogen part of an acid is replaced by a metal. For example, when copper replaces the hydrogen in sulfuric acid, the result is salt copper sulfate. The most common salt is sodium chloride (NaCl) or table salt.

Mixtures. A mixture is a substance made up of elements combined *physically* rather than chemically. The ingredients do not

ELEMENTS AND COMPOUNDS

Matter	Types and Definition	Smallest Particle
Solids Gases Liquids	Elements: Simplest form of matter	Atom: (Cannot be broken down by simple chemical reactions.) About 100 different kinds.
	Compounds: Formed by combination of elements.	Molecule: (Consists of 2 or more atoms chemically combined.) Unlimited kinds possible.

Elements Found in Skin or Hair	Compounds Used on Skin or Hair
Carbon	Water
Nitrogen	Hydrogen peroxide
Oxygen	Ammonium thioglycolate
Sulfur	Alcohol
Hydrogen	Alkalis
Phosphorus	

change their properties as in a compound, but retain their individual characteristics. For example, concrete is a mixture of sand, gravel, and cement. Upon examination, you will notice that although the grains of sand and gravel are held together by the cement, they retain their identity and can be picked apart. Although concrete is a mixture having its own functions, its ingredients never lose their characteristics.

CHEMICAL AND PHYSICAL CHANGES IN MATTER

Matter can be changed in two ways, either through physical or chemical means.

A *physical change* refers to a change in the form (solid, liquid, gas) of a substance without the formation of any *new* substance. For example, ice, a solid substance, melts at a certain temperature and becomes a liquid (water), and water freezes at a certain temperature and becomes a solid (ice). There is no change in the inherent nature of the water; merely a change in its form. An example of a physical change in the cosmetology industry is the physical change in the outside of the hair shaft when a temporary color rinse is applied. The hair has a different appearance because color molecules have been physically added to the surface of the hair. However, there has been no inherent change in the nature of the hair shaft.

A *chemical change* is one in which a new substance or substances are formed, having properties different from the original substances. For example, when you mix hydrogen peroxide into a para dye, a chemical change occurs. The chemical reaction known as oxidation creates color within the cortex of the hair (within the bottle if you are too slow with your application). The chemical reaction between the two has created a new substance (in this case, a color) with its own characteristic properties.

PROPERTIES OF MATTER

Properties of matter refer to how we distinguish one form of matter from another. Substances have two kinds of properties: physical and chemical.

Physical properties refer to characteristics such as density, specific gravity, hardness, odor, and color.

1. *Density* of a substance refers to its weight divided by its volume. For example, the volume of 1 cubic foot (0.03 m^3) of water weighs 62.4 pounds (28.08 kg). Therefore, its density (weight) is 62.4 pounds (28.08 kg) divided by (volume) (0.03 m^3), or water has a density of 62.4 pounds (28.08 kg) per cubic foot (0.03 m^3).

2. *Specific gravity* of a substance is its "lightness" or "heaviness." Using water as the basis for comparison, substances are either more or less dense than water. If "zero" is assigned as the density of water, and if copper is 8.9 times as dense as water, the specific gravity (or relative density) of copper is 8.9.

3. *Hardness* refers to the ability of a substance to resist scratching. A substance will scratch any other substance that is softer. Scientists use the **MOH Hardness Scale** as a basis for comparing the hardness and softness of substances; low numbers indicate softness and high numbers indicate hardness. Some of these ratings might surprise you. For example, the diamond is rated a 10, the average knife blade is rated a 6.2, but asphalt is rated a 1.3.

4. *Odor* helps to identify many substances. For example, the characteristic odor of ammonium thioglycolate, known as the thio odor, helps you identify this product. (Caution: Sniffing products can result in damage to mucous membranes.)

5. *Color* also helps to identify many substances. For example, we easily recognize the colors of gold, silver, and copper. White substances are usually described as colorless.

Chemical properties allow a substance to change and form a new substance. The change is called a *chemical change* or *chemical reaction*. Knowing the chemical properties of a substance allows you to know what happens when that substance is combined with another one. For example, combining 1 atom of carbon with 2 atoms of oxygen produces the gas exhaled by humans and animals known as carbon dioxide (CO_2).

PROPERTIES OF COMMON ELEMENTS, COMPOUNDS, AND MIXTURES

Knowledge about the properties of the most common elements, compounds, and mixtures can help you understand why certain chemical reactions take place.

Oxygen (O) (**OK**-si-jen) is the most abundant element. It can be found either by itself or as one element of a compound. It makes up about 50% of the solid crust of the earth, 20% of the atmosphere, and 89% of water. Oxygen is a colorless, odorless, tasteless, gaseous substance that can be combined with most other elements to form an infinite variety of compounds called oxides.

When a substance is combined with oxygen, the substance is always oxidized. Combining a substance with oxygen creates heat energy. When the rate of reaction is slow and only heat energy is given off, the process is known as *slow oxidation*. Oxidation tints and perm neutralizers are examples of slow oxidizers. When oxygen combines with other substances so rapidly that light energy as well as heat is created, the process is known as *combustion*. Lighting a match or burning wood is an example of *rapid oxidation* or combustion.

Hydrogen (H) (**HEYE**-dro-jen) is a colorless, odorless, and tasteless gas. It makes up about 1% of the earth's crust. In total numbers of atoms, hydrogen is probably the second most abundant element on earth (oxygen is most abundant), and the most abundant element in the *universe*. In the laboratory, hydrogen is prepared by the action of active metals on water or an acid.

Pure hydrogen peroxide (H_2O_2) (pe-**ROK**-seyed) is an oily liquid compound of hydrogen and oxygen. Solutions of 30% are used to bleach fabric, hair, and feathers. Solutions of 12% cause the chemical reaction in oxidation tints, and a solution of 3% is used as an antiseptic.

Oxidizing (**OK**-si-deye-zing) *agents* are substances that readily release oxygen. Hydrogen peroxide releases oxygen, which oxidizes both melanin and artificial pigments found in para dyes. The releasing of oxygen is known as *reduction* and the substance that attracts the oxygen is the *reducing agent*. Thus melanin and artificial pigments are oxidized and the solution left on the outside of the hair shaft is reduced (now missing the extra oxygen element).

Nitrogen (N) (**NEYE**-tro-jen) is a colorless, gaseous element that makes up about 78% of the earth's atmosphere. It is found in nature chiefly in the form of ammonia and nitrates.

Acidity and Alkalinity

You may recall from the chapter on permanent waving that the pH of a solution is a chemical measure of its acidity or alkalinity. The pH scale ranges from zero to 14. (Fig. 25.1) Pure water is considered neutral and represented by the number 7 in the middle of the scale. Recall that if a solution has a pH of less than 7, it has an acid pH. If a solution has a pH of more than 7, it has an alkaline pH. Also remember that an alkaline solution softens and swells hair; an acid solution contracts and hardens hair.

There are meters and other indicators such as *nitrozine paper* available so you can measure the pH of the products you use. If a product is more alkaline, the paper turns dark; if it is more acid, there is not much, if any, change in color.

If you wet hair with water and test the pH balance, it is normally between 4.4 to 4.5; it is slightly acid (remember that 7 is neutral). Shampoos normally have a pH of about 8 (more alkaline); chemical waving solutions have a pH of about 9 (also more alkaline). Color rinses have a pH of about 2; neutralizers about 3

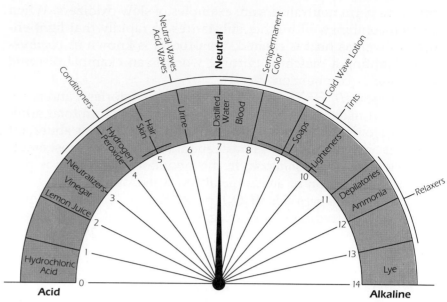

25.1—Average pH values.

(both are more acidic). Until you become familiar with a client's hair and history, and until you are sure of what you're doing, you should try to use solutions that are close to a pH balance of 7. Otherwise, you can unknowingly damage your client's hair.

Chemistry of Water

Water (H_2O) is the most abundant and important chemical on the earth. It is essential to the life process. The human body is made of approximately 70% water, and water covers almost 75% of the earth's surface. Water is a solvent, meaning that it has the ability to dissolve another substance.

WATER PURIFICATION

Fresh water from lakes and streams is purified by sedimentation (a treatment that causes mass to sink to the bottom) and filtration (passing through a porous substance, such as a filter paper or charcoal) to remove suspended clay, sand, and organic material. Small amounts of chlorine are then added to kill bacteria. Boiling water at a temperature of 212° Fahrenheit (100° Celsius) will also destroy most microbic life.

Water can be further treated by distillation, which is a process of heating water so that it becomes a vapor, then condensing the vapor so that it collects as a liquid. This process is often used in the manufacture of cosmetics.

Why is water so important in the cosmetology industry? Although the answer is obvious—water is used for shampooing, mixing solutions, and other functions—it is interesting to learn more about what water is made of. How does water help chemical or other solutions that are used in the salon? Water is made of protons and electrons (also neutrons, but here we are only concerned with protons and electrons), which contain power that gives them electrical charges. Protons are positive charges; electrons are negative charges. If you add a solid particle to water, for example, salt, the positive and negative charges work together to pull apart, or dissolve, the salt. The same process occurs when you combine other solids or liquids with water. Only oil and wax cannot be dissolved with water.

Chemistry of Shampoos

To determine which shampoo will leave your client's hair in the best condition for the intended service you must understand the chemical ingredients of shampoos. Most shampoos have many common ingredients. It is often the small differences in formulation that make one shampoo better for a particular hair texture or condition.

The ingredient that most shampoos have in common, and it usually is number one on the list to show that there is more of it than any other ingredient, is water. Generally, it is not just plain water, but purified or de-ionized water. From there, ingredients are listed in descending order according to the percentage of each ingredient in the shampoo.

CLASSIFICATIONS OF SHAMPOOS

The second ingredient that most shampoos have in common is the *base surfactant* (sir-FAK-tant) or *base detergent*. These two terms, surfactant and detergent, mean the same thing, cleansing or "surface active agent." The term surfactant describes organic compounds brought together by chemical synthesis to create wetting, dispersing, emulsifying, solubilizing, foaming, or washing agents (detergents).

The base surfactant or combination of surfactants determines into which class a shampoo will fall. The base surfactants used in shampoos fall into four broad classifications: *anionic* (an-i-**ON**-ik), *cationic* (**KAT**-i-on-ik), *nonionic* (non-i-**ON**-ik), and *ampholytic* (**AM**-fo-li-tik).

Most manufacturers use detergents from more than one classification. It is customary to use a secondary surfactant to com plement or offset the negative qualities of the base surfactant. For example, an *amphoteric* (**AM**-fo-ter-ik) that is nonirritating to the eyes can be added to a harsh anionic to create a product that is more comfortable to use.

Anionics. Sodium lauryl sulfate and sodium laureth sulfate, which fall into the first classification known as *anionic surfactants*, are the most commonly used detergents. Sodium lauryl sulfate is a relatively harsh cleanser that produces a rich foam. It is suitable for use in hard or soft water because it rinses easily from the hair. Sodium laureth sulfate is also a strong, rich, foaming detergent. However, because it is less alkaline than the lauryl sulfates, it is often used in shampoos that are designed to be milder or less drying to the hair shaft. Other anionics commonly used in shampoos are:

Disodium oleamide sulfosuccinate	Alcohol sulfates
Coconut sulfated monoglycerides	Magnesium salt
Sodium dioctyl sulfosuccinate	Potassium salt
Sodium lauryl isoethionate	Sarcosine
Triethanolamine (TEA) lauryl sulfate	

Cationics. The second classification of detergents or surfactants, cationics, is made up almost entirely of quarternary ammonium compounds or *quats*. Practically all the quarternary compounds have some antibacterial action; therefore they are sometimes included in the chemical composition of dandruff shampoos. Other cationics commonly used in shampoos are:

Benzalkonium chloride
N-2 ethylaminoformylmethylpyridinium

Nonionics. The third classification, nonionics, are valued as surfactants for their versatility, stability, and ability to resist shrinkage, particularly in cold temperatures. They have a mild cleansing action and low incidence of irritation to human tissues. Cocamide (DEA, MEA) is one of the most widely used nonionics in the industry, not only in shampoos but also in lipstick and permanent waving lotions. Other nonionics commonly used in shampoos are:

Diethanolamide	Monoethanolamide
Polysorbate 20 & 40	Sorbitan laurate
Palmitate	Stearate

Ampholytes. The fourth type of cleanser, the ampholyte, is important commercially because it can behave as an anionic or a cationic substance depending on the pH of the solution. The ampholytes have a slight tendency to cling to hair and skin and thus are conducive to hair manageability. They possess germicidal properties that vary between derivatives. Amphoteric surfactants are used in several baby shampoos because they do not sting the eyes. Many amphoterics are identified on the ingredient list by

Amphoteric 1-20. Other ampholytes commonly used in shampoos are:

Cocamidopropyl betaine   Cocamide betaine
Sodium lauraminopropionate
Triethanolamine (TEA) lauraminopropionate

A familiarity with these four classifications of detergents or surfactants and their use in shampoo products will enable you to make a professional decision when selecting a product to use on a client.

Action of Surfactants in Shampoos

A surfactant molecule has two ends: *hydrophilic* (heye-droh-**FIL**-ik) (head) and *lipophilic* (lip-oh-**FIL**-ik) (tail). During the shampooing process the hydrophilic or water-loving end attracts water and the lipophilic or oil-loving end attracts oil. This creates a push-pull process that causes the oils, dirt, and deposits to roll up into little balls that can be lifted off in the water and rinsed from the hair. (Figs. 25.2–25.5)

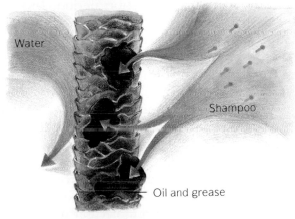

25.2—Tail of shampoo molecules is attracted to hair, grease, and dirt.

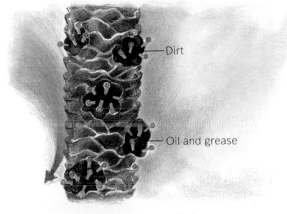

25.3—Shampoo causes grease and oils to roll up into small globules.

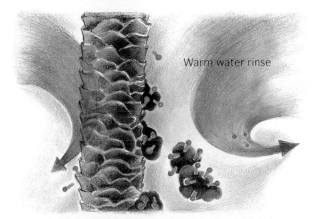

25.4—While rinsing, shampoo heads attach to water molecules and cause debris to roll off.

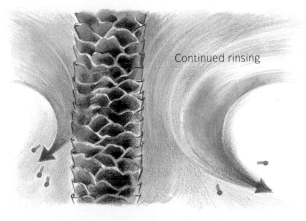

25.5—Thorough rinsing ensures that debris and excess shampoo are washed away.

Other Shampoo Ingredients

Other ingredients are added to the base surfactants to create a multitude of chemical formulations. Moisturizers, oils, proteins, preservatives, foam enhancers, and perfumes are all standard components of shampoo.

CONDITIONERS

The best conditioner is only a temporary remedy for problem hair. It cannot "heal" damaged hair, nor can it improve the quality of the new hair growth. Heredity, health, and diet control the texture and structure of the hair. However, a conditioner is valuable because it can minimize the damage to hair during a cosmetology service, and it can restore luster, shine, manageability, and strength while the damaged hair grows long enough to be cut off and replaced by new hair.

Instant Conditioners

Within the classification of *instant conditioners* fall those products that either remain on the hair for a very short period (1 to 5 minutes) or are left in the hair during styling. Instant conditioners contain humectants to improve the appearance of dry, brittle hair. *Humectants* (hew-**MECK**-tunts) are chemical compounds that absorb and hold moisture from the hair. Sorbitol, ethylene glycol, butylene glycol, and propylene glycol are humectants that work effectively on the hair to temporarily lock moisture into the hair.

Cetyl alcohol and stearyl alcohol, common ingredients in instant conditioners, work as pearlizing agents and lubricants to leave the hair with a glossy finish.

Chemical ingredients of lanolin derivatives, such as acetylated lanolin, lanolin acid, or lanolin oil, are often included in conditioning formulas for fine hair because of their light molecular weight.

Silicone oils, such as simethicone and dimethicone, are effective lubricants and emollients, but they have little staying power and are almost completely removed during the next shampooing.

Most conditioners fall in the pH range of 3.5 to 6.0. Therefore, they have the ability to restore the pH balance after an alkaline chemical treatment. Those conditioners designed primarily to balance pH are considered instant because of their short application time. They generally contain an acid that counteracts the alkalinity of a prior chemical service.

Moisturizers

Moisturizers are a heavier, creamier formulation than instant conditioners, and they also have a longer application time (10 to 20 minutes). They contain many of the same ingredients as instant conditioners but are formulated to be more penetrating and have longer staying power. Some moisturizers incorporate the application of heat, others do not. Stearatkonium chloride is a white paste used in moisturizers to counteract the drying effects of anionic detergents and chemical treatments.

The quarternary ammonium compounds (quats) are included in the chemical formulation of moisturizers for their ability to attach themselves steadfastly to hair fibers and provide longer lasting protection than the instant conditioners.

Protein Conditioners

Proteins are *polymers* (substances formed by combining many small molecules, usually in a long chain-like structure) composed of combinations of any of 23 different amino acids (used to recondition damaged hair), ranging in molecular weight. In the cosmetology industry, hydrolysis (chemical process of decomposition, involving splitting of a bond with the addition of the elements of water) and chemical modification are used to change natural protein into a usable substance. The size of the molecule, the distribution of molecular weights, how much salt the product contains, and how the protein is hydrolyzed all determine a product's effectiveness on the hair.

Setting lotions have protein-based conditioners that are part of the hair setting process. A little water, added during the hair setting procedure, facilitates setting by keeping the hair soft and manageable. This type of conditioner is designed to slightly increase hair diameter with its coating action and to give it body. It is available in several strengths to accommodate the texture, condition, and quality of hair.

Concentrated protein conditioners can be recognized by their brown liquid appearance. They are used to increase the tensile strength of the hair and to temporarily close split ends. These conditioners utilize hydrolized protein (very small fragments) and are designed to pass through the cuticle, penetrate into the cortex, and replace the keratin that has been lost from the hair. They improve texture, equalize porosity, and increase elasticity. The excess conditioner must be rinsed from the hair before setting. Concentrated protein treatments generally are not given immediately after a chemical treatment, because they can alter the freshly completed and desirable rearrangement of protein bonds after a permanent wave, relaxer, or hair coloring.

Packs

Conditioning packs are chemical mixtures of concentrated protein in the heavy cream base of a moisturizer. They penetrate several cuticle layers and are utilized when an equal degree of moisturizing and proteinizing is required.

Other Conditioning Agents

A large variety of conditioning agents in addition to the ones highlighted in this chapter are currently used in cosmetology products. Each one is designed to deal with one or more of the hair and scalp problems that will be encountered in the salon.

Permanent Waving

Permanent waving makes physical and chemical changes in the structure of the hair shaft. Therefore, in order to understand the actions of permanent waving, we will review the composition of the hair and hair bonds.

COMPOSITION OF HAIR

Hair is made of a hard protein called *keratin*. The hair shaft has three layers: the *cuticle, cortex,* and *medulla.* Since permanent hair waving takes place in the cortical layer, you should understand the complex structure of the cortex.

The cortex is composed of numerous parallel fibers of hard keratin, referred to as **polypeptide chains**. These parallel fibers are twisted around one another in a manner resembling the twisting of the fiber strands in a rope.

Peptide Bonds

Each amino acid is joined to another **peptide bond** (end bonds), forming a chain as long as the hair. They are the strongest bonds in the cortex and most of the strength of hair is due to their properties. Peptide bonds are chemical bonds, and if even a few are broken, the hair is weakened or damaged. If too many of these bonds are broken, the hair will break off.

Chemical Bonds

Three types of chemical bonds attract hair proteins to each other. The presence of these bonds or links gives hair the ability to be permanently waved. To become an expert, you should have a working knowledge of these three chemical bonds:

1. Salt bonds called S bonds
2. Hydrogen bonds called H bonds
3. Disulfide bonds called S-S bonds

Salt bonds are formed by the attraction of opposite electric charges. When two atoms of hydrogen are attracted to each other they form a **hydrogen bond**. Both salt and hydrogen bonds help to hold the protein molecules of the hair together. They are relatively weak and can be broken by water. However, because there are thousands of them, they are the main bonds between protein chains and account for most of the hair's resistance to change. (Fig. 25.6)

The **disulfide bond** is formed by the joining of two sulfur atoms. It is the material that surrounds the spiral proteins in the cortex. The number of disulfide bonds is smaller than hydrogen and salt bonds, but they are much more stable.

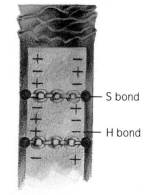

— S bond

— H bond

25.6—Salt and hydrogen bonds.

Changes in Hair Bonds: Wet Waving and Curling

A temporary hair set is produced by physical changes that occur within the hair cortex. The physical changes are a result of using water, stretching techniques, and heat application and are the basis of finger waving, pin curling, roller curling, and blow-dry styling. Because of the nature of these physical changes, you can style hair as frequently as desired.

You can use water alone because it has the ability to break down the hydrogen bonds in the cortex. The hydrogen bonds are held in place by the polypeptide chains, and you must cause these chains to slip before a strong wave can be formed.

Stretching or ribboning the hair strand causes a temporary rearrangement of the chains. Water lubricates the chains so that they can move relative to one another. However, even though the hydrogen bonds are broken, the total amount of movement is very small because the strong disulfide bonds are completely unaffected by the water and continue to resist the slippage of the polypeptide chains.

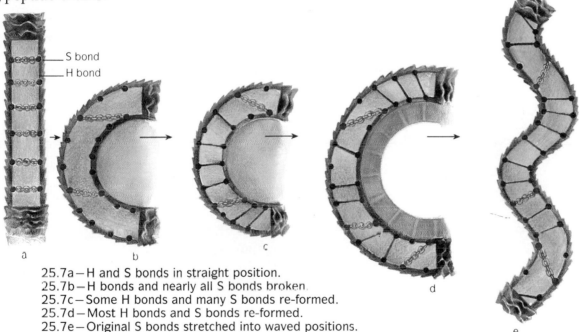

25.7a—H and S bonds in straight position.
25.7b—H bonds and nearly all S bonds broken.
25.7c—Some H bonds and many S bonds re-formed.
25.7d—Most H bonds and S bonds re-formed.
25.7e—Original S bonds stretched into waved positions.

THE PERMANENT WAVING PROCESS

To permanently wave the hair, the disulfide bonds within the cortex must be broken and rearranged. (Fig. 25.7) Permanent waving lotion causes the cuticle of the hair to swell and the imbrications to open, allowing the solution to penetrate into the cortex. The solution breaks the disulfide bonds found within the cortex. Different perm solutions achieve that goal in different ways. In acid waves, also known as neutral waves, heat and tension are used along with the solution to break down the disulfide bonds. In thio solutions (containing ammonium thioglycolate), the chemical is primarily responsible for breaking the bonds. Exo-thermic solutions are those that chemically create heat when Part A is mixed with Part B of the curling solution and the chemical reaction from the heat is primarily responsible for breaking disulfide bonds. However, with all three solutions, breaking the bonds is a physical and chemical action.

Neutralizer

When sufficient processing has taken place, the solution is rinsed from the hair and a neutralizer is applied. The neutralizer, also known as bonding lotion, is an acid solution with a pH between 2 and 6. This solution is a chemical oxidizing agent. This re-oxidation re-forms the disulfide bonds in their new shape and closes the cuticle of the hair shaft. The key ingredient in neutralizers that works to re-form the disulfide bonds is generally either hydrogen peroxide, sodium perborate, or sodium bromate.

Chemical Hair Relaxing (Straightening)

Chemical hair relaxing is the process of straightening excessively curly hair. In this process, the disulfide bonds are broken, which leaves the hair in a relaxed and straightened form. (Fig. 25.8)

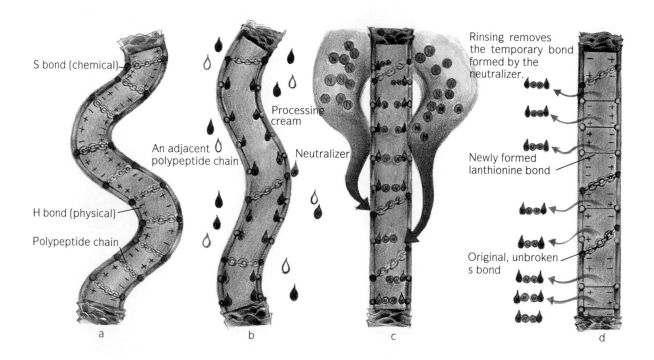

25.8a—Both H and S bonds holding polypeptide chains in position.
25.8b—All H bonds broken and most S bonds broken.
25.8c—Neutralizer fixes hair in a straight position after hair has been relaxed.
25.8d—Straightened hair.

Professional cosmetologists have two types of chemical hair relaxers available for use in the salon: *sodium hydroxide* and *thio*.

Sodium hydroxide works by chemically and permanently altering the disulfide bonds, leaving the hair straightened. Because the bonds are permanently altered, the hair is unfit for other types of permanent waving services. In other words, you will not be able to put curl back in hair that is straightened with sodium hydroxide. The straightened hair must grow out.

Sodium hydroxide relaxers are alkaline in reaction with an approximate pH of 13. These relaxers should be handled with caution because sodium hydroxide is considered a caustic chemical.

SOFT PERMANENT WAVES

A thio cream or gel-based ammonium thioglycolic product is used to straighten the hair by breaking the disulfide bonds. This allows the hair to take on a relaxed and straightened form. After the hair is straightened with the thio relaxer, the hair can be permanently waved in the manner normally used in permanent waving the hair.

The Chemistry of Hair Coloring

Hair color is divided into three classifications: *temporary*, *semipermanent*, and *permanent*. These classifications indicate color fastness or ability to remain on the hair. These characteristics are determined by chemical composition and molecular weight of the pigments and dyes within the products found in each classification.

TEMPORARY HAIR COLORS

Temporary colors are also called certified colors because they contain colors accepted by the government for use in foods, drugs, and cosmetics. Temporary colors for the hair come in various forms, such as color rinses, color sprays, color mousses, and color shampoos. They are available in a wide range of colors and are easily applied.

Temporary colors utilize pigment and dye molecules of the greatest molecular weight. The large size of this color molecule prevents penetration of the cuticle layer of the hair shaft and allows only a coating action on the outside of the strand.

The chemical composition of a temporary color is acid in reaction and makes only a physical change rather than a chemical change in the shaft. This creates a color that is designed to be removed completely with the next shampooing.

SEMI-PERMANENT HAIR TINTS

Two types of semi-permanent colors are available to the professional cosmetologist: *traditional* and *polymer*.

Traditional semi-permanent colors are designed to last 3 to 4 weeks. They utilize pigment and dye molecules that are of a lesser molecular weight than those of temporary colors. These smaller molecules have the physical capability to penetrate the hair shaft somewhat. The chemical composition of semi-permanent colors is mildly alkaline. This makes the hair shaft swell and the cuticle rise, allowing some penetration into the cortex. Traditional semi-permanent colors make a mild chemical change as well as a physical change in the hair shaft.

A polymer is a substance that has long-chain structural units created from the combining of many small molecules. These chains have tensile strength, elasticity, and hardness. Other examples of polymers are vinyl, plastic, and human tissue. Polymer semi-permanent colors are classified as semi-permanent colors because they require no oxidation process, or the addition of an oxidizer for color development. However, the colorfastness of polymer colors differs from traditional semi-permanent colors. The long-chain structure of the polymer inhibits its penetration of the cuticle and ability to adhere to the keratin of the hair shaft. Therefore, heat is applied to deepen the color penetration and extend the colorfastness. (Fig. 25.9)

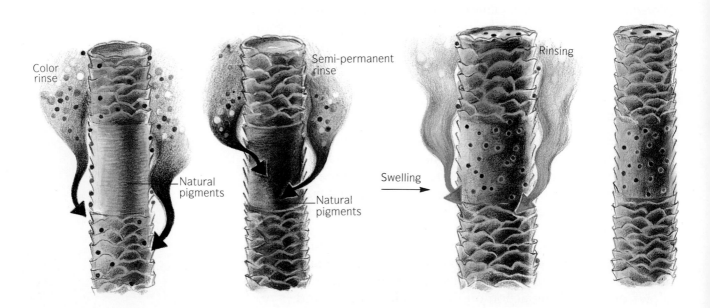

25.9—Action of semi-permanent hair tints.

PERMANENT HAIR TINTS

Four types of products fall within the classification of permanent hair tints: *oxidation tints*, *vegetable tints*, *metallic tints*, and *compound dyes*. (Fig. 25.10)

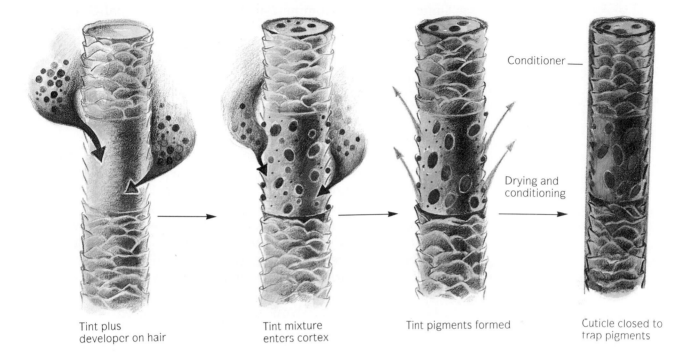

Tint plus developer on hair

Tint mixture enters cortex

Tint pigments formed

Conditioner ___

Drying and conditioning

Cuticle closed to trap pigments

25.10a – Tint and peroxide on hair.
25.10b – Tint mixture enters into cortex.
25.10c – Tint pigments formed.
25.10d – Shrinking of cuticle scales to trap pigment.

Oxidation tints. As a professional cosmetologist, the permanent color you will use most often is known as an *oxidation*, or *aniline derivative*, tint. The pigment and dye molecules of oxidation tints have the lowest molecular weight, the smallest used in the three classifications of hair color.

Oxidation tints are composed of a *base* and *couplers*. The base of an oxidation tint is composed of aromatic (fragrant) compounds obtained almost exclusively from coal. They are synthetic organic ingredients that when mixed with an oxidizer work with the couplers to create artificial pigment. The couplers are ingredients added to obtain certain colors, preserve and stabilize the product, and improve the resulting condition of the hair shaft.

When you mix oxidation tints with the oxidizing agent (hydrogen peroxide), an alkaline reaction creates a chemical process, which causes the cortex to swell. This raising and separating of the cuticle allows the small pigment and dye molecules to enter the cortex and form acid bonds with the keratin chains in the cortex and become part of the hair structure. This formation of acid bonds, rather than affixing to the H-bonds and the S-bonds, leaves the hair free to be permanently waved or relaxed with certain care and precaution.

The Professional Hair Care and Beauty Trades Division of the United Food and Commercial Workers International Union cites studies that indicate some of the chemicals found in oxidation tints do penetrate the skin and can be harmful to health. They advise handling these products with care, which means that wearing gloves during the mixing, application, and removing of oxidation tints is recommended.

Vegetable Tints

In the past many vegetable materials such as logwood, indigo, chamomile, and henna were used as hair coloring ingredients. Both logwood and indigo are also used to color fabric. Apigenin is the pigment distilled from a herb known as chamomile. The chamomile flowers can be ground into a powder and used as a paste to give a lighter, brighter effect to the hair. Although vegetable henna has been used for hair coloring since the days of the early Egyptians, its use is very limited in the modern professional practice of hair color.

Henna owes its hair dying abilities to the presence of a chemical known as *lawsone*. Lawsone is soluble in water and a substantial amount in an acid solution will adhere to the keratin of the hair shaft. Citric or other acids are added to create a pH of 5.5, which is optimum for henna after it is mixed and ready for application.

Henna penetrates into the cortical layer as well as coating the cuticle of the shaft when the pigment molecule of the henna and the S-bonds are combined in the cortex. Henna has a coating action that can process unevenly on hair that has uneven porosity, and it can build up on hair to the point that solutions cannot penetrate properly. Although it is considered permanent, henna eventually fades with shampooing.

Metallic Dyes

Metallic hair dyes make up a small portion of the home hair coloring market and currently are not used professionally. However, it is important for you to be informed of the chemical composition and characteristics of metallic dyes because metals react adversely with the oxidation solutions commonly used in the professional salon.

The colors produced by metallic salts are due to sulfides formed by the reaction between the sulfur in the keratin and the metallic salts, and to the metallic oxides formed by the keratin reducing the metal salts. The metallic salts react with the sulfur of the hair keratin and turn the protein brown.

Metallic salts (lead, silver, copper) have been known to cause headaches, scalp irritation, contact dermatitis, facial swelling, hair breakage and loss, lead poisoning, and can cause bottles of dye to explode. If you do use these dyes, it is important to wash your hands thoroughly because ingestion through oral contact or contamination of food can be fatal.

Compound Dyes

Compound dyes are a combination of vegetable and metallic dyes. Metallic salts are added to the vegetable dyes as a fixative, thus creating a formulation that lasts longer. The addition of metallic salts also creates colors that are new and different from those available with pure vegetable tints. The most common example of this is compound henna, which is the combination of pure vegetable henna and a metallic salt. Like metallic dyes, compound dyes are not used professionally.

Color Removers

Two basic types of products are available to remove artificial pigment from the hair: *oil-based color removers* and *dye solvents*.

Oil-based color removers are products that gently remove color buildup or stain from the cuticle layer of the hair shaft. They make no structural or chemical change in the hair.

Dye solvents are designed to diffuse (break apart) artificial color molecules deposited by aniline derivative tints. However, as a dye solvent lightens the artificial color molecules, it also diffuses the melanin of the hair shaft.

HAIR LIGHTENING

Very simply, the oxidation of melanin in the hair is what causes hair color to lighten. How does this take place? When hydrogen peroxide is added to a bleach formula (the oxidation process), it releases molecules of gas. These molecules of gas are in constant motion. When the bleach formula is applied to the client's hair, the gases crash into the hair melanin with enough force to break apart, or diffuse, the melanin. This action oxidizes the melanin in the hair shaft, making it lighter.

In the salon, three basic classifications of bleach are used: *oil*, *cream*, and *powder*. Each classification has unique uses, abilities, and chemical characteristics.

Oil bleaches are the mildest of the three types and have the least amount of lightening action. Oil bleach is a shampoo-based product containing sulfonated oils (oils treated with sulfuric acid or castor oil) to slow down the bleaching action. These bleaches contain a weak hydrogen peroxide and ammonia solution that creates an alkaline pH strong enough to soften and open the cuticle allowing the bleach to gently lighten the hair.

Cream bleaches are similar to oil bleaches in that both have a shampoo base containing sulfonated oil. However, the cream bleach has other ingredients that make it strong enough to do pastel blonding, yet gentle enough to be used on the scalp. When a cream bleach is mixed for use, it is the addition of protinators or activators containing an alkali such as sodium metasilicate or oxidizers such as urea peroxide, potassium persulfate, and ammonium persulfate that give it the extra lightening power. Cream bleaches have an average pH of 10 and contain a solution of hydrogen peroxide that can be as great as 3%.

Powder bleaches, like cream bleaches, are strong enough to do pastel blonding. Powder bleach is similar to cream bleach in chemical composition, but powder bleach cannot be applied to the scalp because it does not contain the oil and conditioners that make a cream bleach safe for on-the-scalp application. Like oil and cream bleaches, powder bleaches contain ammonia; however, in this instance it is in a dry form. The ammonia begins the oxidation process when it mixes with liquid or cream hydrogen peroxide.

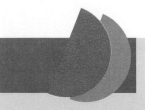

Focus on: Joseph Dallal, Cosmetic Chemist

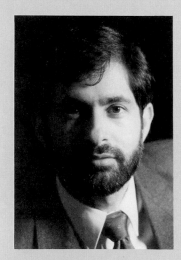

"I mix ingredients together to generate a new type of beauty product, say, a new shampoo or mousse," explains Joseph Dallal, a cosmetic chemist for Zotos International Co. "It's like when you bake a cake. You can choose from among several different types of flour. Some of them will make the cake fluffier and others will make it heavier. Everything that goes into that recipe will affect the cake." Dallal formulates the "recipes" for new products that marketing professionals propose.

Dallal says that he "grew up in a salon," and that working as a cosmetologist launched his desire to improve existing skin and hair care products. "As a stylist, I experienced a lot of frustration. I needed the right tools to do specific jobs. I wanted the perfect shampoo or the perfect conditioner," he explains. "Now, I make those tools."

Equipped with a cosmetology license, an M.S. in chemistry, and a love of cooking, Dallal couldn't be better suited for the challenge of creating today's beauty products. While Dallal says that much of his job involves "trial and error, and combinations of multitudes of ingredients, there's nothing like the magic and creativity you get to see and display, not every day, but once in a while."

TONERS

Toners are permanent aniline derivative colors designed for pre-lightened hair. The difference between a tint and a toner is that the dye load of a toner is less. This creates pale, delicate shades of color used to "tone" pre-lightened hair.

COLOR FILLERS

As a professional cosmetologist, you might use fillers to equalize the porosity of abused or damaged hair and to create a color base in the hair. Fillers are absorbed by the hair according to its porosity; the greater the porosity, the greater the absorption. Filler molecules fill in spaces left in the shaft from prior diffusion of melanin, creating a base to which tint molecules can attach.

Protein fillers are made from inexpensive protein materials such as turkey feathers, scrap leather, and hooves of cattle. These proteins are hydrolyzed into small chains of polypeptides that form protein salt bonds, which will attach to the protein in the hair.

Non-protein fillers are made of oil and water emulsions that are thickened with a mildly acid pH of approximately 3.5 to 4.0. These fillers use cationic compounds as the active ingredient, which cause the product to adhere to the shaft.

Cosmetic Chemistry

Cosmetic chemistry is the scientific study of the cosmetics used in our industry. You will find yourself better equipped to incorporate the art and science of cosmetics into your professional services after you acquire an understanding of the chemical composition, preparation, and use of cosmetics. Cosmetics can be classified according to their physical and chemical nature and the characteristics by which we identify them.

PHYSICAL AND CHEMICAL CLASSIFICATIONS OF COSMETICS

1. Powders
2. Solutions
3. Suspensions
4. Emulsions
5. Ointments
6. Soaps

Powders

Powders are a uniform mixture of insoluble substances (inorganic, organic, and colloidal) that have been properly blended, perfumed, and/or tinted to produce a cosmetic that is free from coarse or gritty particles. Mixing and sifting are used in the process of making powders.

Solutions

A *solution* (so-**LOO**-shun) is an evenly dispersed mixture of two or more kinds of molecules. For example, a solution is made by mixing a solute (for example, a sugar cube) into a solvent (for example, water). A *solute* (**SOL**-yoot) is any substance that dissolves into a liquid and forms a solution. A *solvent* (**SOL**-vent) is any substance that is able to dissolve another substance.

Solutions are clear mixtures of a solute and solvent that do not separate when left standing. Solutions are easily prepared by dissolving a powdered solute in a warm solvent and stirring at the same time. The solute can be separated from the solvent by applying heat and evaporating the solvent. A good solution should be clear and transparent; thus filtration is often necessary if the solution is cloudy.

Water is a universal solvent. It is capable of dissolving more substances than any other solvent. Oils, grain alcohol, and glycerine are frequently used as solvents. Solvents are classified as *miscible* (**MIS**-e-bel) or *immiscible*. Water, glycerine, and alcohol readily mix with each other; therefore, they are miscible (mixable). On the other hand, water and oil do not mix with each other; hence, they are *immiscible* (non-mixable).

The solute can be either a solid, liquid, or gas. For example, boric acid solution is a mixture of a solid in a liquid; glycerine and rose water is a mixture of two miscible liquids; ammonia water is a mixture of a gas in water.

Solutions containing *volatile* (**VOL**-i-til) (easily evaporated) substances, such as ammonia and alcohol, should be stored with lids tightly secured in a cool place to discourage evaporation.

There are three methods of expressing concentration of solutions:

A *dilute* (deye-**LOOT**) *solution* contains a small quantity of the solute in proportion to the quantity of the solvent.

A *concentrated solution* contains a large quantity of the solute in proportion to the quantity of solvent.

A *saturated* (**SACH**-u-rayt-ed) *solution* will not dissolve or take more of the solute than it already holds at a given temperature.

Suspensions

Suspensions are mixtures of one type of matter in another type of matter. The particles might have a tendency to separate on standing, making it necessary to shake or stir the product before use. Some skin lotions, such as calamine lotion, are suspensions. Other examples are whipping cream, salad dressing, clouds, and smoke.

Emulsions

Emulsions (e-**MUL**-shuns) are formed when two or more immiscible (non-mixable) substances, such as oil and water, are united with the aid of a binder (gum) or an emulsifier (soap). If a suitable emulsifier and the proper techniques are used, the resulting emulsion will be stable. A stable emulsion can hold as much as 90% water. Depending on the balance between the liquids and solids, the emulsion may be cream, liquid, or semi-solid in character.

Emulsions are prepared by hand or with the aid of a grinding and cutting machine called a *colloidal mill*. In the process of preparing the emulsion, the emulsifier forms a protective film around the microscopic globules of either the oil or water. The smaller the globules, the thicker and more stable the resulting emulsion.

Emulsions basically fall into two different classes: *oil-in-water (O/W)* and *water-in-oil (W/O)*.

Oil-in-water (O/W) emulsions are made of oil droplets suspended in a water base. In addition to the emulsifier, which coats the oil droplets and holds them in suspension, there may be a number of additional ingredients present that are designed to cause certain reactions in the hair, for example, permanent wave solutions, lighteners (bleaches), neutralizers, and tints.

Water-in-oil (W/O) emulsions are formed with drops of water suspended in an oil base. These are usually much thicker and oilier than the O/W emulsions, for example, hair grooming creams, cleansing creams, and cold creams.

Ointments

Ointments (**OINT**-ments) are semi-solid mixtures of organic substances (lard, petrolatum [vaseline], wax) and a medicinal agent. No water is used. For the ointment to soften upon application, its melting point should be lower than body temperature (98.6° Fahrenheit [37° Celsius]).

Sticks are similar to ointments in that they are a mixture of organic substances (oils, waxes, petrolatum) poured into a mold to solidify. Sticks are firmer and harder than ointments. No water is present. (Examples: lipstick, color crayons.)

Pastes are soft, moist cosmetics that have a thick consistency. They are bound together with gum, starch, and sometimes water. If oils and fats are present, water is generally absent. The colloidal mill assists in the removal of grittiness from the paste. (Example: cream rouge.)

Mucilages are thick liquids containing either natural gums (tragacanth or karaya) or synthetic gums mixed with water. Since mucilages undergo decomposition, a preservative is required. (Example: hair setting lotions.)

Soaps

Soaps are compounds formed when a mixture of fats and oils is fed into a tank of superheated water (which converts the mixture into fatty acids) and then purified by distillation. Potassium hydroxide is mixed with the fatty acids to make soft soap or with sodium hydroxide to make hard soap. During the process of making soap, glycerine is given off as a by-product. A high-quality soap is made from pure oils and fats and does not contain excessive alkalis.

INFORMATIONAL REFERENCES

As a professional cosmetologist, you should become familiar with the United States Pharmacopeia (U.S.P.), a book that defines and standardizes drugs, the Federal Drug Administration (FDA), which also regulates cosmetics and colorings, the Professional Hair Care and Beauty Trades Division of the United Food and Commercial Workers International Union, the health and safety codes of your state, the Material Safety Data Sheets (MSDS) from each manufacturer, and commercially available cosmetic dictionaries. All provide information that is of great importance to you as a professional cosmetologist.

The following are examples of some of the terms used in the cosmetology industry:

Alcohol, also known as grain or ethyl alcohol, is a colorless liquid obtained by the fermentation of starch, sugar, and other carbohydrates. It is no longer used as a skin sanitizer because of current classification as a hazardous chemical due to its ability to kill living tissue.

Alum is aluminum potassium or ammonium sulphate, supplied in the form of crystals or powder. It has a strong astringent action and is used in aftershave and astringent lotions as well as in powder form as a styptic (to stop bleeding).

Ammonia water is ammonia gas dissolved in water. It is a colorless liquid with a pungent, penetrating odor that can be irritating to the eyes and mucous membranes. Ammonia water is used in cosmetology in hair straighteners, aniline and metallic hair dyes, and alone as a 28% ammonia water solution.

Boric acid is used for its bactericidal and fungicidal properties in baby powder, eye creams, mouthwashes, soaps, and skin fresheners. It is a mild healing and antiseptic agent although the American Medical Association warns of possible toxicity. Severe irritation and poisonings have occurred after application to *open* skin wounds.

Ethyl methacrylate is an ester (compound) of ethyl alcohol and methacrylic acid used in the chemical formulation of many sculptured nails. Daily inhalation of fumes is not recommended for health reasons.

Formaldehyde is a colorless gas manufactured by an oxidation process of methyl alcohol. It is used as a disinfectant, fungicide, germicide, and preservative as well as an embalming solution. In the industry, formaldehyde is used in soap, cosmetics, nail hardeners, and polishes. It should be used with caution because National Cancer Institute studies indicate that it is toxic, can lead to DNA damage, and can react with other chemicals to become carcinogenic.

Glycerine is a sweet, colorless, odorless, syrupy liquid formed by the decomposition of oils, fats, or molasses. It is used as a skin softener in cuticle oil, facial creams, and a variety of lotions.

Petrolatum, commonly known as vaseline, petroleum jelly, or paraffin jelly, is a yellowish to white semi-solid greasy mass that is almost insoluble in water. It is used in wax epilators, eyebrow pencils, lipsticks, protective creams, cold creams, and many other cosmetics for its ability to soften and smooth the skin.

Phenylenediamine, derived from coal tar, has a succession of derivatives known to penetrate the skin and believed to cause cancer.

Potassium hydroxide (caustic potash) is prepared by electrolysis of potassium chloride. It may be used for its emulsifying abilities in the formulas for hand lotions, liquid soaps, protective creams, and cuticle softeners.

Quaternary ammonium compounds (quats) are found in many antiseptics, surfactants, preservatives, sanitizers, and germicides. Quats are synthetic derivatives of ammonium chloride. Although quats can be toxic, they are considered safe in the proportions used in the industry.

Sodium bicarbonate (baking soda) is a precipitate made by passing carbon dioxide gas through a solution of sodium carbonate. The resulting white powder is used as a neutralizing agent and (when mixed in shampoo) to remove hair spray buildup.

Sodium carbonate (soda ash or washing soda) is found naturally in ores and lake brines or seawater. It is used in shampoos and permanent wave solutions. Sodium carbonate absorbs water from the air.

Witch hazel is a solution of alcohol, water, and powder ground from the leaves and twigs of the Hamamelis virginiana. It works as an astringent, local anesthetic, and skin freshener. Because of the alcohol content it should not be applied directly to an open wound or the delicate membranes of the eye. (See *alcohol*.)

Zinc oxide is a heavy white powder that is insoluble in water. It is used cosmetically in face powder and foundation creams for its ability to impart opacity.

COSMETIC BODY CLEANSERS

Cosmetics that are designed to cleanse and beautify the skin, hair, and nails are important to the industry. To provide clients with professional services, you need an understanding of these products designed to remove dirt, hair, or foreign odors from the skin. The classifications of these products are soaps, depilatories, and epilators.

Kinds of Soaps

There are two methods of making soap: *traditional* and *synthetic*. *Traditional soap* is a mixture of various types of fatty acids and sodium salts manufactured through a process of adding alkalies to the fats with glycerol. The *synthetic* process is a chemical combination of oils and fatty acids.

The soaps currently used in the beauty industry fall into three classifications: deodorant, beauty, and medicated.

Deodorant soaps include a bactericide that remains on the body to kill the bacteria responsible for odors. The most common antiseptic and antibacterial agent is probably triclocarban. Triclocarban, often listed in the ingredients as TCC, is prepared from aniline. Aniline additives have been known to increase the skin's sensitivity to the sun, which can inflame some types of skin.

Beauty soaps are intended for the more delicate tissues of the face. They are more acid in pH, less drying to the skin, yet able to remove dirt and debris from the skin's surface. Many beauty soaps are transparent and contain large quantities of glycerine. Other beauty soaps contain larger amounts of oils that leave an emollient film on the skin.

Medicated soaps are designed to treat skin problems such as rashes, pimples, and acne. Many contain small percentages of cresol, phenol, or other antiseptics. Resorcinol is often used as a drying agent in medicated products designed to treat oily conditions. The strongest medicated soaps can only be obtained with a physician's prescription.

Depilatories

Depilatories are preparations used for the temporary removal of superfluous hair by dissolving it at the skin line. Depilatories contain detergents to strip the sebum from the hair and adhesives to hold the chemicals to the hair shaft for the 5 to 10 minutes necessary to remove the hair. During the application time swelling accelerating agents such as urea or melamine expand the hair, helping to break hair bonds. Finally, chemicals such as sodium hydroxide, potassium hydroxide, thioglycolic acid, or calcium thioglycolate destroy the disulfide bonds. These chemicals turn the hair into a soft, jelly-like mass of hydrolyzed protein that can be scraped from the skin. Although depilatories are not commonly used in salons, you should be familiar with them in case your clients have used them.

Epilators

Epilators remove the hair by pulling it out of the follicle. Two types of wax are currently used for professional epilation: cold and hot. Both products are made primarily of resins and beeswax. Beeswax has a relatively high incidence of allergic reaction; therefore it is advisable to give a small patch test of the product to be used. Recently, electrical apparatus made for the home market has become available.

COSMETICS FOR SKIN AND FACE

The cosmetic industry has made available a vast array of products designed to improve the condition and appearance of the skin.

Creams

The creams you will be using for professional skin treatments fall into four main categories: *cleansing*, *wrinkle treatments*, *moisturizers*, and *massage cream*.

The action of **cleansing cream** is, in part, caused by the oil content of the cream, which has the ability to dissolve other greasy substances. Older formulas, such as cold cream, contain relatively few ingredients: vegetable or mineral oil, beeswax, water, preservatives, and emulsifiers. The new cleansing formulations are much more complicated and may contain additional de-greasers such as lemon juice, synthetic surfactants, emollients (oils), and humectants (water retainers).

Wrinkle treatments are designed to conceal lines on aging skin in two ways. One is with a crease-filling capacity and the other is through a plumping up of the tissues. Among the many possible ingredients in these treatments are hormones, hyaluronic acid, and collagen. Some are made of herbs and other natural ingredients; others are entirely synthetic.

Moisturizing creams are designed to treat dryness. They contain humectants, which create a barrier that allows the natural water and oil of the skin to accumulate in the tissues. This barrier also works to protect the skin from air pollution, dirt, and debris. Moisturizers contain a variety of emollients, ranging from simple ingredients such as peanut, coconut, or a variety of other oils to more complex chemical compounds such as cetyl alcohol, cholesterol, dimethicone, or glycerine derivatives.

Massage creams are used to help the hands glide over the skin. They are formulations of cold cream, lanolin or its derivatives, and possibly casein (a protein found in cheese).

Lotions

Lotions are used professionally in a variety of hair and facial treatments. The lotions you will work with generally are available in clear or lightly tinted solutions.

Cleansing lotions serve the same purposes as cleansing creams but are of a lighter oil content. They come in formulations for dry, normal, and oily skin conditions. Some ingredients common to cleansing lotions are cetyl alcohol, cetyl palmitate, and sorbitol combined with perfumes and colorings to enhance their marketing value.

Astringent lotions are designed to remove oil accumulation on the skin. The alcohol content of the product also "irritates" the skin, causing it to swell slightly and appear to "close" the pores. Astringent lotions contain a large percentage of alcohol and small percentages of some or all of the following: alum, boric acid, sorbitol, water, camphor, and perfumes.

Freshener lotions are similar to astringent lotions; however, they are designed to be gentler for dry to normal skin types. The formulation of a freshener typically includes some or all of the following: witch hazel, alcohol and camphorated alcohol, citric acid, boric acid, lactic acid, phosphoric acid, aluminum salts, menthol, chamomile, and floral scents.

Eye lotions are generally formulas of boric acid, bicarbonate of soda, zinc sulfate, glycerine, and herbs. They are designed to soothe and brighten the eyes.

Medicated lotions are prescribed by a physician for skin problems such as acne, rashes, or other eruptions.

Suntan lotions are designed to protect the skin from the harmful ultra violet rays of the sun. They are rated with a sun protection factor (SPF) that enables sunbathers to calculate the time they can remain in the sun before the skin begins to burn. Suntan lotions are emulsions that might contain para-aminobenzoic acid (PABA), a variety of oils, petrolatum, sorbitan stearate, alcohol, ultra violet inhibitors, acid derivatives, preservatives, and perfumes.

COSMETICS FOR MAKEUP

Face Powder

Two forms of face powder are widely used in the salon: *loose* and *compact (cake)*. Both types have the same basic composition; compact powders are simply compressed and held together with binders so the cake will not crumble.

Face powder consists of a powder base, mixed with a coloring agent (pigment) and perfume. A good face powder for normal skin should possess the following qualities:

1. *Slip*—gives a smooth feel to the skin. This quality is gained primarily (35% to 79%) by the talc content, but zinc stearate or magnesium stearate may be added for additional slip.
2. *Covering power*—the balance between opacity (covering defects and skin shine) and transparency (allowing the

natural appearance of the skin to show through). The two ingredients that provide the balance in most powders are zinc oxide and titanium dioxide.

3. *Adherency*—determines how long the powder will remain on the face without needing to be touched up. Talc, zinc stearate, magnesium stearate, kaolin, and chalk have adhesive qualities.

4. *Bloom*—ability to impart a velvet-like appearance to the skin. Starches and chalk are used to create bloom.

5. *Other ingredients*—include bactericides, color, and perfume. Bactericides are added to inhibit growth of bacteria and preserve the product. The colors listed on the ingredient list should be FD&C (Food, Drug, and Cosmetic) or D&C (Drug and Cosmetic) approved, indicating that the colors have been certified by the Food and Drug Administration. Perfumes are added to increase the marketability of the product.

CAUTION

▶ *Although talc is generally considered safe for use in powders, the FDA has received reports of tissue swelling upon use. Talc has also been linked to coughing, vomiting, pneumonia, and even ovarian cancer when inhaled. Miners of talc frequently suffer from a lung disease called talcosis.*

Foundation Makeup

The purpose of foundation makeup is to improve the appearance of the complexion by blending skin tones, covering blemishes, and creating a smooth, healthy glow. Many foundations contain barrier agents such as UV inhibitors, cellulose derivatives, and silicone to protect the complexion from light rays (artificial and natural), the wind and cold, and from dirt and debris.

Cream foundations are predominantly water, mineral oil, stearic acid, cetyl alcohol, propylene glycol, triethanolamine, lanolin derivatives, borax, and insoluble pigments. Foundations may also contain surfactants (detergents), emulsifiers, humectants, perfume, and preservatives such as paraben. The formulation of this product is generally suited for dry to normal skin and gives good coverage.

Liquid foundations are suspensions of organic and inorganic pigments in an alcohol and water solution. Most liquid foundations must be shaken before use, but bentonite is added to help keep the product blended. The formulation of this product is generally suited for clients with oily to normal skin conditions desiring light to natural-looking coverage.

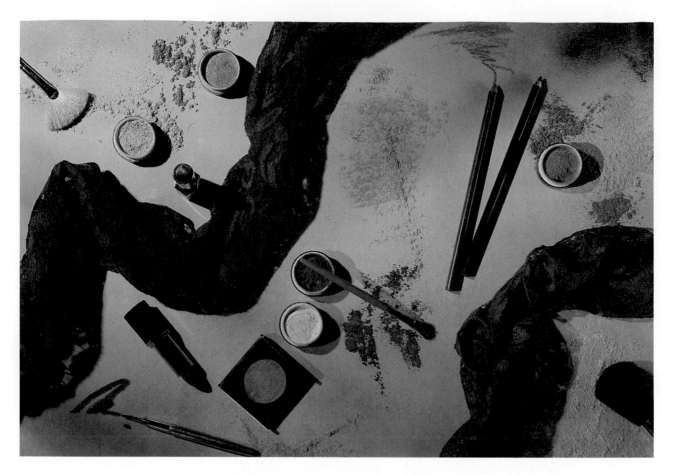

25.11—There is a variety of cosmetics available on the market.

Cheek Color (Blush)

Cheek color is available in powder and cream form.

Powder cheek color is simply compact or cake powder with coloring added. The pigment ranges from 5% to 20% of the product.

Cream cheek colors fall into two categories: oil-based and emulsions. The oil-based formulations are combinations of pigments dispersed in an oil or fat base. Blends of waxes (carnauba wax and ozokerite) and oily liquids (isopropyl myristate and hexadecyl stearate) create a water-resistant product. In addition, cream cheek colors contain water, thickeners, and a variety of surfactants or detergents that enable particles to penetrate the hair follicles and cracks in the skin.

Lip Color

Lip color is available in a variety of forms: creams, glosses, pencils, gels, and sticks. All are formulas of oils, waxes, and dyes. Castor oil is the primary ingredient in lipsticks, accounting for approximately 65% of the product. Other oils used are olive, mineral, sesame, cocoa butter, petroleum, lecithin, and hydrogenated vegetable oils. Waxes commonly included in the ingredients are paraffin, beeswax, carnauba (also used in car waxes), and candelilla wax. Bromic acid, D&C Red No. 27, D&C Orange No. 17 Lake, and related dyes are examples of those often used as coloring agents.

Eye Makeup

Eye pencils consist of a wax (paraffin) or hardened oil base (petrolatum) with a variety of additives to create color. They are available in both soft and hard form for use on the eyebrow as well as the upper and lower eyelid. According to the American Medical Association, eye pencils should not be used to color the inside border of the eyes because this can lead to infection of the lacrimal duct, tearing, blurring of vision, and permanent pigmentation of the mucous membrane lining inside the eye.

Eye shadows are available in cream and powder form. The cream shadows are water-based with oil, petrolatum, thickener, wax, perfume, preservatives, and color added. Water-resistant shadows have a solvent base such as mineral spirits. Powder shadows are composed much the same as pressed face powder and powdered cheek color.

Mascara is available in tube and wand applicators. Both are polymer products that include water, wax, thickeners, film-formers, and preservatives in their formulation. The pigments in mascara must be inert (unable to combine with other elements) and usually are carbon black, carmine, ultramarine, chromium oxide, and iron oxides. Coal tar dyes are not permitted. Some wand mascaras contain rayon or nylon fibers to lengthen and thicken the hair fibers.

CAUTION

▶ *Apply mascara carefully. The most common injury with mascara is poking the eye with the applicator.*

Eyeliners are available in liquid and cake form as well as the pencil form described earlier. In the ingredient list you will find alkanolamine (a fatty alcohol), cellulose, ether, polyvinylpyrrolidone, methylparaben, antioxidants, perfumes, and titanium dioxide.

Eye makeup removers fall into two categories: oil-based and non-oil-based. Oil-based removers are generally mineral oil with a small amount of fragrance added. Non-oil-based removers are a water solution to which acetone, boric acid, oils, lanolin or lanolin derivatives, and other solvents have been added. Because most eye makeup products are water-resistant, plain soap and water is less effective for removal.

Cosmetics for eye and face makeup comprise an important segment of the beauty industry. As a professional cosmetologist, you will be called upon to use, recommend, and sell these cosmetics.

Miscellaneous Cosmetics

Greasepaint is a mixture of fats, petrolatum, and a coloring agent and is used for theatrical purposes.

Cake or *pancake makeup* is generally composed of kaolin, zinc, talc, titanium oxide, mineral oil, fragrances, precipitated calcium carbonate, finely ground pigments, and inorganic pigments such as iron oxides. Cake makeup is used to cover scars and pigmentation defects.

Masks and *packs* are available to serve many purposes and skin conditions—deep cleansing, pore reduction, tightening, firming, moisturizing, wrinkle reduction. Clay masks typically contain varying combinations of kaolin (china clay), bentonite, purified siliceous (fuller's) earth or colloidal clay, petrolatum, glycerine, proteins, SD alcohol, and water. The prime ingredients typically found in peel-off masks are SD alcohol 40, polysorbate-20, and polymers such as polyvinyl alcohol or vinyl acetate.

Scalp Lotions and Ointments

Scalp lotions and ointments usually contain medicinal agents for the purpose of correcting a scalp condition such as itching and flakiness. An astringent lotion may be applied to the scalp before shampooing to control oiliness as well as the itching and flakiness of dry scalp conditions. Medicated lotions and ointments for severe scalp conditions must be prescribed by a physician.

Hair Dressings

Hair dressings give shine and manageability to dry or curly hair. They may be applied to either wet or dry hair. Such dressings typically consist of lanolin or its derivatives, petrolatum, oil emulsions, fatty acids, waxes, mild alkalies, and water.

Styling Aids

As a professional cosmetologist, you will utilize a variety of styling gels and mousses. Both of these products are typically polymer and resin formulations designed to give the hair body and texture. Many incorporate the same ingredients found in hair sprays (see below) but add moisturizers and humectants, such as cetyl alcohol, panthenol, hydrolyzed protein, quats, or a variety of oils to the ingredient list.

Hair Sprays

Hair spray is used to hold the finished style. Many new formulations for hair spray contain a variety of polymers, such as acrylic/acrylate copolymer, vinyl acetate, crotonic acid copolymer, PVM/MA copolymer, and polyvinylpyrrolidone (PVP), and plasticizers such as acetyl triethyl citrate, benzyl alcohol, and silicones as stiffening agents. Additional ingredients might include silicone, shellac, perfume, lanolin or its derivatives, vegetable gums, alcohol, sorbitol, and water.

CAUTION

▶ *Careless use of hair spray can cause eye and lung damage and throat irritation.*

Success Spotlight

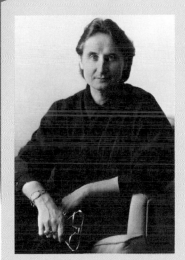

Many hairdressers who care about their industry go on to change it for the better.

Horst Rechelbacher, chairman and founder of the Aveda Corporation, began his hairdressing career in Austria and came to the United States after winning every major hair design award worldwide. He established his first Horst and Friends salon in Minneapolis in 1965.

Dedicated to the belief that there must be a balance between the body and mind and that each individual has a responsibility to preserve the environment, Horst began conducting extensive research on plant and flower essences to determine how nature could be utilized to benefit the body and the mind. The result is his line of environmentally responsible, aromatherapy skin, hair, and body products.

Says Horst, "We are committed to increasing the consumer's awareness of the devastating effects synthetic ingredients have on our environment. Chemically produced petroleum derivatives contribute to ozone depletion, acid rain, and birth defects."

To continue his research, Horst founded the International Aromatherapy Research Foundation, a nonprofit organization that supports research on the activities of plant and flower essences as well as environmental protection and preservation. Driven by a desire to share his knowledge with others, he also founded the Horst Education Center for Cosmetology, which offers basic and advanced courses in hair, skin, and nail care.

Review Questions

CHEMISTRY

1. Why is it important to understand basic chemistry to be successful as a cosmetologist?
2. What is the difference between organic and inorganic chemistry?
3. List the three forms of matter.
4. Define physical change and give one example.
5. Define chemical change and give one example.
6. What is pH?
7. List the four classifications of shampoo.
8. What are polypeptide chains?
9. List the three types of chemical bonds in the cortex.
10. What changes occur in the hair cortex during permanent waving?
11. Define the following terms as they relate to oxidation tints: base, coupler, oxidizer.
12. List the six physical and chemical classifications of cosmetics.
13. Why must you be concerned with the application of concentrated alcohol on the skin?
14. What causes hair removal when using a depilatory?
15. List the four main types of creams you will be using as a professional cosmetologist.
16. What is the action of an astringent?
17. What are some of the common chemical ingredients in foundation makeup?

26

THE SALON BUSINESS

LEARNING OBJECTIVES

After completing this chapter, you should be able to:

1. List some facts you need before opening a beauty salon.
2. Discuss financial considerations involved in operating a beauty salon.
3. Explain the importance of maintaining accurate business records.
4. Explain the importance of good business operation and personnel management.
5. Discuss the principles and practices of good selling.
6. Explain the importance of advertising.

Introduction

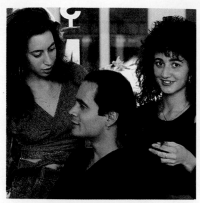

26.1—Active salon managers.

Numerous management opportunities exist in the field of cosmetology. Many cosmetology school graduates want to advance themselves and become owners or managers of salons. However, only if you are adequately prepared to manage a business will you be able to realize your ambitions. (Fig. 26.1)

Starting your own business is a big responsibility and not a step to be taken without serious planning. A knowledge of business principles, bookkeeping, business laws, insurance, salesmanship, and psychology is crucial to the cosmetologist who aspires to be an owner and/or manager of a salon. This chapter covers some of the areas you must know about before becoming an owner/manager of a business.

What You Should Know About Opening a Salon

When planning to open a salon, give careful consideration to every aspect of running a business, including location, written agreements, business regulations, laws, insurance, salon operation, record keeping, and salon policies.

LOCATION

A good location is one that has a population large enough to support the salon. When possible, the salon should be located near other active businesses, such as restaurants, department stores, or specialized clothing stores, shoe stores, and other fashion-related shops or supermarkets. People are drawn to shopping areas where they can make one stop serve several purposes, and unless you can afford to do a great deal of advertising, it is difficult to operate a successful salon in a low traffic area.

In general, the location you select should reflect your target market. If you are targeting a high-income client, your location should reflect that. If you plan to appeal to middle-income clients, you should consider a high-traffic area with access to public transportation.

Study the Area
Determine the area's demographics. Find out about the size, income, and buying habits of the population. Talk to other business owners to see how well they think a salon would do in the area.

Be Visible
The salon should be clearly visible and eye catching to attract the attention of people walking or driving by.

Parking Facilities

When selecting a site for a new business, or when planning to take over an established business, you must consider parking facilities. People hesitate to patronize a business that is inconvenient to reach during bad weather. Convenience of parking should be a major consideration. If your salon is open for evening service, the parking area should be well lighted. In larger cities, consider locating the salon near public transportation to attract clients who do not drive or for easy access when the weather is bad.

Competition

Avoid too much direct competition in the immediate area. It is better to locate in an area where yours is the only salon of its type. Salons can be located near each other, provided that each has a different clientele. For example, an up-scale salon can operate close to a budget salon and both may be successful because they attract different markets.

WRITTEN AGREEMENTS

Written agreements for building alterations and repairs will prevent disputes over who must pay for what.

Study the Lease

Before signing a *lease*, be certain you understand all provisions that pertain to the landlord and to the tenant. The lease should provide for alterations that must be made by the landlord. Most leases provided by the landlord are written in favor of the landlord. To protect your interests, hire a lawyer to help with your negotiations.

BUSINESS PLAN

It is very important that you develop a business plan before you open a salon. It is a necessary tool to obtain financing and to provide a blueprint for future growth. The plan should include a general description of the business and the services it will provide; a statement of the number of personnel to be hired; their salaries and other benefits; an operations plan that includes your price structure, expenses such as equipment, supplies, repairs, advertising, taxes and insurance, and a financial plan that includes a profit and loss statement. If you are uncertain about developing a business plan, consult a professional.

In addition, it is important to have enough working capital when you open a salon. It often takes time to build a clientele, so you must have enough money available for your expenses.

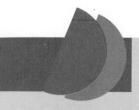

Focus On: Carol Phillips, Retail Specialist

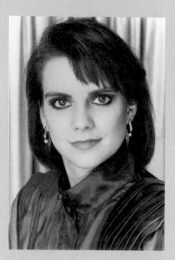

Like many resourceful entrepreneurs, when Carol Phillips encountered a problem, she turned it around into a dynamic opportunity. Her ambition to boost her salon's profits led her into an exciting new career as a retail specialist. "I had to find a way to bring in more revenue to the salon," Phillips recalls. "I couldn't do any more services. You only have two hands and two legs so you can only do so many services in a given day. I was maxed out where I was." So Phillips explored new ground.

"I decided to increase retail sales," she says. "I really investigated how to market products. I read everything about selling I could get my hands on, and I observed people all the time." Phillips's homework so successfully paid off, she later gave up the salon and built a career from the marketing knowhow she had personally uncovered. Now she travels around the country teaching salons and manufacturers how to increase retail sales.

"My experience is what's most valuable," notes Phillips. "I spent 12 years in the trenches." From that experience, she defines how to rise above the crowd: "It's not that you have to do something one thousand percent better than everyone else. It's that you have to do one thousand things one percent better than everyone else."

REGULATIONS, BUSINESS LAWS, AND INSURANCE

When running a business you must comply with local, state, and federal regulations and laws.

Local regulations usually cover building renovations (local business codes).

Federal law covers Social Security, unemployment compensation or insurance, and cosmetics and luxury tax payments. OSHA requires that ingredients of cosmetic preparations (including permanent wave solutions and hair tints) be displayed prominently for clients. OSHA distributes MSDS sheets for this purpose.

State laws cover sales taxes, licenses, and employee compensation.

Income tax laws are covered by both the state and federal governments.

Insurance covers malpractice, premises liability, fire, burglary and theft, and business interruption. Also, check into Key Man Insurance (an insurance policy that safeguards against the loss of work of an important employee or yourself) and disability policies and make sure you are covered for everything your lease demands.

TYPES OF SALON OWNERSHIP

A salon can be owned and operated by an *individual*, a *partnership*, or a *corporation*. Before deciding which type of ownership is most desirable, you should be acquainted with the relative merits and shortcomings of each.

Individual Ownership

1. The proprietor is owner and manager.
2. The proprietor determines policies and makes decisions.
3. The proprietor receives all profits and bears all losses.

Partnership

1. Ownership is shared (not necessarily equally) by two or more people. One purpose of this type of arrangement is to have more capital available for investment.
2. The abilities and experience of each partner make it easier to share work and responsibilities and to make decisions.
3. Each partner assumes each other's unlimited liability for debts.

Corporation

1. Ownership is shared by three or more people called *stockholders*.
2. A *charter* is required by the state.
3. A corporation is subject to taxation and regulation by the state.
4. The management is in the hands of a board of directors who determine policies and make decisions in accordance with the corporation's charter.
5. The division of profits is proportionate to the number of shares owned by each stockholder.
6. The stockholders cannot lose more than their original investment in the corporation.

Purchasing an Established Salon

An agreement to buy an established salon should include the following:

1. A written purchase and sale agreement to avoid any misunderstandings between the contracting parties.
2. A complete and signed statement of inventory (goods, fixtures, etc.) indicating the value of each article.
3. If there is a transfer of a note, chattel mortgage, lease, and bill of sale, the buyer should initiate an investigation to determine if there is any default in the payment of debts.
4. Identity of owner.

5. Use of salon's name and reputation for a definite period of time.
6. A statement that the seller will not compete with the new owner within a specified distance from the present location.
7. Additional guidance provided by your lawyer.

Drawing Up a Lease
1. Secure exemption of fixtures or appliances that might be attached to the salon so that they can be removed without violating the lease.
2. Secure an agreement about necessary renovations and repairs, such as painting, plumbing, fixtures, and electrical installation.
3. Secure an option from the landlord to assign the lease to another person. In this way, the obligations for the payment of rent are kept separate from the responsibilities of operating the business.

PROTECTION AGAINST FIRE, THEFT, AND LAWSUITS
1. Keep the premises securely locked.
2. Purchase liability, fire, malpractice, and burglary insurance.
3. Do not violate the medical practice law of your state by attempting to diagnose, treat, or cure a disease.
4. Become thoroughly familiar with all laws governing cosmetology and with the sanitary codes of your city and state.
5. Keep accurate records of the number of workers, the amount of salaries, lengths of employment, and Social Security numbers required by various state and federal laws that affect the social welfare of employees.

▶ NOTE: Ignorance of the law is no excuse for its violation.

BUSINESS OPERATION
The owner or manager must have business sense, knowledge, ability, good judgment, and diplomacy. Smooth salon management depends on:

1. Sufficient investment capital.
2. Efficiency of management.
3. Good business procedures.
4. Cooperation between management and employees.
5. Trained and experienced salon personnel.

If there is failure in one or more of these categories, you probably will have difficulty staying in business.

Allocation of Money

As a good business operator you must always know where your money is being spent. A good accountant and accounting system are highly valuable.

The following figures may vary in different localities. In large towns and cities items such as rent might run higher, while in small towns rent might be lower and utilities and telephone higher. The figures are suggested merely as a general guide.

Average Expenses for Salons in the United States

(Based on total gross income)	Percent
Salaries and commissions (including payroll taxes)	53.5
Rent	13
Supplies	5
Advertising	3
Depreciation	3
Laundry	1
Cleaning	1
Light and power	1
Repairs	1.5
Insurance	.75
Telephone	.75
Miscellaneous	1.5
Total expenses	85
Net profit	15
	100%

Clearly, the largest expense items are salaries, rent, supplies, and advertising. The first three merit your closest attention. Advertising can be adjusted at your discretion.

THE IMPORTANCE OF RECORD KEEPING

Good business operation requires that you have a simple and efficient record system. Proper business records are necessary to meet the requirements of local, state, and federal laws regarding taxes and employees. Records are of value only if they are correct, concise, and complete. Bookkeeping includes keeping an accurate record of all income and expenses. Income is usually classified as receipts from services and retail sales. Expenses include rent, utilities, insurance, salaries, advertising, equipment, and repairs. A professional accountant is recommended to help keep records accurate. Retain check stubs, canceled checks, receipts, and invoices.

All business transactions must be recorded for the following reasons:

1. To determine income, expenses, profit, or loss.
2. To assess the value of the salon for prospective buyers.

3. To arrange a bank loan or financing.
4. For reports on income tax, Social Security, unemployment and disability insurance, accidents, and for percentage payments of gross income required in some leases.

Weekly Records

A weekly or monthly summary helps to:

1. Make comparisons with other years.
2. Detect any changes in demands for services.
3. Check on the use of materials according to the type of service rendered.
4. Control expenses and waste.

Daily Records

Keeping daily records enables the owner or manager to know just how well the business is functioning. Each expense item affects the total gross income. Accurate records show the cost of operation in relation to income. Keep daily sales slips, appointment book, and a petty cash book for at least six months. Payroll book, canceled checks, and monthly and yearly records are usually held for at least seven years. Service and inventory records are also important to keep.

Purchase and Inventory Records

Purchase records help to maintain a perpetual inventory that can be used to:

1. Prevent overstock of needed supplies.
2. Prevent running short of needed supplies.
3. Help establish the net worth of the business at the end of the year.

Keep a running inventory of all supplies. Classify them according to their use and retail value. Those to be used in the daily business operation are *consumption supplies*. Those to be sold to clients are *retail supplies*.

Inventory records can tell you which merchandise is selling most quickly and which items do not sell well. You will then be able to judge how much of each product to order so that it can be used or sold within a reasonable period of time. It is better to have slightly more than enough supplies. Try to plan major purchases of supplies around times when dealers offer special prices.

Service Records

A service record should be kept of treatments given and merchandise sold to each client. A card file system or memorandum book kept in a central location should be used for these records.

All service records should include the name and address of the client, date of each purchase or service, amount charged, products used, and results obtained. Also, note the client's preferences and tastes.

PLANNING THE SALON'S LAYOUT

The layout of a salon should be well planned to achieve maximum efficiency. Most professional product suppliers will be happy to help you plan your layout, usually at a reasonable fee, or perhaps for no fee at all. (Fig. 26.2)

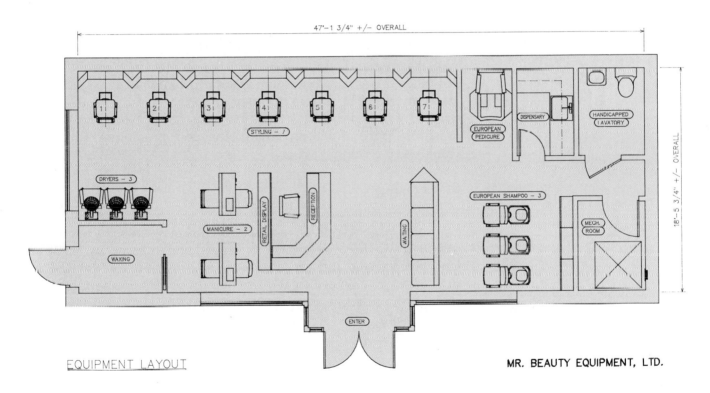

26.2—Salon blueprint.

To obtain maximum efficiency when planning the physical layout of a salon, you should consider the following:

1. Flow of operational services to and from the reception area.
2. Adequate aisle space.

3. Space allotment for equipment.
4. Furniture, fixtures, and equipment chosen on the basis of cost, durability, utility, and appearance. The purchase of standard and guaranteed equipment is a worthwhile investment.
5. A color scheme that is restful and flattering.
6. A dispensary.
7. Adequate storage space.
8. A clean restroom with a toilet and basin.
9. Good plumbing and sufficient lighting for satisfactory services.
10. Good ventilation, air conditioning, and heating.
11. Adequate clothing closet and changing area for clients.

Operating a Salon

Clients who visit your salon should feel that they have been well taken care of and should look forward to their next visit. To accomplish this goal, your salon needs to be well organized and smoothly run. The factors to consider about operating your salon efficiently on a day-to-day basis are your personnel, policies and practices, price structure, advertising and promotion, and the "look" of the salon.

PERSONNEL

The size of your salon will determine the size of your staff. For example, large salons have receptionists, hair stylists, manicurists, hair washers, colorists, masseurs and masseuses, people who give facials, and those who do waxing and electrolysis. A smaller salon will have some combination of these personnel who are able to perform more than one service. For example, in a smaller salon, the stylist might also be the colorist and give permanents.

Hiring Your Staff

The success of a salon depends on the quality of the work done by the staff. A satisfied client returns for more services and recommends the salon to others. When interviewing potential employees, you should consider their personality, level of skill, personal grooming, and the clients they will bring with them.

SALON POLICIES AND PRACTICES

It is important that all salon personnel are aware of policies and practices in order to maintain a smooth day-to-day operation.

Pricing of Services

Cost of services is generally established according to the location of the salon and the type of clientele you expect to serve. A price list should be posted in a place where it can be seen by all clients—probably at the reception desk.

The Reception Area

First impressions count, and since the reception area is the first thing clients see, you should make your reception area attractive, appealing, and comfortable. Remember that your receptionist, phone system, dressing area, and retail merchandise may be located in this area. You should also have a supply of business cards with the address and phone number of the salon on the reception desk. Most important to you, this is also the place where the client's financial transactions are handled. (Fig. 26.3)

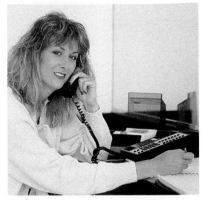

26.3—Salon receptionist.

The Receptionist

Second only in importance to your cosmetologists is your receptionist. A good receptionist is the "quarterback" of the salon. This is the first person seen by the arriving client. The receptionist should be pleasant, greet each client with a smile, and call him or her by name. Efficient service creates goodwill, confidence, and satisfaction. Favorable impressions begin with the courteous reception of the client. These impressions last as long as the client obtains the desired results from salon services.

The receptionist handles many important functions including answering the phone, booking appointments, informing the stylist that a client has arrived, preparing the daily appointment information for the cosmetologists, recommending other services, and reminding the client of retail products.

The receptionist should be especially attentive on the hour and then every 15 minutes after the hour because these are the times clients are scheduled to arrive. Incidental duties and activities such as cleaning, maintaining inventory and daily reports, personal calls, or any other reason to be away from the desk should be carried out during the slowest periods of the hour.

Booking Appointments

Booking appointments must be done with care, because services are sold in terms of time on the appointment page. Appointments must be scheduled so that there is the most efficient use of the time of all salon personnel. A client should not have to wait for a service and a cosmetologist should not have to wait for the next client.

The size of the salon determines who books the appointments. This can be done by a full-time receptionist, the owner or manager, or any of the cosmetologists working in the salon.

A receptionist with a pleasing voice and personality is a valuable asset to the beauty salon. In addition, she must have:

1. An attractive appearance.
2. Knowledge of the various beauty services, their cost, and how much time they require.
3. Unlimited patience with both clients and salon personnel.

Appointment Book

The use of an appointment record helps the cosmetologist arrange working time to suit the client's needs. The salon appointment book accurately reflects what is taking place in the salon at a given time. The appointment schedule allows the cosmetologist to see how many clients will be coming in during the day and how much time is needed to deliver the appropriate services. In most salons, the receptionist prepares the appointment schedule for staff members; in smaller salons, however, each person may prepare his or her own schedule. (Fig. 26.4)

26.4—Appointment book.

USE OF THE TELEPHONE IN THE SALON

An important part of the salon business is handled over the telephone. Good telephone habits and techniques make it possible for the salon owner and cosmetologist to increase business and improve relationships with clients and suppliers. With each call, you have a chance to build the salon's reputation by providing high-caliber service.

The telephone can be used to:

1. Make or change appointments.
2. Seek new business, or find out why you've lost a client.
3. Remind clients of needed services.
4. Answer questions and provide friendly service.
5. Handle complaints to the client's satisfaction.
6. Receive messages.
7. Order equipment and supplies.

Business in the salon can be promoted effectively over the phone, provided there is:

1. Good planning.
2. Good telephone usage.

Good Planning

Good planning consists of assigning the right person to a telephone task and providing the necessary information with which to perform the task. A reliable substitute should be trained to make outgoing and answer incoming calls when the regular person is not in.

The phone is usually located at the reception desk since this is where the salon appointment book is located. Because it can be noisy at the reception desk, outgoing business calls to clients and suppliers should be made at a quiet time of the day or from a telephone placed in a quieter area of the salon.

Provide a comfortable seat by the phone. There should also be an appointment book, client's record cards, pencil or ball-point pen, and paper pad readily accessible. An up-to-date list of frequently-called telephone numbers and a recent telephone directory should also be available.

The person using the telephone should:

1. Have a pleasant telephone voice. Speak clearly, use correct grammar, and put a "smile" in his/her voice.
2. Show interest and concern when talking with a client or a supplier.

3. Be polite, respectful, and courteous to all, even though some people test the limits of your patience.

4. Be tactful. Do not say anything to irritate the person on the other end of the phone.

5. Plan what is to be said during the call. Make a list of the main points you want to discuss. Knowing what you want to say helps you to project an image of confidence and efficiency. It is also useful to jot down key points of the other person's responses or questions. That can help you address yourself to the speaker's concerns and interests.

Incoming Phone Calls

Incoming phone calls are the lifeline of a salon. Clients usually call ahead for appointments with a preferred cosmetologist, or they might call to cancel or reschedule an appointment. The person answering the phone, usually the receptionist, should develop telephone skills to handle the different types of incoming calls. As mentioned, always answer the phone with a smile in your voice, speak clearly, use correct grammar, concentrate on listening to the person you are speaking with, and be polite, respectful, and tactful. In addition, here are some guidelines to remember when answering the telephone:

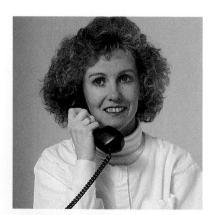

26.5—The telephone is an important part of the salon business.

1. When you answer the phone, say, "Good morning (afternoon or evening), Milady Salon. May I help you?" Some salons also require that you give your name to the caller. The first words you say tell the caller something about your personality. Let that person know that you're glad he or she called. (Fig. 26.5)

2. Answer the phone promptly. Nothing is more irritating than calling a place of business and having to wait four or five rings before somebody answers the phone. On a multi-line system, when a call comes in while you are talking on another line, ask to put the person on hold, answer the second call, and ask that person to hold while you complete the first call. Take callers in the order that they phone.

3. If you do not have the information requested by the caller, you can do one of two things: put the caller on hold and get the information or offer to call the person back with the information as soon as you have it.

4. Do not talk with someone standing nearby while you are speaking with someone on the phone. You are doing a disservice to both clients.

Booking Appointments by Phone

1. When booking appointments, you should be familiar with all services and products available in the salon and their costs.

2. Be fair when making assignments. Do not schedule six appointments for one cosmetologist and two for another unless, of course, a client has requested a particular cosmetologist. Assign four clients to each cosmetologist.

3. If someone calls asking for an appointment with a particular cosmetologist at a particular day and time and that technician is not available then, there are several ways to handle the situation:

   a) If the client regularly uses one cosmetologist, suggest other times the cosmetologist is available.

   b) If the client cannot come in at any of those times, suggest another cosmetologist.

   c) If the client is unwilling to try another cosmetologist, offer to call the client if there is a cancellation at the desired time.

Handling Complaints by Telephone

Handling complaints, particularly over the phone, is a difficult task. The caller is probably upset and short-tempered. Try to use self-control, tact, and courtesy, no matter how trying the circumstances may be. Only then will the caller be made to feel that he or she has been fairly treated.

Remember that the tone of your voice must be sympathetic and reassuring. Your manner of speaking should make the caller believe that you are really concerned about the complaint. Do not interrupt the caller. Listen to the entire problem. After hearing the complaint in full, you should try to resolve the situation quickly and effectively. The following are suggestions for dealing with some problems. If other problems arise, follow the policy of the salon or check with the owner/manager for advice.

1. Tell the unhappy client that you are sorry for what happened and explain the reason for the difficulty. Tell the client that the problem will not happen again.

2. Sympathize with the client by saying that you understand and that you regret the inconvenience suffered. Express thanks that the person called this matter to your attention.

3. Ask the client how the salon can remedy the situation. If the request is fair and reasonable, check with the owner/manager for approval.

4.   If the client is dissatisfied with the results of a service, suggest a visit to the salon to see what can be done to remedy the problem.

5.   If a client is dissatisfied with the behavior of a cosmetologist, call the owner/manager to the phone.

Selling in the Salon

As more products are added to salon operations, selling is becoming an increasingly important responsibility of the cosmetologist. The cosmetologist who is equally proficient as hairstylist and salesperson is most likely to be the one to succeed in business. Advising clients about the proper products to use in their beauty regimen will not only add dollars to your income, but will better enable the clients to maintain the look you worked so hard to achieve.

No attempt is made here to cover all aspects of selling, but if you use this material as a basis upon which to build, effective selling techniques will become part of your repertoire of skills.

To be successful in sales you need ambition, determination, and a good personality. The first step in selling is to sell yourself. Clients must like and trust you before they will purchase beauty services, cosmetics, skin care items, shampoos and conditioners, or other merchandise.

Every client who enters the salon is a prospective purchaser of additional services or merchandise. The manner in which you treat that person lays the foundation for suggestive selling. Recognizing the needs and preferences of clients makes the intelligent use of suggestive selling possible. (Fig. 26.6)

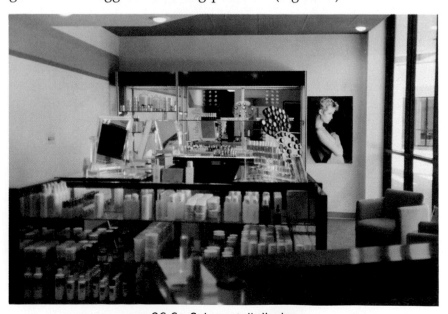

26.6—Salon retail display.

SELLING PRINCIPLES

To become a proficient salesperson you must understand and be able to apply the following principles of selling:

1. Be familiar with the merits and benefits of each service and product.
2. Adapt your approach and technique to meet the needs of each client.
3. Be self-confident.
4. Generate interest and desire, which are the steps leading to a sale.
5. Never misrepresent your service or product.
6. Use tact when selling to a client.
7. Don't underestimate the client or the client's intelligence.
8. To sell a product or service, deliver a sales talk in a relaxed, friendly manner and, if possible, demonstrate its use.
9. Recognize the right psychological moment to close any sale. Once the client has offered to buy, quit selling—don't oversell, except to praise the client for the purchase and assure her that she will be happy with it.

TYPES OF CLIENTS

The cosmetologist who is most likely to be successful in selling additional services or merchandise to clients is one who can recognize the many different types of people and knows how to deal with each type.

The following material describes seven of the most common types you are likely to meet and suggests ways each type might be treated.

1. *Shy, timid type.* Make the client feel at ease. Lead the conversation. Don't force the conversation. Be cheerful.
2. *Talkative type.* Be a good, patient listener. Tactfully switch the conversation to beauty needs.
3. *Nervous, irritable type.* Does not want much conversation. Wants simple, practical hairdo and a fast worker. Get started and finished as quickly as possible.
4. *Inquisitive, over-cautious type.* Explain everything in detail. Show him or her facts—sealed bottles, brand names. Ask for the client's opinion.
5. *"Know-it-all" type.* Suggest things in question form. Don't argue with this person. Offer compliments.
6. *Teenager.* Usually interested in current fashions. Give special advice on hair care and other beauty needs.

7. *Mature* (60 and older). Be extra courteous. Suggest hairstyles that give this person a younger look without looking too young (and foolish).

THE PSYCHOLOGY OF SELLING

Each person who enters a salon is an individual with specific wants and needs. No matter how good a beauty service or product may be, you will find it difficult to make a sale if the client has no need for it. Thus, your first task is to determine whether the client has a need for or an interest in a service or product.

Motives for Buying

What are the motives that prompt clients to purchase services and products? Very often the motivations are vanity, personal satisfaction, and esthetic gratification. In our society people try to look youthful with a trim figure, fresh complexion, and a contemporary hairstyle.

Helping Your Client Decide

If a client is doubtful or undecided about a service or a product, help the decision along with honest and sincere advice. For example, if a client is thinking about coloring her hair and she already has had a permanent, you might advise her about the extra care that is needed with both treatments.

It is important that you tell the client about the beauty service and what it can mean in terms of results and benefits. Always keep in mind that the best interests of the client should be your first consideration. Careful consideration will acquaint you with the client's needs, and those needs can be fulfilled to the complete satisfaction of the client as well as to your financial advantage.

SELLING PRODUCTS

Many salons offer a wide range of products from jewelry to cosmetics. In order to satisfy the varied needs and desires of clients, the salon should stock a wide range of inventory. The person in charge of these accessories must be familiar with all products and their comparative merits.

Advertising

Advertising includes all activities that promote the salon favorably. Advertising must attract and hold the reader's, listener's, or viewer's attention and create a desire for the service or product.

A pleased client is the best form of advertising. Some salons hire a public relations firm rather than develop their own advertising, but this is expensive.

An advertising budget should run about 3% of your gross income. Plan at least 6 months to a year ahead, and concentrate most of your advertising on traditionally slow periods. Also, plan for holidays and special yearly events. Here are some suggested ways to advertise:

1. Newspapers.
2. Direct mail for closer contact with the potential client.
3. Classified advertising in the yellow pages of your telephone book is relatively inexpensive. For a yellow pages display ad, consult with your suppliers as to the availability of *co-op advertising* with certain major product lines.
4. A window display attracts passersby.
5. Radio advertising is more expensive, but is very effective.
6. TV is a dramatic, but expensive, medium of advertising.
7. Personal public appearances are an excellent means of advertising, especially at women's and men's clubs, church functions, political gatherings, charitable affairs, and on TV and radio talk shows.
8. Contacting clients who have not been in the salon for a while and inviting them back can be very effective.
9. Telemarketing your products and services can also be very effective, and can be done by stylists with "down time."
10. Taped promotions shown on a VCR in the salon can also be developed.

Review Questions

THE SALON BUSINESS

1. What things should be considered when opening a beauty salon?
2. Under what three types of ownership may a beauty salon be operated?
3. What purpose do accurate records serve?
4. What two types of supplies make up a beauty salon's inventory?
5. Why is the reception area of a beauty salon important?
6. How will the use of good telephone techniques help a salon?
7. What are the main principles and practices of good selling?
8. Define advertising.
9. What is the best form of advertising?

Glossary/Index

Secondary color, 278
Semi-peremanent hair coloring, 278
Semi-stand up curls, 131
Sensitivity, 278
Sensory nerves, carry impulses or messages from sense organs to the brain, 477
Serratus anterior (ser-RAT-us an-TEER-ee-or), muscles which assist in breathing and in raising the arm, 475
Seventh (facial) cranial nerve, is the chief motor nerve of the face, 479
Shade, 278
Shadow wave, 108
Shampoo
    highlighting color, 252
    selecting, 75
Shampooing
    chemical hair relaxing and, 289-290
    chemically treated hair, 78
    described, 74
    draping for, 68
    materials and implements for, 75
    pre-perm, 200
    procedures, 76-78
    water and, 74
Shampoos
    chemistry of, 513-516
    color, 81
    conditioning, 80
    dry, 81
    hairpieces and, 81
    highlighting, 81
    medicated, 80
    surfactants actions in, 515
    types of,
        acid-balanced, 79
        pH and, 79
        wigs and, 81
Shaping, is a section of hair that is molded into a design to serve as a base for a curl or wave pattern, 116
Shaving, 456-457
Shears
    haircutting, thinning with, 89-90
    holding, 87
    thinning, thinning with, 89
Sheen, 278
Shoes, feet care and, 12
Shortwave method of hair removal, 453-456
Shoulder, muscles of, 475
Shoulder girdle, made up of the clavicle and scapula, 468
Side parts, 160
Single end paper wrap, 208
Single halo perm wrap, 203
Single-process color, 278
Singling hair, 93
Sinks, sanitizing, 36-37
Sinusoidal current, is similar to the faradic current and is used during scalp and facial manipulations, 496
    application of, 497
    caution when using, 497
Sitting, correct posture for, 16
Skeletal (SKEL-e-tahl) system, is the phys-

ical foundation of the body, the bones, 465, 466-469
Skin, 487
    color, 437
    described, 434
    disorders of, 440-441
    elasticity of, 437
    functions of, 439
    glands of, 438-439
    histology of, 435-439
    hypertrophies of, 449
    lesions of, 440-441
        secondary, 442
    nerves of, 436-437
    nourishment of, 436
    pigmentation, definitions concerning, 447-448
Skin disease, any infection of the skin by an objective lesion, 442
Skip waves, 130
Smaller ocipital nerve, located at the base of the skull, affects the scalp and muscles of that region, 479
Soaps, are compounds mixtures of fats and oils purified by distillation, 530, 532
Soda ash, is found naturally in ores and lake brines or sea water, 531
Sodium bicarbonate, a precipitate made by passing carbon dioxide gas through a solution of sodium carbonate, 531
Sodium carbonate, is found naturally in ores and lake brines or sea water, 531
Sodium hydroxide, chemical hair relaxing and, 283, 286-292
Sodium hypochlorite (SOH-di-um HY-po-chlor-it), a disinfectant used to sanitize implements, 33
    described, 33-34
Soft curl permanent, 295-299
Soft pressing, 306-308
Softening agent, 278
Solute (SOL-yoot), is any substance that dissolves into a liquid and forms a solution, 528
Solution (so-LOO-shun), is an evenly dispersed mixture of two or more kinds of molecules, 278, 528
Solvent (SOL-vent), is any substance that is able to dissolve another substance, 278, 528
Specialist, 278
Specific gravity, of a substance is its "lightness" or "heaviness" using water as the basis for comparison, 510
Spectrum, 278
Sphenoid (SFEEN-oid) bone, joins together all the bones of the cranium, 466
Spinal cord, anatomy of, 477
Spiral curls, thermal waving/curling, 175
Spiral wrap for perms, 205
Spirilla, curved or corkscrew-shaped organisms causing diseases such as syphilis, 27
Spot lightening, 278
Square base pin curls, 119

Stabilizer, 278
Stack perm wrap, 206
Stage, 278
Stain, an abnormal discoloration remaining after the disappearance of moles, freckles, or liver spots, 442
Stain remover, 278
Stains, abnormal brown skin patches, having a circular and irregular shape, 447
Stance
    men, 15
    women, 15
Stand up curls, 130-131
Staphylococci, pus-forming organisms that grow in bunches or clusters causing abscesses, pustules, and boils, 26
Steamers, 499
Steatoma (stee-ah-TOH-mah), is a subcutaneous tumor of the sebaceous gland, 445
Sterilization (ster-i-li-ZAY-shun), the process of making an environment germ-free by destroying all bacteria whether they are beneficial or harmful, 24, 32
    described, 32
    methods of, 32-33
Sternum (STUR-numn), the breastbone and cartilage that connects the ribs to the sternum, 468
Straight back perm wrap, 204
Strand test, 278
Stratum corneum (STRAT-um KOHR-nee-um), is the outer layer of the skin, 435
Stratum germinativum (STRAT-um jur-mi-nah-TIV-um), skin which is composed of several layers of different-shaped cells, 435
Stratum granulosum (STRAT-um gran-yoo-LOH-sum). skin that consists of cells that look like distinct granules, 435
Stratum lucidum (STRAT-um LOO-si-dum), skin that consists of small, transparent cells through which light can pass, 435
Stratum mucosum (STRAT-um myoo-KOH-sum), skin which is composed of several layers of different-shaped cells, 435
Streptococci, pus-forming organisms that grow in chains which cause infections such as strep throat, 26
Striated muscles, voluntary muscles which are controlled by will, 469
Styling lotions, blow-dry styling and, 182
Submental (sub-MEN-tahl) artery, supplies the chin and lower lip, 484
Sudoriferous (soo-dohr-IF-er-us)
    disorders of, 446
    sweat glands, 438
Suntan lotions, 534
Supercilia (soo-per-SIL-ee-a), hair of the eyebrows, 48
Superficial temporal (TEM-po-rahl) ar-

052546000

APPROXIMATE CONVERSIONS TO METRIC MEASURES

Symbol	When You Know	Multiply by	To Find	Symbol
LENGTH (speed)				
In	inches	2.5	centimeters	cm
ft	feet	30	centimeters	cm
MASS (weight)				
oz	ounces	28 grams	g	
lb	pounds	0.45	kilograms	kg
	short tons (2000 lb)	0.9	tonnes	t
VOLUME				
tsp	teaspoon	5 milliliters	ml	
tbsp	tablespoon	15 milliliters	ml	
fl oz	fluid ounces	30 milliliters	ml	
c	cups	0.24	liters	l
pt	pints	0.47	liters	l
qt	quarts	0.95	liters	l
gal	gallons	3.8	liters	l
TEMPERATURE (exact)				
°F	Fahrenheit temperature 32	5/9 after subtracting	Celsius temperature	°C